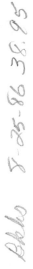
WITHDRAWN

Nursing Administration of Psychiatric-Mental Health Care

Christina L.S. Evans, RNC, MSN, CNA
Sharon K. Lewis, RN, MA, CNA

Kingswood Hospital
Ferndale, Michigan

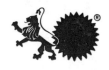

AN ASPEN PUBLICATION®
Aspen Systems Corporation
Rockville, Maryland
Royal Tunbridge Wells
1985

Library of Congress Cataloging in Publication Data

Evans, Christina L.S.
Nursing administration of psychiatric-mental health care.

"An Aspen publication."
Includes bibliographies and index.
1. Psychiatric nursing — Management. I. Lewis, Sharon K.
II. Title. [DNLM: 1. Mental Health Services — organization &
administration — nurses' instruction. 2. Psychiatric Nursing —
organization & administration. WY 160 E92n]
RC440.E85   1985   362.2'1'068   85-6082
ISBN: 0-87189-099-2

Editorial Services: Martha Sasser

Library of Congress Catalog Number 85-6082.
ISBN: 0-87189-099-2

Printed in the United States of America

2   3   4   5

Dedicated to

the following family members

whose support was instrumental

in the completion of this text:

Timothy Evans;

Louis, Doris, and Millie Sieloff;

William and Althea Evans;

and

Helen and Franklin Lewis.

Table of Contents

Preface

The purpose of this book is to provide guidelines and practical assistance to nurses responsible for the administration of psychiatric–mental health nursing care. Drawing from principles of nursing administration and the specialty of psychiatric–mental health nursing, the authors hope to give support and direction to nurses engaged in the administration of this often-isolated clinical specialty. Although this book is not exhaustive in its treatment of the subject, it does provide a theoretical and practical framework for the psychiatric–mental health nursing administrator—whether a veteran or a newcomer to the field. The topics covered address practical areas that often face the psychiatric nursing administrator. With the large number of psychiatric–mental health programs in existence—and increasing daily—today's nursing administrator needs resource tools that address the unique aspects of psychiatric–mental health nursing.

Numerous nursing administration and nursing management books are available, but none of them is directed to the specialty area of psychiatric–mental health nursing. As a result, the idea for this book came into being.

Christina L.S. Evans
Sharon K. Lewis

Chapter 1

Foundation for Psychiatric–Mental Health Nursing Administration

THE ADMINISTRATIVE CHALLENGES

Psychiatric–mental health nursing presents continuing challenges to the nurses practicing in that field; it presents, however, even greater challenges to those nurses charged with administering that department. They must correct behaviors that often cannot be directly observed, and they must provide quality nursing care to a client population that often cannot define its own health care problems. In addition, psychiatric–mental health client populations differ from other specialty populations; therefore, general nursing administration tools, problem solving strategies, and techniques cannot be used without substantial modification.

Added to these inherent challenges are the problems that arise when nurses assume new positions—career changes for which they are not fully prepared. This is often the case with nonclinical nursing positions. For example, psychiatric–mental health nursing administrators frequently move up the executive ladder primarily through promotions based on their clinical expertise rather than on their management abilities. Many nurses have failed in these management positions because they had little, if any, preparation for their new roles or because their skills did not lie in the management area. Even today, psychiatric–mental health nurses wishing to improve their financial position often choose to enter a nursing management career track rather than continue working in clinical areas for which they are better suited or qualified. This choice can mean disaster for the nurse who is not prepared for the challenges of the administrator's role. The areas of service and education, often viewed in the past as being at odds with each other, are now viewed as needing closer communication to bridge the gap between the philosophical ideals of nursing education and the stark realities the professional nurse faces upon entry into practice.

Today's psychiatric–mental health nursing administrator is faced with the problems of labor relations, unionization, strikes, computerization, rapidly changing technology, multi-million-dollar budgets, staffing problems, financial cutbacks, and consumerism. Within that context, this nurse-administrator is charged with the grave responsibility of assuring that quality nursing care is provided to the health care consumer in the most humane, cost-effective, and efficient manner. As mentioned previously, the psychiatric–mental health client population differs from other nursing populations in distinct ways (e.g., the longer length of stay and the abstract nature of nursing interventions). Furthermore, no substantial body of nursing administration knowledge exists to aid the psychiatric–mental health nursing administrator in assuring the quality of care.

Obviously, preparation for this challenge is a necessity. Fortunately, leadership and management courses are filtering into nursing curriculums—even in basic nursing programs—which will better prepare nurses for future psychiatric–mental health management positions. Graduate programs in nursing administration, with emphasis on psychiatric–mental health nursing, now assist those nurses who wish to follow nursing management careers. This combination of administration and psychiatric–mental health nursing theory aids the nurse-administrator in integrating administrative strategies into the psychiatric–mental health setting. Workshops and seminars addressing topics from basic management principles to the most sophisticated administrative functions are finally available to nurses.

To provide ongoing support, professional networking (the process of establishing professional contacts and building and maintaining groups) is beginning to occur among psychiatric–mental health nursing administrators. Through professional organizations on a local, state, regional, and national level, a network of resources is being provided. In the face of the uncertain financial future of the health care delivery system, these organizations are forging the future for psychiatric–mental health nursing administrators, as well as for professional nursing.

NURSING ADMINISTRATION AND THE NURSING PROCESS

The processes involved in administration are planning, organizing, directing, and controlling. In psychiatric–mental health nursing administration, these processes can be facilitated through using components of the nursing process (assessing, planning, implementing, and evaluating). The nurse-administrator continually uses the nursing process, either consciously or unconsciously, while conducting the business of the nursing department. In order to assist psychiatric–mental health nursing administrators in further integrating the nursing process as a part of their practice, this text uses a nursing process format.

However, before the nursing process can be integrated into the administrative process, the psychiatric–mental health nursing department must have a theoretical foundation upon which the nursing process can be applied. This foundation consists of the department's philosophy, its relevant practice standards, and the organizational plan in which the department exists.

Role of a Psychiatric Nursing Philosophy

To administer effectively the practice area of psychiatric–mental health nursing, the nurse-administrator uses several documents as the basis for the management process. The purpose or mission statement and the philosophy of the psychiatric–mental health nursing department are two of the documents that provide a foundation for all nursing activities within that setting. Such documents are vital for the dynamic growth of the nursing service. In any setting, from a single nurse's private practice to a department comprised of hundreds of employees, the nurse-administrator must assess these documents in the light of the current client population and nursing practice.

Based on reality, the purpose or mission statement defines the societal reasons for the existence of psychiatric–mental health nursing within the setting and must be consistent with the institution's overall purpose. This document should, therefore, address the population being served and the manner in which specific nursing care is delivered (Rowland & Rowland, 1980). Because the document is used as a guideline for establishing policies, procedures, and protocols to be used in the daily delivery of care, generalities should be avoided in formulating the purpose or mission statement. General statements are too broad and are soon ignored. A realistic and specific document defines daily practice and becomes an integral part of each nurse's delivery of care.

The statement of departmental philosophy includes the basic beliefs that guide the administration and the practice of psychiatric–mental health nursing and reflects the purpose of that practice. To be useful, this document must also be based on reality. The philosophy expands concepts delineated in the purpose by including the beliefs and values associated with the provision of the nursing care. These beliefs include the type of care required by specific client populations and the academic and clinical preparation needed by the providers of such care. This document also provides the direction for future departmental changes, growth, and adjustments of staff composition that may be necessary to meet the demands of changing client populations or societal pressures. By delineating beliefs and values concerning climates of practice, research, administration, nursing students, and professional relationships (within nursing and between nursing and other disciplines), the statement of philosophy serves not only to define psychiatric–mental health nursing practice but also to clarify the role and practice of nursing for other health care disciplines.

Role of Psychiatric–Mental Health Nursing Standards

Standards serve as a basis for most aspects of the nursing management process, from the recruitment of staff to the planning of programs. The psychiatric–mental health nursing department of any health care organization needs guidelines and direction to assist the nurse-administrator in providing the highest quality nursing care in the most humane, cost effective, and efficient manner. These nursing standards provide the nurse-administrator with the tools necessary to administer and to effectively evaluate the quality of care being provided. Various accrediting, licensing, and professional bodies (such as the Joint Commission on the Accreditation of Hospitals, state mental health or public health departments, Medicare or Medicaid, American Nurses' Association, third party payers, and insurance companies) establish regulations that specify the minimum level of quality of care the health care organization must provide. By using these standards, the nurse-administrator can create and maintain a nursing practice that provides quality care.

A dual set of professional standards, those for nursing service administration and those for psychiatric–mental health nursing practice, provides guidance for the psychiatric–mental health nursing administrator (see Appendix 1-A for the psychiatric–mental health nursing standards). The standards form a base from which psychiatric–mental health nurse administrators evaluate not only the effectiveness of the administration of their department but also the specific care their staff provides. Nurse-administrators' participation in the formulation of these standards, when feasible, confirms the philosophy of care these nurses espouse. It is important, therefore, that nurse-administrators provide their expertise to the professional organization when accrediting bodies seek professional feedback on proposed standards before the standards are included in their accrediting process. This participation gives the discipline of nursing a voice in the setting of standards for nursing that are applied by nonnursing organizations.

These standards serve as basic standards for any psychiatric–mental health setting. However, the criteria for each standard must be modified to apply specifically to each setting. Additional clinical standards relating to the delivery of care to specific client populations (e.g., schizophrenic clients) should also be developed. For ease in applicability and for consistency, these standards should be documented in a format similar to that of the other standards.

Formal Organizational Plans

Within any organization, the organizational plan (also known as the organizational structure) illustrates the management hierarchy and the lines of authority. The overall concepts of such formal organizational plans are not reviewed in depth here because other administrative texts discuss this topic thoroughly. However, the psychiatric–mental health nursing administrator should be familiar and comfortable with these concepts and able to freely utilize them. The administrator can then review and critique the current organizational structure to determine if it is as clear, concise, and efficient as possible, in order to meet the needs of the client population. It is important that this structure be reviewed annually in order to reflect changes in practice. (For example, lines of authority may change when the department decentralizes.) The current structure can serve as a resource tool as well as to orient new members of the department.

An accurate organizational chart or plan is a useful tool for planning and delineating policy or organizational changes. Relationships between nursing positions or divisions must be reviewed and clarified when necessary to decrease confusion and a source of stress. Such a review should assess the strengths and deficiencies existing within the organization and should serve to clarify relationships with other disciplines or departments (Rowland & Rowland, 1980).

If the psychiatric–mental health nursing component exists as a subsystem within a larger nursing department, the same concepts apply. Psychiatric–mental health nursing as a specialty area needs to be continually in contact with other nursing areas to prevent isolationism. Isolation may lead to fewer confrontations, but it also results in decreased support and assistance from other nurses.

Administrative roles within the psychiatric–mental health nursing area must be at the same hierarchical levels in the organizational structure as are those in other areas of nursing. This demand for parity also applies to other disciplines and departments with which psychiatric–mental health nurses interact. Unless the equality exists on paper, the psychiatric–mental health nurse is at an immediate disadvantage in the management of the nursing area and the delivery of client care. Such inequality creates undue frustration and stress, which has an impact on not only the staff but, ultimately, client care. The discipline of psychiatric–mental health nursing is often identified as the leader in the delivery of client care. Without an organizational structure to support this, however, the concept is only theory.

The nursing organizational structure should also be reviewed as it relates to other components in the larger structural unit. For the psychiatric–mental health nursing component of the organization to be fully integrated into that organization, the nursing department or division must be aware of, assess, and communicate with all other components of the total organization. This integration requires that the psychiatric–mental health nursing administrator be hierarchically located on the same level as all other major department leaders. The psychiatric–mental health nursing administrator position title also must be consistent with the titles of other department leaders. For example, if the medical chief is designated as the vice president for medical affairs, the equivalent nursing title would be vice president for nursing affairs.

Nurses at all levels should be familiar with the structure of the overall organization and with the roles of its various members. The psychiatric–mental health nursing department must be aware of the activities between and within other departments and must communicate freely and comfortably with all other departments. Activities of one department invariably have an impact on others. The nursing department must be kept informed if improvements in the planning and the cooperative efforts involved in organizational changes and modifications are to be effected. Through collaborative efforts with all departments and disciplines, psychiatric–mental health nursing becomes equal, rather than a subordinate, in the delivery of quality patient care.

Representation on Hospital-Wide Committees

One of the major roles of the psychiatric–mental health nursing administrator is as a spokesperson for nursing. In the past, hospital committees, as well as medical staff committees, were exclusive groups. Now, however, these committees play an important role in assuring that the organization complies with Joint Commission on the Accreditation of Hospitals' (JCAH) quality assurance standards and, as such, need representation from all disciplines of the treatment team. When nurses are not represented at these meetings, and when decisions affecting nursing are made without consideration of their impact on the nursing department or the staff, client care is affected.

Communication between nurses and physicians must be open and honest if mutual respect is to be fostered. Establishment of a joint practice committee can be instrumental in fostering collaborative practice between nurses and physicians. The National Joint Practice Commission, established by the American Medical Association and the American Nurses' Association (ANA) to promote professional respect and collaboration between nurses and physicians, developed guidelines for the establishment of joint practice in the hospital setting. These guidelines can be helpful to psychiatric–mental health nursing administrators if they wish to explore this method for enhancing nurse-physician relationships.

The psychiatric–mental health nursing administrator is responsible for ensuring opportunities for the appointment of nurses to key hospital and medical staff committees. Once nursing is represented on such committees, however, each nurse must be committed to active participation. Through this participation, the psychiatric–mental health nursing department can have a voice in determining the direction the organization takes. The nurse-administrator can then establish appropriate goals and objectives for the psychiatric–mental health nursing department or division that are congruent with the organization's goals. Assessment of nursing and client needs, long range planning, and the implementation of change can then be more easily accomplished because psychiatric–mental health nursing has greater control of its future.

REFERENCES

American Nurses' Association. (1984). *Standards of psychiatric and mental health nursing practice*. Kansas City, Mo: Author.

Rowland, H.S., & Rowland, B.L. (1980). *Nursing administration handbook*. Rockville, Md: Aspen Systems Corporation.

Appendix 1-A
Psychiatric–Mental Health Nursing Standards

The American Nurses' Association Division on Psychiatric–Mental Health Nursing Practice developed standards (1982) for the provision of psychiatric and mental health nursing. The following document presents the revised standards.

Standard I. The nurse applies appropriate therapy that is scientifically sound as a basis for decisions regarding nursing practice.

Standard II. The nurse continuously collects data that are comprehensive, accurate, and systematic.

Standard III. The nurse utilizes nursing diagnoses and/or standard classification of mental disorders to express conclusions supported by recorded assessment data and current scientific premises.

Standard IV. The nurse develops a nursing care plan with specific goals and interventions delineating nursing actions unique to each client's needs.

Standard V. The nurse intervenes as guided by the nursing care plan to implement nursing actions that promote, maintain, or restore physical and mental health; prevent illness; and effect rehabilitation.

Standard V-A. The nurse uses psychotherapeutic interventions to assist clients in regaining or improving their previous coping abilities and to prevent further disability.

Standard V-B. The nurse assists clients, families, and groups to achieve satisfying and productive patterns of living through health teaching.

Standard V-C. The nurse uses the activities of daily living in a goal-directed way to foster adequate self-care and the physical and mental well-being of clients.

Standard V-D. The nurse uses knowledge of somatic therapies and applies related clinical skills in working with clients.

Standard V-E. The nurse provides, structures, and maintains a therapeutic environment in collaboration with the client and other health care providers.

Standard V-F. The nurse utilizes advanced clinical expertise in individual, group, and family psychotherapy; child psychotherapy; and other treatment modalities to function as a psychotherapist, and recognizes professional accountability for nursing practice.

Standard VI. The nurse evaluates client responses to nursing actions in order to revise the data base, nursing diagnoses, and nursing care plan.

Standard VII. The nurse participates in peer review and other means of evaluation to assure quality of nursing care provided for clients.

Standard VIII. The nurse assumes responsibility for continuing education and professional development and contributes to the professional growth of others.

Standard IX. The nurse collaborates with other health care providers in assessing, planning, implementing, and evaluating programs and other mental health activities.

Standard X. The nurse participates with other members of the community in assessing, planning, implementing, and evaluating mental health services and community systems that include the promotion of the broad continuum of primary, secondary, and tertiary prevention of mental illness.

Standard XI. The nurse contributes to nursing and the mental health field through innovations in theory and practice and participation in research.

Source: From *Standards of psychiatric and mental health nursing practice* (pp. 3–19) by American Nurses' Association, 1982, Kansas City, Mo: Author. © 1982 by the American Nurses' Association. Reprinted by permission.

Chapter 2

Role and Function of Power Within the Psychiatric– Mental Health Organization

The concept of power and its impact on the health care structure has finally been given attention in nursing circles. As nursing strives for its professional identity and as psychiatric–mental health nursing administrators seek to make changes in their organizations, it becomes evident that a knowledge of power is essential. As a group, nurses are beginning to see how power can be used as a positive means of creating changes (Hendricks, 1982). Before we can expect to exert influence in the administrative arena, we need to have an understanding of power and its function in management.

ASSESSMENT OF POWER

Webster's New World Dictionary (1975) defines *power* as "the ability to do, act, or produce . . . to control others; to influence" (p. 585). Rollo May (1972) refers to power as an ability to facilitate or to prevent change. The concept of power can be divided into three parts: authority, power bases, and influence. These three elements together are the most important aspects of an effective manager. Authority gives one the right and the responsibility to take action, to carry out activities, and to make final decisions (Kraegel, 1980). As Byrd (1974) states, "power is the ability to control the behavior of other people. Authority gives you the legal right but power is the muscle" (p. 126).

Influence is the result of the appropriate use of power. It is the "power of a person . . . to produce an effect upon others, often indirectly or intangibly" (Doubleday, 1975, p. 368). In order to exert influence, one must have power.

Power stems from three different bases: personal power, interpersonal-social power, and organizational power. Personal power stems from the individual's feeling of self-worth and a strong self-concept (Claus & Bailey, 1977). A personal power base is gradually developed over time as the person comes to a deeper and

9

greater self-knowledge (Culbert, 1980). Personal power can be cultivated through ongoing personal and professional development aimed at those areas that need the most attention. For example, the psychiatric–mental health nursing administrator with only little knowledge and experience in budgets can broaden and strengthen that personal power base through mastery of appropriate accounting classes. Likewise, the nurse-administrator who is fearful of speaking before others and who gradually moves from speaking before small groups to larger audiences, can considerably solidify the personal power base through a better self-concept.

The interpersonal-social power base depends on interactions with others. The greater the nurse-administrator's ability to gain cooperation from others, the stronger the interpersonal-social power base. The nurse-administrator who is able to promote group cohesiveness and to facilitate participation in decision making within the group has sound interpersonal-social power. Interpersonal techniques may be used to influence a group to work together effectively by seeing the group as a synergistic whole in which the sum is greater than the parts (Claus & Bailey, 1977). Through this process of shared decision making, change is more easily accepted and successfully effected. Unlike the directive, authoritarian approach, it requires the risk of delegation of power.

The organizational power base is built into the organizational structure and is inherent in the position one holds within the organization. The power of a unit clerk is far less than the power of a nursing supervisor because of the relative position each has within the organizational framework. This power base changes when a person is promoted or demoted, or when the organizational structure is altered in some way. For instance, if a nursing supervisor is promoted to the Director of Nursing, that person gains more power through the change in position. Inasmuch as a nursing supervisor (by virtue of the organizational structure) does not have power equal to the director of nursing, any supervisor wishing to influence the decisions of the director of nursing would need to use personal or interpersonal-social power bases.

NEED FOR POWER

Nursing has been a female-dominated profession, and so nurses have experienced the same frustration in realizing their potential as have women in general in our society. Women have been involved in an age-old socialization process in which men have maintained and controlled the greatest influence. In health care, physicians have controlled, to a great degree, the role of nurses in providing that care. Nurses in the psychiatric–mental health field, like all nurses, have been exposed to the difficulties perpetuated by a predominantly male physician group. The evolution of psychiatric–mental health nursing practice into a viable, expanded therapeutic role is directly dependent on the perceptions of nurses as professional care givers with a valuable contribution to make to client care (Grissum & Spengler, 1976). Having an understanding of the role of women in our society and the perceptions female nurses have as women in a male dominated health care system, the psychiatric–mental health administrator can better prepare for changes in psychiatric nursing practice. By assisting nurses to identify themselves as professionals and by articulating to physicians the role of psychiatric–mental health nursing, other professionals and the administration of the organization can set the groundwork for improved quality care, nursing autonomy, and increased job satisfaction.

Historically, psychiatric–mental health nursing has been influenced by a variety of other disciplines, but primarily by psychiatrists. By examining any typical mental health care organization, a person can easily see the power and the influence psychiatrists have over most (if not all) professional disciplines comprising the interdisciplinary treatment team. Who really controls nursing practice—nursing or psychiatry? Sadly, much of the psychiatric–mental health nursing staff must consult the psychiatric staff before implementing policies and procedures that are related to nursing practice. As long as nurses continue to delegate responsibilities for their own practice to others, they will not be able to make significant progress in modifying nursing as a profession.

The psychiatric–mental health nurse plays a vital part in the provision of the interdisciplinary care. As a member of the interdisciplinary treatment team, the nurse is not only responsible for the nursing care provided to clients, but is on the firing line to articulate directly nursing's unique perspective of holistic mental health care. Members of other disciplines, including physicians, are not always accustomed to nurses' taking the initiative in aspects of health care that are not task oriented. Relying on the therapeutic relationship, the psychiatric–mental health nurse uses the nursing process to provide nursing care to clients. Fostering a collegial relationship with persons in other disciplines requires a knowledge of and a respect for the skills required by each discipline.

Whether recruited into administrative positions through promotion or hired specifically, nurses are given tremendous responsibility and only promises of power (Storlie, 1982). As time goes on, frustration and dissatisfaction can arise if the psychiatric–mental health nursing administrator faces apparent lack of success when attempting to enhance the image and position of nursing among other professions. This feeling of powerlessness allows the stress of the position to take its toll. As a result, many nurse-administrators burn out and become disillusioned by the reality of the powerlessness of nursing.

Powerlessness is experienced not only by the psychiatric–mental health nursing administration but also by nurses at every level within the system. It contributes greatly to the high turnover of nurses, and is the single, most-cited factor of nurses' dissatisfaction. Given a measure of power to exercise control over psychiatric–mental health nursing practice, nurses are often their own worst enemy. The cohesiveness seen among psychiatrists is lacking in psychiatric–mental health nursing. Nurses either overcontrol—thereby stifling colleagues—or they ignore each other by going separate and ineffectual ways. Nurses have heard the cry to become assertive, but then they use the assertiveness against each other, undermining colleagues at every turn (Storlie, 1982). Unless nurses wish to continue to be told by others how psychiatric–mental health nursing is to be practiced, we must, as Storlie states, "demand the right to define and control our own practice" (p. 17). More importantly, the nurse-administrator must recognize the reality and the necessity of power (Claus & Bailey, 1977).

USES OF POWER

Planning: Influencing Others

Claus and Bailey (1977) state, "power is the *source* of influence, whereas influence is the result of the proper use of power" (p. 21). The effective leader takes action that influences the group to set and to reach goals. Goals are essential for the upward progress of any organization, department, or individual (see Chapter 5). Goals provide a focus, a source of identity, and motivation for the group. Used as a basis for performance evaluation, they also provide measurable outcome criteria. Realistically, however, goals can only be accomplished in and through others. Consequently, it is essential that the psychiatric–mental health nursing administrator be able to influence others in order to meet established goals.

Working with people usually involves conflict. Through effective leadership, the nurse-administrator can use the necessary power to influence those in conflict to minimize the conflict as much as possible, thus allowing the group to continue forward. Conflict resolution will be successful when trust exists between the nurse-administrator and those engaged in conflict. If such trust exists, the nurse-administrator has several mechanisms of influence that may be helpful. The most obvious means of influence is coercion, whereby a person is forced to comply with demands. Although coercion may be necessary in extreme situations, it is risky and may well cause the conflict to worsen.

Another method of exerting influence is by the use of similar interests. "When a relationship or an interaction between two people involves interests that are similar, influence can be expressed in forms that would be impossible when interests are divergent or at odds with each other" (Claus & Bailey, 1977, p. 32). This similar interest may be used to foster collaboration to accomplish the task at hand. For example, both the psychiatric–mental health nurse and the psychiatrist desire to provide high quality client care. It is this similar interest that provides the nurse with a power base when negotiating with the psychiatrist on issues of client care.

Likewise, conflicting interests may be used to exert influence by giving the appearance of having the same goal and working together for resolution that handles both interests. For example, the nurse-administrator does not wish the nursing supervisor to be required to admit clients after the admission office closes. The admission clerk does not want to refuse admission to clients at any time. The nursing administrator may express concerns about the problem of the nursing supervisor producing an incomplete admission process because of the lack of time and may explore the need to simplify the admission process. This exploration might lead to a discussion of the scheduling of admissions. The result could be an expansion of admission hours in which the nursing supervisor would provide support for the admission clerk, who would be available extended hours.

Rewards can also be very effective as a means of influence—if they are used in a supportive, judicious manner. For example, a nursing supervisor working on a special project may be rewarded through additional time off, if this is economically feasible. A formal acknowledgment can also be used as a reward. This may be accomplished in several ways: for example, an article about the person or the person's contributions could be published in the organization's newsletter, or recognition could be given at staff meetings with peers and other managers.

Coalitions, as a means of influence, are essential in today's complex psychiatric–mental health care settings. A coalition is a group of people who join together for the purpose of advancing a particular idea or striving towards a common goal. It is impossible for the nurse-administrator to have enough power to be able effectively to exert influence in all areas essential to the advancement of psychiatric–mental health nursing practice. Joining forces with other nurses, department heads, and professionals provides a stronger power base that can be difficult to overcome. Coalitions simply use the previously mentioned principle of similar interests on a larger scale.

Another means of influence is persuasion. The nurse-administrator can use persuasion to induce another to accept a change in behavior, viewpoint, or direction without exercising power in a more direct and confrontational manner. This method can be very effective. When conflict is high, however, persuasion can easily be perceived suspiciously as manipulation, in the same way that a reward can be viewed as a bribe.

Implementation: Communication as a Tool

Although persuasion can be successfully used, there are times when direct use of power is more effective and less time consuming. For example, the psychiatric–mental health nursing administrator influences others through displays of expertise, setting high standards, attending to growth opportunities for subordinates, and maximizing relations between the nurse-administrator and others. However, this direct influence can be accomplished only when communications are at an optimum. Open communication is essential in settling arguments and misunderstandings, resolving conflicts, establishing clearly defined goals, and expressing one's point of view in an effort to increase organizational power. The person who maintains open lines of communication is seen as influential and can more easily influence others.

The more opportunities the nurse-administrator takes to enhance open communication channels, the greater is the chance of success for effective leadership as these opportunities strengthen the administrator's realm of influence. Attention should be paid to participation in staff and board meetings; formal and informal contacts with nurses; interactions with psychiatrists, department heads, therapists; memberships on committees; and participation in inservice programs. All of these activities provide countless opportunities for the psychiatric–mental health nursing administrator to become visible, known, and accepted as an interested and responsive administrator (Claus & Bailey, 1977).

Communication is accomplished verbally or in written form. Because verbal communication encourages immediate feedback, it is often the quickest and most effective means of communication. Written communication is formal and less personal, but it does provide a permanent record for future reference. However, it does not provide a means for an immediate response and, in many cases, requires and expects *no* response. Although both forms are frequently used by the administrator, verbal communication is the more effective approach.

Through open communication, mutual respect develops between the psychiatric–mental health nursing administrator and subordinates and peers. Only then—after a solid rapport and mutual respect is established—can the nurse-administrator take the risks involved in the delegation of authority without fear of loss of personal power. When delegating authority and responsibility to a subordinate, the administrator assumes that the subordinate is competent and will use the power associated with that authority and responsibility in a constructive and appropriate manner. Through the sharing of power, the administrator can gain great cooperation from subordinates. Keeping power to oneself, on the other hand, can give rise to competition, power struggles, and conflict. It is virtually impossible to do personally everything that needs to be done. Through delegation of responsibilities and the power necessary to execute those responsibilities, the nurse-administrator can gain more. As Ganong and Ganong (1980) state, "the exercise of power requires organization plus the capability of delegating" (p. 193). Delegating power is difficult, however, for many nurses because the acquisition of that power was an arduous process, usually eked out in small portions along the ladder. Even though it may seem easier to do something than to delegate it, the growth potential for subordinates, when such responsibility and power are delegated, yields greater rewards in the long run.

Nursing can also gain more power through the use of coalitions. This gain may come about as the nursing department joins forces with other departments to share goals, concerns, and program planning. In this way, the psychiatric–mental health nursing program can have greater influence over elements affecting delivery of psychiatric–mental health care. Coalition formation can be effectively used through all levels of the nursing organization—from the staff nurse to the nurse administrator.

EVALUATION

The effective psychiatric–mental health nursing administrator needs to claim and to use all the power sources available. Power is inherent in every organizational structure, but it is not distributed evenly among all managers. Without power, the nurse-administrator's ability to influence others is minimized. Having power requires, however, the associated skill to use it effectively to influence others for the promotion of one's own interests. Influence can be accomplished through several ways, but the basis ultimately rests in open communication. Through communication, the nurse-administrator reinforces strengths and becomes visible, trusted, and accepted. As a consequence the administrator's power is increased. The more power is gained, the more that power should be shared with subordinates. Sharing of power increases cooperation and advancement towards common goals. Underlying all, however, is the need for all psychiatric–mental health nurses to seek cohesiveness collaboratively as a professional group, accepting and acknowledging whatever power an individual person might have rather than challenging and undermining each other. Through this united stand, the psychiatric–mental health nursing administrator can represent these professionals and make a greater impact on the health care system in which they all practice.

REFERENCES

Byrd, R.E. (1974). *A guide to personal risk taking*. New York: AMACOM.

Claus, K.E., & Bailey, J.T. (1977). *Power and influence in health care*. St. Louis: Mosby.

Culbert, S.A. (1980). *The invisible war: Pursuing self interests at work*. New York: J. Wiley.

Doubleday dictionary. (1975). New York: Doubleday.

Ganong, J.M., & Ganong, W.L. (1980). *Nursing management*. Rockville, Md.: Aspen Systems.

Grissum, M., & Spengler, C. (1976). *Womanpower and health care*. Boston: Little, Brown & Co.

Hendricks, D.E. (1982). The power problem. *Journal of Nursing Management, 13*(10), 23–24.

Kraegel, J.M. (Ed.). (1980). *Organization-environment relationships*. Rockville, Md.: Aspen Systems.

May, R. (1972). *Power and innocence: A search for the sources of violence*. New York: W.W. Norton.

Storlie, F.J. (1982). Power, getting a piece of the action. *Journal of Nursing Management, 13*(10), 15–18.

Webster's New World Dictionary. (1975). New York: Wm. Collins & World Publishing Co.

Chapter 3

Licensing and Accreditation

OVERVIEW

Today's psychiatric–mental health care organization, like all health care organizations, is bombarded with myriad regulatory surveys throughout the year. Tighter controls over the health care dollar, and a quality care focus for health care spending, have prompted third party payers to scrutinize health care practices carefully. Local, state, and federal regulations that prompt economical health care spending and ensure client safety and human rights have also placed increasing demands on health care providers. The psychiatric–mental health organization has frequent on-site visits from voluntary agencies (such as the JCAH) and mandatory regulatory agencies (such as state departments of mental health). In addition, the paperwork required to support and to justify an organization's compliance with regulatory requirements has greatly increased. The importance of such compliance cannot be underestimated. The very existence of most health care organizations depends on the approval of and recognition by certain regulatory agencies.

Because of the impact of regulatory noncompliance, the psychiatric–mental health nursing administrator has a great responsibility to ensure that all standards related to psychiatric–mental health nursing are known, understood, and met by the department. Some of the regulatory bodies that directly or indirectly have an impact on psychiatric–mental health nursing include:

- state and local fire marshals
- state Department of Mental Health
- state Department of Public Health
- Medicare (federal)
- Medicaid (federal and state)
- Office of Substance Abuse Services (OSAS)

17

- Joint Commission on Accreditation of Hospitals (JCAH)
- Blue Cross and other third party payers
- state Department of Licensing and Regulation (governing nursing licensure)
- National Institute of Mental Health (NIMH)

In some instances, all or part of the organization may be under review at any given time.

ASSESSING COMPLIANCE WITH REGULATORY STANDARDS

Before the psychiatric–mental health nursing administrator can assess the nursing department's compliance with regulatory standards, relevant standards must be known and understood. It is the responsibility of the nurse-administrator to obtain all necessary documents that define the standards affecting psychiatric–mental health nursing care. Copies of the state public health and mental health codes, with associated administrative rules, are available from those state departments. If the organization provides substance abuse treatment, or serves Medicare or Medicaid clients, regulations governing these clients are available from OSAS and from Medicare and Medicaid review offices located in each state. Usually, the administrator or chief executive officer has this information, which is shared with the nurse-administrator when separate copies are not supplied. Facilities being surveyed by JCAH for accreditation may be reviewed under either the consolidated standards or the Accreditation Manual for Hospitals (AMH). In many instances, most regulatory bodies have similar or closely related standards. Comparisons of standards can enable administrators to identify areas of similarity and difference. Before making any survey, the nurse-administrator should also review the reports of the previous survey in order to identify those areas that need attention before the next survey occurs.

If state licensure is necessary and licensure requirements are not met, compliance with other regulatory standards is an exercise in futility. Without the appropriate licenses, health care services may be legally terminated. Many regulatory bodies mandate that state licenses, where necessary, be acquired. In cases in which licensure requirement standards exceed those of other regulatory bodies, the state requirements must be met. For example, JCAH (1983) states, "Multidisciplinary case conferences shall be regularly conducted to review and evaluate each patient's treatment plan and his or her progress in attaining the stated treatment goals and objectives" (p. 73). If the state mental health code requires case conferences at least every 30 days, JCAH also expects regular case conferences to be held at least every 30 days. The psychiatric–mental health organization must comply with all relevant state laws. Likewise, when the requirements of another regulatory body exceed state requirements, the psychiatric–mental health organization must comply with the other regulatory body's requirements if it wishes to be approved by that body. For example, JCAH (1983) states, "Appropriate attention shall be paid every fifteen minutes to a patient in restraint or seclusion, especially in regard to regular meals, bathing, and use of the toilet" (p. 79). If state licensing requirements are 30 minutes instead of JCAH's 15 minutes, JCAH requirements must be met if accreditation is desired.

The JCAH surveys hospitals and other facilities on a voluntary basis. JCAH accreditation was instituted as a mark of excellence for those hospitals and facilities that chose to comply with JCAH standards of care. With the increased establishment of psychiatric–mental health programs across the country, JCAH established standards for psychiatric facilities in 1969 and implemented those standards in 1970. Although JCAH accreditation is voluntary, Blue Cross (the largest independent third party payer) and other third party payers require JCAH accreditation for reimbursement eligibility. Thus, in practice, JCAH accreditation is not strictly voluntary.

PLANNING FOR SITE SURVEY

The consolidated standards "are applicable to all of a hospital's/facility's services, units, programs, and settings that provide services to psychiatric and substance abuse patients" (JCAH, 1983, p. vii). Among the criteria for survey eligibility are the following:

- Be in compliance with applicable federal, state and local laws and regulations, including any requirements for licensure;
- Maintain facilities, beds, and/or services that are available to individuals and their families over a continuous 24-hour period, 7 days a week, or maintain services to individuals and their families that are available on a regularly scheduled basis less than 24 hours a day; [This criterion includes inpatient, residential, outpatient, and partial hospitalization.]
- Have a governing body and an organized professional staff whose primary function is the diagnosis, treatment, and/or rehabilitation of persons evidencing psychiatric, mental health, alcoholism, and/ or drug abuse problems. (JCAH, 1983, p. xi)

The standards, which are divided into four sections, are summarized as follows:

The first section, "Hospital/Facility/Program Management," includes . . . governing body, professional staff organization, personnel, and quality assurance. The second section, "Patient Management," concerns the implementation and documentation of intake, assessment, treatment plans, and special treatment procedures. The third section, "Patient Services," covers various components of the service delivery system (anesthesia, dental, emergency, etc.). The fourth section . . . , "Physical Plant Management," [is] related to . . . safety, sanitation, and therapeutic environment. (JCAH, 1983, p. vii)

Psychiatric–Mental Health Nursing Accreditation Committee

The approach of the JCAH consolidated standards is interdisciplinary and holistic. Consequently, there are no separate standards labelled "Nursing Services." Standards that are related to nursing are integrated throughout the manual. The AMH has, however, a lengthy section related to nursing services, but it has fewer specific standards addressing psychiatric–mental health care in particular. Regardless of the manual of standards under which the facility is being surveyed, the psychiatric–mental health nursing administrator needs to become familiar with all the standards and must identify those that need to be addressed by nursing.

A nursing accreditation committee may be useful for the purpose of "involving staff year round in following JCAH guidelines [while] generat[ing] enthusiasm for improving the operating quality of the facility as well as avoiding the last minute rush of preparing for a survey" (Salmore, 1982, p. 41). The psychiatric–mental health nursing accreditation committee could be established as a permanent departmental committee. Meetings would be scheduled on a regular basis, and membership would include management and staff level employees. The committee would review each standard related to nursing, and would assess the department's current compliance status. (The committee could also conduct its own annual survey—as well as one a few weeks before a scheduled survey—to evaluate compliance.) The nursing committee would make recommendations to the nurse-administrator for corrective measures, procedural changes, educational needs, and so forth. Responsibility for implementing these recommendations would then be delegated to the appropriate nursing committees or staff. The nurse-administrator would be a member or a liaison between the accreditation committee for nursing and the committee for the organization.

By promoting staff participation, this procedure would provide a greater acceptance of any changes within the psychiatric–mental health care delivery system that are necessary for JCAH compliance. The resultant familiarity with JCAH standards would reduce the anxiety all staff members feel when a survey occurs, and the survey process would be more meaningful and personal to the staff.

JCAH Accreditation Process

A psychiatric–mental health nursing administrator's first experience of a JCAH survey can be anxiety-producing and frightening. In addition to providing adequate preparation for the survey, a review of the actual survey process may assist the nurse-administrator to overcome undue anxiety. Before the on-site visit, the organization makes application for a survey. All necessary eligibility requirements must be met before the JCAH schedules a survey. JCAH then gives notice a minimum of 30 days before the actual survey date. In preparation for the site visit, "JCAH requires a facility to post, in a public place on its premises, the official JCAH announcement of the date of survey and of the opportunity for a public information interview" (JCAH, 1983, p. xiii). This announcement must be posted 4 weeks before the survey is conducted so that interested and concerned persons in the community may have an opportunity to provide the JCAH surveyor with information about the organization.

The length of time established for the survey is dependent on profile information submitted to JCAH by the hospital or the organization.

The nurse-administrator may act as a liaison for the nursing department to the surveyor for the review of psychiatric–mental health nursing policies and procedures, the review of current (or closed) case records, the tour of the organization, and the summation conference at the close of the survey. The nurse-administrator also attends the two workshops the surveyor presents for the staff in order to assist them in the improvement of client care.

These workshops are the medical record–client management conference and the quality assurance conference. Both workshops focus on current practices in the organization and on those areas in which improvement can or should be made. They provide the staff with the opportunity to discuss client care concerns with the surveyor and to explore alternative methods of dealing with those concerns. When feasible, concrete and objective suggestions given by the surveyor can then be put into practice in order to help the organization in its attempts to improve compliance with JCAH standards. Because these workshops can be valuable as an educational tool, the role of the surveyor can be more readily seen to be that of an evaluator and facilitator rather than a criticizer and manipulator.

The JCAH surveyor allows the nurse-administrator to make on-the-spot changes in noncompliant or inadequate policies and procedures to bring the nursing department into compliance with a standard. Thus, recognition is given when the nurse-administrator attempts to correct or to improve deficient compliance.

At the final summary conference (open to all staff members), the surveyor discusses each standard and the related findings. Areas of minimal or noncompliance are reviewed, and acknowledgement is given for any acceptable measures instituted by the organization to bring the organization into compliance. In addition, the persons in attendance at the summation conference are given an opportunity to discuss the surveyor's comments and to clarify unclear areas.

The surveyor then submits a report of the findings from the site survey to the JCAH Board of Commissioners. The board, not the surveyor, is responsible for the decision to grant or to withhold accreditation. In the event a nonaccreditation decision is reached, the organization can appeal the decision. Guidelines for appeal are available from the JCAH.

JCAH Standards Affecting Psychiatric–Mental Health Nursing

Under the consolidated standards, JCAH (1983) requirements for psychiatric–mental health nursing include a written plan of nursing services and the provision of such services by a registered nurse who is responsible to "plan, assign, supervise, and evaluate nursing care" (p. 18). Other areas of the standards are indirectly related to psychiatric–mental health nursing practice within the context of the interdisciplinary treatment team. As a member of the interdisciplinary treatment team, nursing must also comply with these standards. Three important areas pertinent to nursing include treatment plans, special treatment procedures, and staff development. (Quality assurance, a fourth major component of the JCAH standards, is discussed in Chapter 16.)

Treatment Plans

Because of the nursing process approach to client care, the discipline of nursing has more experience than any discipline in the identification of client needs and in the establishment of care plans in a specific and objective manner. The nursing care plan for psychiatric–mental health clients must be individualized for each client's specific needs while interfacing and integrating with the overall inter-disciplinary treatment plan. The psychiatric–mental health nursing administrator, in conjunction with staff development and other care-giving disciplines, is faced with the challenge of determining a method whereby treatment goals and objectives for each client are specific, realistic, time-limited, and measurable. Furthermore, specific treatment interventions, which specify the staff responsible for the implementation of the intervention, must be indicated for each goal and objective. In addition, the frequency of each intervention and outcome measures, which indicate achievement of treatment goals and objectives, must be specified.

Written goals, objectives, interventions, and outcome measures for the discontinuation of treatment have been problematic in many psychiatric–mental health settings. The nurse-administrator can assist the treatment team by providing resources for staff education in treatment planning and assistance in designing and formulating treatment planning forms that facilitate the planning process. Psychiatric–mental health care deals with intangible, sometimes imperceptible, behaviors that must be identified in concrete, measurable, and behavioral terms. Identification of such behaviors is an essential assessment skill required of the psychiatric–mental health nurse practitioner.

Documentation in the clinical record must focus on client problems and the treatment; client response and progress must also be written in measurable terms. Because documentation is of great importance, the nurse-administrator must be alert to problems encountered by the treatment team and must provide whatever assistance is necessary to improve the quality of documentation and to resolve client care problems.

Special Treatment Procedures

Another area in which the JCAH standards affect nursing is that of special treatment procedures. JCAH (1983) carefully outlines them.

> Treatment procedures that require special justification shall include, but not necessarily be limited to, the following:
>
> a. the use of restraint;
> b. the use of seclusion;
> c. the use of electroconvulsive therapy and other forms of convulsive therapy;
> d. the performance of psychosurgery or other surgical procedures for the intervention in or alteration of a mental, emotional, or behavioral disorder;
> e. the use of behavior modification procedures that use painful stimuli;
> f. the use of unusual medications and investigational and experimental drugs;
> g. the prescribing and administering of drugs for maintenance use that have abuse potential (usually Schedule II drugs) and drugs that are known to involve a substantial risk or to be associated with undesirable side effects; and
> h. research projects that involve inconvenience or risk to the patient.
> (p. 77)

Special treatment procedures require detailed, specific policies and procedures that insure compliance with this standard.

The nurse-administrator needs to be involved in the development of organizational policies and procedures to insure coordination and interfacing of approaches. Again, staff education and the development of flow charts, special forms, and the like are necessary. Nursing has great responsibility for the care of clients who undergo special procedures. It is imperative, then, that the nursing staff have the knowledge, the skills, and the tools to provide that care safely and in a professional, caring manner.

Staff Growth and Development

Staff growth and development is concerned with three specific areas: (1) orientation of new employees, (2) staff development programs to prepare the staff for promotions and new responsibilities, and (3) continuing education aimed at keeping the professional staff up-to-date with new developments and skills (JCAH, 1983, p. 43). If the organization has a separate staff development department, the nurse-administrator would be responsible only for the articulation of psychiatric–mental health nursing education needs to that department. Collaboration and cooperation between departments is essential if the needs of the staff and the JCAH standards are to be met. Inservice and orientation content needs to be reviewed, and selected content needs to be included on a routine basis. This content would include such items as cardiopulmonary resuscitation training, therapeutic milieu concepts, physical crisis intervention, client safety precautions, fire and disaster drills, therapeutic approaches, psychological assessment, and psychopharmacology.

Programs that update staff knowledge on policy and procedural changes, leadership skills, and professional networking also contribute to the staff's preparation for increased responsibility or promotions. The use of workshops and seminars outside the organization—especially in conjunction with ANA and state nurses' associations—assist the staff in fostering expertise in their practice areas, and promote professionalism. These programs, in turn, reward the organization as the quality of staff performance improves.

Staff development is essential in most efforts to improve quality care, particularly when specific quality assurance studies have identified problem areas. Educational programs are a valid and an available means of aiding the staff to overcome and to resolve client care problems. Whether a simple review of existing policies and procedures is warranted or the implementation of a complex new system is needed, staff development personnel provide skills and expertise in the promotion of quality care. The nurse-administrator needs qualified, committed clinicians who can provide the staff development the nursing department needs.

Additional Focus of Regulatory Bodies

In addition to JCAH, other regulatory bodies focus on such issues as staffing patterns, RN-to-client ratios, and RN-to-other nursing personnel ratios. Although these standards may not identify determined staff numbers and staff mix, they do emphasize this area of concern. Safety, security, and sanitation are also often scrutinized by these accrediting and regulatory bodies. Clearly, then, any psychiatric–mental health care agency providing service to a client population of often suicidal, regressed, and psychotic persons must have crucial concerns for safety, security, and sanitation. The physical plant needs to provide the appropriate setting for the type of program and the client population being served. For example, a nursing unit that treats acutely suicidal clients needs to have an adequate staff to provide the level of supervision these clients require. In addition, policies and procedures related to special precautionary measures—including 1:1

supervision, monitoring of dangerous or potentially dangerous items, and the freedom to leave the unit—need to be defined. Furthermore, because the standards of many regulatory bodies may be stated in broad terms, the nurse-administrator needs to translate them into specifics for the individual organization. Ambiguities do exist, as do occasional conflicts in standards, from one regulatory body to another. This problem is yet another challenge for the psychiatric–mental health nursing administrator.

IMPLEMENTING MEASURES TO IMPROVE COMPLIANCE

Whether preparing for an on-site visit by a regulatory body or implementing recommended changes as a result of a survey, the nurse-administrator has several resources available. A nursing accreditation committee (mentioned above) is a useful tool for preparing the staff and the department for an on-site visit. Other psychiatric–mental health committees can also be used to provide ongoing assessment, planning, implementation, and evaluation of compliance with relevant regulatory body standards.

For example, the nursing department policy and procedure committee, as a standing committee with representation from all levels of the staff, could be a useful tool in assuring compliance with standards of the many surveying bodies. Scheduled meetings should include the regular review of the nursing department's policies and procedures. In addition, changes that reflect current practice or that effect an improvement in practice must be made in existing policies and procedures. Recommendations made by regulatory bodies that require policy and procedure changes, additions, or deletions would be referred by the nurse-administrator to this committee for implementation. As in the case of all committees, use of staff level personnel allows input from those persons most directly affected by changes in policies and procedures. Implementation of changes is, therefore, smoother because the staff has had opportunity to review those changes and shares responsibility for them. As new programs are planned, the department's policy and procedure committee can be involved in setting new policies and establishing new procedures.

The chairperson of the policy and procedure committee needs access to all standards that affect specific areas of nursing care. For example, if the members of the committee are working on a policy and procedure related to client contraband, they must know the state mental health code and the administrative rules about client rights and safety, as well as JCAH standards on clients' rights. In addition, some sensitive areas (such as contraband issues) may require legal clarification before a policy and procedure may be implemented.

Another important psychiatric–mental health nursing committee is the nursing quality assurance (QA) or nursing audit committee. Like the policy and procedure committee and the accreditation committee, the QA committee concerns itself with methods that improve the quality of the psychiatric–mental health nursing care provided to the client population. Findings of the QA committee are often referred to the policy and procedure committee for corrective measures that involve modifications of procedure. The QA committee also has a strong reliance on staff development for educational programs. These programs provide the staff with the necessary level of knowledge required to resolve the problem identified by the QA committee. The function of the QA committee is discussed in depth in the chapter on quality assurance.

A clinical privileges committee for psychiatric–mental health nursing is another useful tool in maintaining and improving quality care standards. The committee on credentials, composed of registered nurses at all levels, has the responsibility of reviewing the clinical practice of a licensed nurse as measured against predetermined standards. The review process, often a component of a career-ladder program, is peer review. Each nurse is required to submit documentation of clinical achievement during the review period. Documentation of educational requirements, necessary for certain privileges, must also be submitted. The committee on credentials determines whether the nurse should be continued at the same level or a different level of practice. For instance, a nurse who wishes to co-lead group therapy may need a BSN degree and a certain number of hours of group process or therapy classes before being considered eligible for certification. Once certified, the nurse would be eligible to function as a co-therapist in group therapy. Each nurse's employment record would contain specific certification information related to the type of practice the nurse would be allowed to perform. More information about this concept as it relates to clinical career ladders is included in the chapter on staff development.

EVALUATING DEPARTMENTAL COMPLIANCE WITH STANDARDS

The psychiatric–mental health nursing administrator should not rely on survey reports as the sole means of evaluating the department's compliance with the standards of the regulatory body. A proactive approach can aid the department in functioning at a much higher level of compliance and with less of the stress and panic associated with the appearance of a surveyor. Periodic review of the standards with the staff and a scheduled monitoring system can also be most helpful. (Even such basic public health standards as those regarding the storage of dirty linen can be neglected if not monitored.) Routine monitoring at the unit level can avoid risks and can reduce last minute cleanups and increased workload for the nursing staff. Furthermore, a mock survey done before the JCAH visit can provide an evaluation of the department's overall compliance and the time needed to make the necessary corrections.

REFERENCES

Joint Commission on Accreditation of Hospitals. (1983). *Consolidated standards manual/83 for child, adolescent, and adult psychiatric, alcoholism, and drug abuse facilities*. Chicago: Author.

Salmore, R. (1982). JCAH is coming. *Journal of Nursing Management, 13*(7), 41–42.

Chapter 4

Legal Issues and the Psychiatric–Mental Health Nursing Administrator

The nursing profession has always been faced with legal constraints, and the specialty of psychiatric–mental health nursing is no exception. Whether it is the objectivity of the charting, the seclusion or restraint of a client, or the administration of medication to a psychotic client who refuses it, the psychiatric–mental health nursing administrator is continually confronted with questions and concerns of a legal nature. These circumstances necessitate that the nurse-administrator be well versed in the local, state, and federal rules and regulations that affect the delivery of psychiatric–mental health nursing care and their application to the particular organization and department. By using this knowledge base, the nurse-administrator serves as a resource for the staff regarding both current daily practices and future program planning.

ASSESSMENT OF LEGAL ISSUES

Whether done as an annual review or before the opening of a new program, the legal issues affecting the department, the staff, and the client population should be thoroughly assessed in order to develop a comprehensive plan to address those issues. Departmental needs may include such areas as overall liability insurance; risk management programs, which would include incident reporting and medication administration systems; comprehensive quality assurance programs; and policies and procedures covering areas in which legal issues arise. Staff needs may be related to organizational or to client needs, or may be unique unto themselves. Such needs may include individual liability insurance (for both management and staff); knowledge regarding Nurse Practice Acts and mental health codes; experience in commitment and court proceedings; documentation guidelines; and relevant information about the legal constraints on daily nursing practice. Should the organization have differing levels of staff (such as clinical specialists, staff nurses,

29

and paraprofessionals), each group needs to be assessed separately in order to determine their differing needs.

The legal issues related to the psychiatric–mental health client population vary with the population. The definitions of client rights, which may differ from state to state, must be communicated to each client in a concise and comprehensible fashion. This communication must be documented. (See Appendix 4-A for a listing of client rights.) The abuse of psychiatric–mental health clients is another area that must be addressed within the organization and department through careful definition, investigative approaches, and corrective measures—including disciplinary actions. Guidelines for the above areas may be found within rules and regulations external to the organization but may need to be tailored individually to the specific setting.

Admission and Discharge Processes

The admission and discharge processes are always a legal concern within a psychiatric–mental health setting. Definitions of voluntary and involuntary admissions must be readily available and thoroughly reviewed. Nursing staff involved in the admitting process must be familiar with the required procedures. There are certain forms that *must* be signed before admission. If these forms are not properly signed and treatment is instituted for the patient, the admission may not be legal and the application of such treatment plans may place the staff in legal jeopardy. In addition to improperly signed forms, other situations may constitute illegal admissions in various states. The admitting nursing staff should be educated about these situations. The consequences of such illegal admissions for the admitting nursing staff must be assessed and incorporated into the department's plan for the legal support of the staff.

The discharge process in psychiatric–mental health nursing includes a discharge against medical advice that is similar to that in other specialty areas. However, in many settings, the client must give notice that he or she wishes to be discharged. The organization, then, has a specified amount of time to honor that request. For example, in Michigan, the amount of time is three working days. During this time, the staff are to assess whether the client can safely be discharged or whether commitment proceedings should be instituted. Should the client be capable of sufficient self-care and pose no danger to self or others, discharge may be indicated.

Client Records: Confidentiality

An issue directly related to psychiatric–mental health clients is the confidentiality of client records. Confidentiality of patient information is important in all nursing areas, as this is a basic principle of nursing's code of ethics. In addition, various legislation supports this principle by declaring illegal the disclosure of client information without the involved client's consent. Hence, all health care organizations need to have confidentiality policies and procedures that apply to all persons within that setting.

Confidentiality of client treatment information becomes an even more crucial issue when the client population is involved in treatment for any type of substance abuse. In these situations, based on federal law, "the identity, diagnosis, prognosis or treatment" (Federal Register, 1975, p. 27803) of a person receiving treatment for substance abuse *must be* kept confidential. In many psychiatric–mental health organizations, clients—although admitted for psychiatric–mental health problems—also have additional problems with substance abuse. Hence, it is often more efficient to treat all clients in the same confidential manner than to have two sets of confidentiality standards. It is crucial, in whatever setting, to maintain client confidentiality by discussing client information only with those staff essential to the client's treatment and insuring that those staff understand and respect the confidentiality of the information.

PLANNING TO ADDRESS LEGAL ISSUES

After a careful assessment of department, staff, and client issues that have legal implications, an overall plan should be developed to address the identified issues. This overall plan, hereafter referred to as the nursing department's legal protection plan, includes those documents and activities that focus on the legal protection of clients and staff. The documentation and activities included vary with individual departments and organizations and are based upon identified needs and client populations.

An informed staff is crucial for the development of an appropriate plan. If a few knowledgeable staff are not available within the department or organization, the nurse-administrator may wish to establish a contract with outside consultants to provide the necessary expertise. Staff involved in the plan's component, which addresses the maintenance of confidential records, should include not only those from the nursing department but also from the risk management, the quality assurance, the medical records, and the admitting departments—as well as the hospital's legal counsel.

Any plan developed should include extensive policies and procedures designed to address defined goals and objectives while recognizing the legal uncertainties of the practice environment. Such organizational policies should include, but not be limited to, those involving documentation, client rights, restraints or seclusion, admission and discharge processes, photographing, fingerprinting, tape recording, informed consent, personal and property searches, restrictions of mail, telephone usage, and release of information to the news media. In conjunction with the development of these documents, in-service training should be planned and repeated on a regular basis to facilitate the staff's awareness and understanding of such issues. These in-service training programs should be available to all shifts and all staff members—part-time as well as full-time. By involving as many staff members as possible, the nurse-administrator provides a work environment that fosters a knowledgeable and concerned staff.

Organizational Protection

Any legal protection plan must address all areas of treatment that have legal implications for the organization, the staff, and the clients. To provide protection for the overall organization, a detailed risk management program with well-defined quality assurance mechanisms—similar to those in other health care organizations—could be established by the organization. Such programs would identify potential legal problems and would develop strategies to prevent their occurrence. In addition, insurance policies should be a component of the overall plan to provide needed protection should a problem occur. Such insurances should include worker's compensation, unemployment compensation, professional liability, and general liability. The psychiatric–mental health nurse administrator could be helpful to administration in defining the parameters and the necessary components of such a program.

In addition, the psychiatric–mental health nursing department of the organization must also include knowledge of the relevant Nurse Practice Act in its legal protection plan. "A nurse who engages in activities beyond the legally recognized scope of practice runs the risk of prosecution for violating the state medical practice act, and the [organization] that employs the nurse could also be held criminally responsible for aiding and abetting the illegal practice of medicine" (Rowland & Rowland, 1980, p. 124). Hence, it is important that nursing administration be familiar with all the components of the relevant Nurse Practice Act. The application of the act to the psychiatric–mental health setting may not require extensive consultation. However, it is crucial for the nurse-administrator to understand fully the ramifications of the Nurse Practice Act and its relevant application to the particular setting. If the setting includes a variety of levels of nurses (i.e., clinical nurse specialists, staff nurses, licensed practical nurses, licensed vocational nurses, and licensed psychiatric attendant nurses), the nurse-administrator must make certain that all levels of practice conform with the practice act.

Staff Protection

Two areas of concern in terms of the legal protection of the staff include liability insurance and the quality of the documentation of care. Hence, any plan that attempts to provide legal protection for staff must address these two areas.

Liability insurance may be handled in a variety of ways. The organization may provide basic coverage for all employees or may recommend that each staff carry an individual policy. Whichever plan is ultimately selected, the nurse-administrator should examine it carefully to determine its applicability to both the psychiatric–mental health setting and the practice needs of the staff, and should ensure that the staff members clearly understand what the organization provides and the extent of their own responsibility.

Proper documentation is essential for the legal protection of the staff. "Proper recording of the facts of a [client's] illness, symptoms, diagnosis, and treatment is one of the most important functions in [providing] modern [health] care" (Rowland & Rowland, 1980, p. 127). Nursing documentation is often included in legal proceedings for three basic reasons: (1) "the nurses' notes hold the only clue as to whether . . . orders were carried out and what the results were. (2) Nurses' notes are [generally] the only notes written with both time and date and strictly in chronological order. . . . (3) They [nurses' notes] . . . offer the most detailed information regarding the [client]" (Kerr, 1975, p. 34). Hence, it behooves the nurse-administrator to expect and to require proper documentation by all nursing staff on all clients.

Charting should reflect the continuity of care (Kerr, 1975) and should include all relevant data and information about nursing interventions in order to provide an accurate, comprehensive picture of a client's care. Kerr also suggests avoiding generalized terms. This is particularly important in psychiatric–mental health nursing. Documentations must be objective and descriptive of behavior in order to portray a client's condition adequately and accurately. Generalities, biases, and deductions do not provide the specific information needed by other professionals to plan and to revise care.

Client Protection

Many legal issues have an impact on clients. In psychiatric–mental health nursing, client rights, confidentiality of records or release of information, and client abuse are particularly important. "The full implementation of clients' rights frequently is the responsibility of psychiatric personnel, specifically psychiatric nurses" (Wilson & Kneisl, 1979, p. 721). In many circumstances, the client may be unaware of rights that have been established to protect persons or may be unable to question occurrences that impinge on legally identified rights. Nursing staff, thus, have an obligation to understand the rights of clients and to aid in their protection. (A list of the rights of clients has been included in Appendix 4-A, and other lists are available in the literature.)

Confidentiality of client records is identified as a major client right. Today's technology makes it increasingly difficult to ensure a client's confidentiality routinely. The psychiatric–mental health nursing organization must have detailed policies and procedures that address this area and define both confidentiality and any related actions that must be taken to preserve that client confidence. A system for the release of information is one of those related actions that serve to protect a client's confidentiality, and requests for the release of such information are usually referred to the organization's medical records department. Clients and staff must be aware that information cannot be provided to others without a formal release of information from the client involved. Through this mechanism, the confidentiality of the client's treatment record can be protected, inasmuch as the client determines who will receive information. Routine in-service training and educational efforts directed to these areas of concern can increase the staff's awareness of the importance of these activities.

The abuse of clients is an unacceptable occurrence in any setting. In psychiatric–mental health settings, clients may be vulnerable to various types of abuse. To create a milieu that fosters safety, policies and procedures should exist to define abusive activities, to delineate a reporting system for suspected abuse should it occur, and to determine corrective actions for those staff members who are abusive. As in the case of confidentiality, the provision of regular in-service training can reinforce, to all staff, the great importance of ensuring the professional treatment of clients.

In discussing client abuse, the staff members often confuse abuse with treatment against the client's wishes. This concern is often expressed in psychiatric–mental health nursing settings, because clients are frequently confused and refuse treatment in their confusion. The Task Force on Behavior Therapy makes the following recommendations for determining the appropriateness of treating a client against his or her verbal wishes:

1. The client must be judged to be dangerous to [self] or others.
2. Those administering treatment [must believe] that it has a reasonable chance to benefit the [client] and those related. . . .
3. [The client] must be judged to be incompetent to evaluate the necessity of treatment. . . .
4. The [client] should not be deceived. [The client] should be informed as to what will be done, . . . the reasons for it, and its probable effects. (Stuart & Sundeen, 1983, p. 526)

Policies and procedures must also direct the staff to keep the client informed, and these policies and procedures should be reviewed on a regular basis with all the staff. Through these efforts, the staff can continue to provide therapeutic care while protecting themselves and the client from abuse or legal action.

IMPLEMENTING A LEGAL PROTECTION PLAN

The implementation of the plan designed above requires the careful organization and cooperation of many staff members. The detailed delineation of the persons involved, as well as the activities for which they are accountable, can do much to ensure the successful implementation of the plan. During orientation, the plan can be reviewed with each staff member to facilitate understanding and cooperation. Periodically held during the year, in-service training that reviews components of the legal protection plan (such as confidentiality issues) can enable all staff members to keep current in this area.

Medication Administration

The major activity areas of any plan designed to improve legal protection vary among organizations. However, the areas of medication administration, malpractice protection, commitment proceedings, and research are relevant to almost every psychiatric–mental health organization. In terms of medication administration, client consent and the prevention of medication errors are of major importance to the psychiatric–mental health nursing department. "The common law in this country has long held that medical treatment performed without the [client's] consent constitutes a battery (unconsented touching). In the past twenty-five years, this has changed to a requirement for the [client's] *informed* consent, thereby expanding the provider's potential liability" (Bassuk, Schoonover, & Gelenberg, 1983, p. 401). Although the bulk of the responsibility for obtaining a client's consent falls to the prescribing physician, the nurse often becomes involved as a monitor of this process, or in instances when the medication must be administered against the client's consent. Should the psychiatric–mental health nursing department be involved in the monitoring of the client's consent to treatment, meetings should occur that facilitate an understanding of what is to be monitored, and how this monitoring is to be done. Through such clarification, the departments of medicine, nursing, and pharmacy can collaborate to protect client interests.

"One of the most intensely debated issues in psychiatry . . . is the [client's] right to decline treatment, particularly psychoactive medications" (Bassuk et al., p. 404). Psychiatric–mental health nurses are placed in a double bind as the hospitalized client's right to receive appropriate treatment often conflicts with the right to refuse such treatment. "The right to refuse medications is not absolute. The courts recognize that in an emergency the clinician can administer medications without the client's consent" (Bassuk et al., p. 404). It is crucial, therefore, for the nursing staff to understand the definition of *emergency* specific to the locality as established by the state Mental Health Code. Departmental policies and procedures must address this issue specifically, and in detail, to provide a sound basis for this aspect of psychiatric–mental health nursing practice.

Client education is also a valuable and essential mechanism to increase a client's knowledge and awareness of the medications being received. Through client teaching, the nurse provides information to improve the client's knowledge of side-effects, interactions, and situations in which the physician should be contacted. This increase in knowledge can do much to facilitate the client's safety and progress and to decrease the nurse's legal risks.

The prevention of medication errors is another major priority in any nursing setting. It is no different in psychiatric–mental health organizations. Specific detailed policies and procedures can, again, do much to decrease errors. When coupled with regular in-service training, this approach can serve to decrease errors substantially. When errors do occur, the staff should report them through a defined reporting system. In this manner, the underlying causes of medication errors can more easily be determined and steps taken to correct them—e.g., procedural changes, staff education, or employee counselling.

Malpractice

Malpractice is a major concern of all nurse-administrators. It can be defined as the

> negligence or carelessness of professional personnel. The four elements
> of negligence are: (1) a standard of due care under the circumstances;
> (2) a failure to meet the standard of due care; (3) the foreseeability of
> harm resulting from failure to meet the standard; and (4) the fact that the
> breach of this standard proximately causes the injury to the plaintiff. The
> standard of care is determined by deciding what a reasonably prudent
> person acting under similar circumstances would do. (Rowland &
> Rowland, 1980, pp. 133–134)

In psychiatric–mental health nursing, "the most common causes of malpractice suits against nurses are negligence in the areas of suicide [and elopement] precautions and assisting in electroconvulsive therapy" (Stuart & Sundeen, 1983, p. 531). In order to aid the nursing staff in decreasing their vulnerability in this area, educational efforts can stress several points.

- "The nurse is responsible for reporting pertinent information about [the client] to . . . co-workers involved in [that client's] care." (Stuart & Sundeen, 1983, p. 531). This report should be made through both oral and written communications.
- Documentation in the medical record must be comprehensive.
- Nursing staff must maintain the confidentiality of client care information.
- Care must be given in a thorough and attentive fashion. Through inattention or the haphazard delivery of care, the client is placed at risk and the nurse may be found to be negligent.

- Nursing care implemented must meet standards of psychiatric–mental health nursing practice.

- The nurses must "know the laws of the state in which [they] practice, including the rights and duties of the nurse as well as the rights of the [clients]." (Stuart & Sundeen, 1979, p. 283)

By adhering to these guidelines and related policies and procedures, the nursing staff can provide consistent quality care without risk of negligence.

Commitment (Involuntary Hospitalization)

Clients enter into treatment through a variety of mechanisms. Psychiatric–mental health nurses must be informed and comfortable with each of the mechanisms to protect the client, themselves, and the organization. Again, the policies and procedures of both the organization and the department must address these mechanisms in a clear and detailed manner to provide sufficient information to the nursing staff. The content of such policies and procedures, and related educational efforts, should include the different types of admissions (formal, informal, voluntary, involuntary) and the points of difference between them. Generally, the more restrictive types of admission processes can occur only if the client is a danger to self or others, or is unable to care for basic needs. The processes involved in each admission mechanism must also be regularly reviewed with all nursing staff. Figure 4–1 illustrates the process involved in the involuntary commitment process.

The role assumed by the staff must be clearly delineated and reviewed so that the staff is comfortable in assuming its role. In addition, support mechanisms must be provided that foster a comfortable environment in which the nursing staff can participate in the specific admission mechanism required by a client. For example, a knowledgeable nurse may be designated to accompany an inexperienced nurse who may be required to attend court proceedings on behalf of a client. Staff members would know that this support is available, and this knowledge would serve to increase their self-confidence as they participate in this legal process. The admission of a client into a psychiatric–mental health treatment program is a stressful one. Through proper implementation of an organized plan to decrease this stress, the client, the staff, and the organization are protected.

Research

Research in clinical settings is increasing and should continue to increase in order to further clinical knowledge in psychiatric–mental health nursing. However, research that directly involves clients requires policies and procedures specifically related to the research process. Such policies should include the

Figure 4–1 Diagrammatical Model of the Involuntary Commitment Process

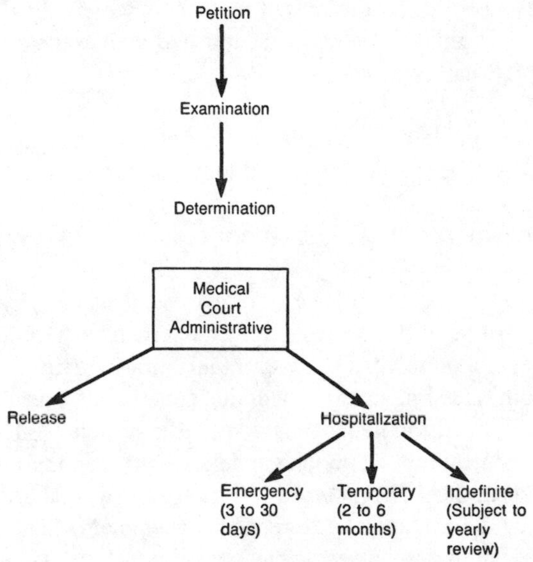

Petition

↓

Examination

↓

Determination

```
            ┌──────────────────┐
            │     Medical      │
            │     Court        │
            │  Administrative  │
            └──────────────────┘
           ↙                    ↘
    Release                  Hospitalization
                          ↙        ↓        ↘
                   Emergency   Temporary   Indefinite
                   (3 to 30    (2 to 6     (Subject to
                   days)       months)     yearly
                                           review)
```

Source: From *Principles and Practice of Psychiatric Nursing,* (2nd ed.) by G.W. Stuart & S.J. Sundeen, 1983, St. Louis: C.V. Mosby Co. © 1983 by C.V. Mosby Co. Reprinted by permission.

formation of a research committee, which oversees the obtaining of consents, the informing of clients, and the purpose of the study. The nurse involved in research must "be aware of the individual's rights and of [the nurse's] share in the responsibility of preserving them" (Rowland & Rowland, 1980, p. 133). Such awareness is fostered and supported by appropriate policies and procedures, but the nurse should also refer to the American Nurses' Association (ANA) publication *The Nurse in Research: ANA Guidelines on Ethical Values* for further clarification. Research should not occur within an organization unless a program has been implemented that protects the client, the staff, and the organization. (For additional information on research, refer to Chapter 18.)

EVALUATION

As is the case with any program, an evaluative mechanism must be incorporated into the initial design. The psychiatric–mental health nursing administrator must not assume that the program has been a success if there have been no legal actions taken against the organization or if lawsuits that have gone to court have been won by the organization. The goals and objectives of the program and its components must be reviewed on an annual basis to determine whether they have been attained. Adjustments must be made to reflect not only goal attainments but also changes that have occurred in the legal and psychiatric–mental health nursing environment. As cases continue to be heard in court and related verdicts are finalized, the nursing practice environment will change. A program designed to legally protect an organization, its staff, and its client population must also change to reflect practice realities. All components of the program may not need to be altered simultaneously, but the overall program needs to be reviewed on an annual basis to ensure a safe environment for all.

REFERENCES

Bassuk, E.L., Schoonover, S.C., & Gelenberg, A.J. (1983). *The practitioner's guide to psychoactive drugs.* New York: Plenum Medical Book.

Federal Register. (July 1, 1975). *Statutory authority—drug abuse, confidentiality of patient records,* 40 (27), p. 27803.

Kerr, A.H. (1975). Nurses notes: That's where the goodies are! *Nursing 75, 5*(2), 34–41.

Rowland, H.S., & Rowland, B.L. (1980). *Nursing administration handbook.* Rockville, Md: Aspen Systems.

Stuart, G.W., & Sundeen, S.J. (1979). *Principles and practice of psychiatric nursing.* St. Louis: C.V. Mosby.

Stuart, G.W., & Sundeen, S.J. (1983). *Principles and practice of psychiatric nursing,* (2nd ed.). St. Louis: C.V. Mosby.

Wilson, H.W., & Kneisl, C.R. (1979). *Psychiatric nursing.* Menlo Park, CA: Addison-Wesley.

Appendix 4-A

Patient Rights

National League for Nursing

NLN believes the following are patients' rights which nurses have a responsibility to uphold.

Patients have the right to:

- health care that is accessible and that meets professional standards, regardless of the setting.
- courteous and individualized health care that is equitable, humane, and given without discrimination as to race, color, creed, sex, national origin, source of payment, or ethical or political beliefs.
- information about their diagnosis, prognosis, and treatment—including alternatives to care and risks involved—in terms they and their families can readily understand, so that they can give their informed consent.
- informed participation in all decisions concerning their health care.
- information about the qualifications, names, and titles of personnel responsible for providing their health care.
- refuse observation by those not directly involved in their care.
- privacy during interview, examination, and treatment.
- privacy in communicating and visiting with persons of their choice.
- refuse treatments, medications, or participation in research and experimentation, without punitive action being taken against them.
- coordination and continuity of health care.
- appropriate instruction or education from health care personnel so that they can achieve an optimal level of wellness and an understanding of their basic health needs.

- confidentiality of all records (except as otherwise provided for by law or third party payer contracts) and all communications, written or oral, between patients and health care providers.
- access to all health records pertaining to them, the right to challenge and to have their records corrected for accuracy, and the right to transfer of all such records in the case of continuing care.
- information on the charges for services, including the right to challenge these.
- be fully informed as to all their rights in all health care settings.

Source: From *Nursing administration handbook* by H.S. Rowland & B.L. Rowland, 1980, p. 139. Rockville, Md.: Aspen Systems. © 1980 by National League for Nursing. Used by permission.

Chapter 5

Departmental Planning

FUNCTION OF PLANNING

Management has four functions: planning, organizing, directing, and controlling. By far the most elementary management function is planning. *Planning* is a systematic process that provides purpose and direction to the department. This process focuses on the future and encompasses such activities as assessing strengths and weaknesses of the department, defining problems, setting goals and objectives, identifying opportunities, and devising strategies to achieve the established goals and objectives (Ganong & Ganong, 1980). In psychiatric–mental health nursing administration, as in many other administrative areas, the planning function is often forgotten. Day-to-day crises seem to be foremost in the nurse-administrator's mind, leaving little time designated for planning activities. So many things need attention each day that time for planning becomes a luxury. Breaking out of this crisis mentality is difficult but necessary if the department is to progress. The other three management functions of organizing, directing, and controlling are meaningless if goals are not established.

Once the organization's mission statement has been defined and the philosophy of psychiatric–mental health nursing has been written, departmental planning can begin. Organizational goals set the stage for the planning of a period of five to ten years. From these long-range goals, the organization, department, service, or unit can set short-term objectives, focusing on one to three years. Setting objectives focuses attention on areas in which change is necessary and desirable. The overall organizational goals and objectives form the framework within which departmental objectives are developed. All objectives need to be in synchronization with organizational goals and must interface with each other. When combined as a whole, each department or service must have objectives that together support the organization's goals (W. Stevens, 1978). The planning process further requires constant evaluation and periodic modification in plans to allow for flexibility in meeting the ever-changing needs of the organization.

PURPOSE OF PLANNING

If support and understanding of organizational goals do not exist, chaos and confusion become the norm. It is necessary, then, to have formal, clearly defined plans in order to proceed smoothly toward the goals. Failure to plan appropriately can sabotage the best of efforts.

Health care has not always been viewed as a business. With the impetus for improved management techniques becoming more evident, health care organizations are being forced to reevaluate the effectiveness of their management styles. Accrediting bodies, insurance carriers, and others are placing greater emphasis on productivity, improved quality of care, lower costs, and future planning. Health care agencies are now compelled to adopt management techniques previously used in a predominantly industrial context. Through a well-defined process of planning, organizing, directing, and controlling, objective measures of productivity can be developed. A scientific approach to management also provides objective means for assessing management and employee performance. The scientific approach is a more systematic, objective method of management that provides clearer definitions of the management process as established through a problem-solving approach.

The day-to-day crisis orientation may keep the organization afloat, but it cannot facilitate its growth. Without planning for desired changes, the health care organization cannot remain competitive in a marketplace in which competition for services and personnel is keen. Failure to plan makes change a slow, difficult, and haphazard process during which the staff become complacent or frustrated. Nothing dampens enthusiasm faster then chaos and thwarted efforts.

ASSESSMENT OF RESOURCES

Before defining objectives, the psychiatric–mental health nursing administrator must have a thorough understanding of the mission and goals of the organization as well as a realistic assessment of the department's current operation. Knowledge of the capabilities of the staff is essential so that changes can be adjusted to the strengths of employees. This technique is also helpful in preparing the staff for possible future advancement.

In addition to an awareness of internal resources, the nurse-administrator must be cognizant of the health care community in which the organization exists. Health care resources outside the organization may be available and, therefore, of benefit not only to the organization but to the consumer as well. The use of outside resources, moving from within the health care organization into the environment, is known as "boundary spanning." The use of boundary spanning broadens the scope of the nurse-administrator's alternatives for problem resolution by fostering a sharing with health care professionals outside the bounds of the organization. Mutual sharing benefits both participants and strengthens the networking bonds so vital for supporting all nursing administrators (Kraegel, 1980). Any number of possibilities exist for the exchange of ideas and services. For example, a free-standing psychiatric hospital with a well developed physical crisis intervention program might offer a staff development program on physical crisis interventions to the emergency room staff of a nearby general hospital in exchange for phlebotomy or CPR training for their staff.

PLANNING AS FORMULATING DEPARTMENTAL OBJECTIVES

When objectives are defined, all factors that might have an impact on the outcome of the objective must be considered. This consideration includes such variables as existing services, staffing patterns, client census information, new services, budget constraints, and so forth. Objectives need to be realistic and attainable, not grandiose. Likewise, they must not be so effortless that they do not provide some challenge. They need to be written in measurable, behavioral terms that are clear and concise and accompanied by related activities necessary for the accomplishment of each objective. (See Exhibit 5–1 for examples.) Target dates need to be stated so that activities can be planned in an organized fashion. Designated persons should be responsible for the coordination and the implementation of each objective within a certain time frame (Gillies, 1982). Because everyone involved in achieving the objectives must understand what the objectives mean, it is beneficial to have copies of departmental objectives available for review and reference. Whenever possible, the nursing staff should be included in the planning process.

Exhibit 5–1 Examples of Departmental Objectives

Revise and implement job (performance) descriptions and performance evaluation tools that reflect ANA Standards for Psychiatric–Mental Health Nursing by July 198_____.

Within fiscal year 198_____, present four in-service programs for nonclinical hospital staff geared to increasing their understanding of their roles in the therapeutic milieu.

Develop and implement two on-unit [client] programs on 2S and three on-unit [client] programs on 5N by May 198_____.

Source: Reprinted with permission of Kingswood Hospital, Ferndale, Michigan.

PROBLEMS OF CHANGE

The management of change is the most challenging and frustrating responsibility of nursing administrators. How to manage and to control change is a basic problem. Any organization that remains the same becomes stagnant and ineffective. Change is, therefore, not only necessary but desirable (Drucker, 1964). Today, change is more complex and rapid because of the explosion of technological advances, rapid social changes, and an increased demand by consumers for new or expanded services (Gillies, 1982). Managing change requires an adjustment of the organization to meet the needs of an ever-changing environment.

Change always causes disruption, but careful planning can minimize problems. It is the task of the psychiatric–mental health nursing administrator to foster a climate within which change can take place as painlessly as possible.

PLANNING FOR CHANGE

The nurse-administrator must first carefully assess the environment. People affected by the change must be involved in the planning. To discuss the proposed changes at length, meetings should be held with those involved. Remember that all changes produce unexpected, unforeseen, and somewhat undesirable side-effects, even though the desired result is achieved. Careful planning, continuous monitoring of the process, and open lines of communication with staff are essential.

Concessions to the staff may be necessary to balance their needs in relation to the needs of the organization. As Warren Stevens (1978) states, "If the change is properly conveyed, then adjustment will occur and accommodation can be achieved through a series of trade-offs" (p. 109). Keep in mind that most failures in effecting change are due to personnel problems. The more involved the group is in the planning, implementing, and assessment of the change, the fewer the roadblocks. For example, if an education program for clients on psychotropic medications is desired, the psychiatric–mental health nursing administrator can introduce the subject to the head nurse and the client education or staff development coordinator for exploration. Through a series of meetings, this core group would develop the essential objectives of the proposed program. When the program looks feasible and plans need to be developed for its implementation, the head nurse then takes the program to the staff. Members of the staff are selected to work with the head nurse and client education or staff development coordinator to work out the details of the program. Members of the project report to the rest of the staff on a periodic basis, seeking input into the particulars of the program. Personnel responsible for the actual program presentation to clients need to be involved in the development of the program to whatever extent is possible. Scripts of the program can be circulated to the staff and trial presentations can be made amongst the staff to work out the problems before the program is introduced to clients. Involving the staff in such a project generates enthusiasm, a sense of worth, and ownership of the change.

After implementation of the client education program, a periodic review of its effectiveness should be carried out. Staff appraisal of the program is essential, using the information to modify the program as necessary. Through such a process, staff members have greater control of their work and the new program becomes a worthwhile project.

RESISTANCE TO CHANGE

Because people are most comfortable with the status quo, even changes that result in obvious improvements can be difficult to implement. It is important to involve all levels of the staff who will be affected by the change. When they are not involved in planning for change, the staff tend to be more resistant and to perceive the change as being forced upon them. The more involvement staff have, the more they will incorporate the change into their expectations, thus claiming the change as their own. It is essential, therefore, that the psychiatric–mental health nursing administrator control the rate and number of changes within the work environment to keep the disruption of the status quo to a minimum. Any change may be placed on a continuum—from that requiring minimal modification to that requiring a major project. As the change becomes greater, increased resistance can be anticipated (W. Stevens, 1978; B. Stevens, 1980).

Successful change is effected on three levels.

1. The change agent experiences altered behavior (the individual person adopts the change).
2. The altered behavior of the change agent affects the behavior of others in the environment (others adopt the change).
3. The combined altered behavior of everyone involved affects the entire system (the entire group accepts the change).

According to Lewin (1951), in order to effect a change, the change process passes through three stages.

1. unfreezing the forces of the status quo (employees see the benefits of a new way)
2. implementation of the change
3. refreezing the forces to stabilize the new system as part of the routine (giving positive reinforcement or other benefits or rewards)

This process occurs by loosening the stable present state, introducing the change, and then creating a new stable state. It is a means of creating order from chaos (Gillies, 1982).

In some instances, unrest can be used to loosen the status quo. Ideas can be introduced informally, slowly, and on an individual basis. Key persons can then be approached and the links between the department's objectives and their personal goals reinforced. Positive reinforcement should then be provided and support should be built for the change among the staff.

Change in any form causes feelings of insecurity among staff. These feelings are common among health care employees because of the fragmentation and the diverse job responsibilities inherent in their roles. The health care system retains the control for decision making, often making the staff feel like automatons. The way change is presented by the principal change agent can cause resistance from the remainder of the staff. Cliques form and peer pressure can create an effective barrier to change. Employees who sulk can cause more damage than the most verbal opponents.

TACTICS FOR CHANGE

With all these barriers, how can the psychiatric–mental health administrator reduce resistance? The climate must be conducive to change. This objective is accomplished by giving the staff more control over the decision-making process. Meetings should be conducted frequently and open communication maintained. Innovative ideas should be rewarded, and assignments should be made that provide for scheduled blocks of time in order to promote creative thinking. Misperceptions can cause resistance; so explain, explain, explain!

The nurse-administrator may also seek out persons and convince them of the value of the proposed change. The employees with the greatest influence should be consulted and won over. They, in turn, will become change agents. Change can be implemented first with the most receptive people, regardless of their place in the organizational hierarchy. Attention should be focused upon the cliques. If they cannot be persuaded of the benefit of the change, the nurse-administrator should divide and conquer. By trying to see the viewpoint of opponents, compromises can be facilitated when appropriate. The nurse-administrator must continue to state clearly and often the change that is expected.

The nurse-administrator has another tool available, which is the least effective—force. The power of the position can be used to impose a change. However, hostility, anger, and low morale, as well as possible failure, can occur as a result. (Chapter 2 discusses power in more detail.)

Consultants can often be very effective in altering the attitudes and the behavior of higher level employees. In conjunction with the consultant, the nurse-administrator delineates the activity plan (what the change is and why it is necessary), as well as the logistical plan (how to make the change and when it will be accomplished). Above all, however, the nurse is advised to meet, speak, and listen to all those involved in the change process (Gillies, 1982).

MANAGEMENT BY OBJECTIVES

One approach to change that can be very effective is management by objectives (MBO). MBO is a systems approach to management that sets short-term objectives, directs activities towards their attainment, and measures the achievement of the objectives. The MBO approach is future-oriented. It relies on explicit, attainable, measurable, and timely actions established for the objectives, activities, and measures. With MBO, change is expected and planned. Surprises are minimized, and the focus is on results (McConkey, 1975).

In MBO, objective setting is made routine among employees at different levels. Thus it facilitates risk taking. With MBO, mistakes are permitted. It allows the supervisor and the subordinate to negotiate objectives. Crisis orientation and day-to-day thinking are minimized, and the focus is on longer-term changes. MBO can be very effective with the nurse practitioner and clinical specialist because it allows more individualized freedom, autonomy, and decision making. It is a participative management style that looks more to results than to daily performance.

If the psychiatric–mental health nursing administrator feels the need to control very closely, the MBO approach can be very disruptive if maintained too rigidly. Latitude is needed for the unexpected.

When used appropriately, MBO results in an increase in the effectiveness of planning, a higher probability that activities will be delegated to subordinates, and an increase in employees' self-direction, accountability, and initiative (McConkey, 1975).

MANAGING TIME

Time is a problem for everyone. It is our scarcest resource. Yet, we all have the same number of hours in our days. Why is it, then, that some people are so productive while others never seem to get their jobs done? Planning and using time wisely is the key. Day-to-day activities can get out of control and overrun us if time is not planned. The best use of time is in planning—the nurse-administrator must think things through before acting.

To make better use of time, the psychiatric–mental health nursing administrator needs to assess current use of time. For example, a log may be kept for one week, including an entry every 15 minutes regarding current tasks. This log facilitates the identification of patterns. All the non-essential work listed should be assessed. Check all the people who did not need to be seen. How often did interruptions occur? Decide what must be achieved and how to do it. Delegate all non-essential tasks to subordinates. Remember the 80/20 law, which states that 80 percent of the value of work results from 20 percent of what is done.

Organize tasks by their priority. A useful method for many people is the composition of a list of urgent or important items and a list of items to be done at random. At the end of the day, review what was accomplished and prepare a new list for the following day. By focusing on specific activities, the most urgent and important matters can be accomplished. The non-essentials that are not addressed for a period of time should be eliminated or should be delegated to a subordinate. Leading time wasters include—

- lack of planning
- lack of priorities
- overcommitment
- management by crisis
- haste
- paperwork and reading
- indecision
- failure to delegate
- routine and trivia
- visitors
- telephone calls
- meetings

When going through the mail, the secretary should weed out all the non-essentials. Look through memos, letters, and other paperwork only once, and make a decision about each item immediately. Try to eliminate as much routine work and trivia as possible. Discontinue reports and other paperwork for two weeks. After two weeks, determine what needs to be reinstated. The remainder should be eliminated.

The psychiatric–mental health nursing administrator who feels the necessity to do everything ends up controlling nothing. Learn to delegate, and to maximize subordinates' strengths. It is not time-effective to evaluate the performance and quality of the staff on a daily basis—do it once a year. Modify the open door policy if it causes problems. Establish times when you are available or blocks of time when you are not available. Shut the door periodically, and do not accept calls for a certain length of time (Schmied, 1979). Set limits on intrusions.

When confronted with many projects or tasks, start with the most difficult. Once that task is completed, the remaining work can be more easily finished. When there is a recurrent crisis, evaluate its cause and take steps to correct it.

Look at the times of the day when you are at your best, and schedule your most demanding work during that time. In this way, you can have the energy to complete your most demanding work and can utilize your less productive times for less strenuous activities (Drucker, 1977). The mark of success of the nurse administrator is how that person contributes to the success of the organization.

PLANNING AND THE BUDGET

The budgetary process is a tool for the planning, monitoring, and controlling of costs. Budgetary planning requires setting objectives creatively and realistically assigning them priorities. Careful attention is given to detailing the activities required to meet the objectives and how each objective fits into the overall organizational goals. From this detailed planning and analysis, cost estimates are established.

The budgetary process stimulates thinking in advance. It also leads to specificity in the planning and the addressing of such issues as volume and type of services, revenue, number and type of personnel required, furniture, supplies and equipment needed, and other costs. This process benefits the overall organization because of the thinking process involved. According to Schmied (1979), planning, budgeting, and forecasting—known as the "financial triangle"—are interdependent and essential to the realistic attainment of objectives. (See Chapter 7 for further information.)

PROGRAM PLANNING

At least annually, each program should be evaluated through a review of its long-range objectives. Comparisons of costs and benefits should be made. Can alternative programs that will satisfy the program goals be initiated at lower costs? Is there a demand or a need for the program? If not, can it be eliminated? The population served varies over time; therefore, program evaluation and planning must assess the changing needs of the society it serves. Modifications in programs should evolve from this analysis, and so the planning process continues.

When looking at program changes, allow for creativity. Many an absurd-sounding idea blossoms in a creative atmosphere and provides an innovative approach to a different problem. Use a brainstorming approach to problems, and assess the value of every idea before discarding it.

REFERENCES

Drucker, P.F. (1964). *Managing for results*. New York: Harper & Row.

Drucker, P.F. (1977). *People and performance: The best of Peter Drucker on management*. New York: Harper & Row.

Ganong, J.M., & Ganong, W.L. (1980). *Nursing management*. Rockville, Md: Aspen Systems.

Gillies, D.A. (1982). *Nursing management: A systems approach*. Philadelphia: W.B. Saunders Co.

Kraegel, J.M. (Ed.). (1980). *Organization-environment relationships*. Rockville, Md: Aspen Systems.

Lewin, K. (1951). *Field theory in social science*. New York: Harper & Row.

McConkey, D.D. (1975). *Management by objectives for nonprofit organizations*. New York: Amacom.

Rowland, H.S., & Rowland, B.L. (1980). *Nursing administration handbook*. Rockville, Md: Aspen Systems.

Schmied, E. (Ed.). (1979). *Maintaining cost effectiveness*. Rockville, Md: Aspen Systems.

Sisk, H.L. (1973). *Management and organization*. Cincinnati, Ohio: Southwestern Publishing.

Stevens, B. (1980). *The nurse as executive* (2nd ed.). Rockville, Md: Aspen Systems.

Stevens, W. (1978). *Management and leadership in nursing*. New York: McGraw-Hill.

Chapter 6

Unionization

OVERVIEW OF LABOR MOVEMENTS IN HEALTH CARE

The labor movement in the United States has been a recognized force in business and industry for several decades. Organized labor has been well established in its representation of blue-collar factory workers seeking improved economic factors for the labor force. These factors include such things as wages and salaries, benefits, and working hours. In the health care industry, however, organized labor is quite new. The voice of unions in the professional activities of health care providers has been recognized only since 1974. In that year, the National Labor Relations Act (NLRA) was amended, and health care agencies were removed from their exempt status. This meant that employees of the health care industry had the right to organize. In 1975, the National Labor Relations Board (NLRB) recognized nurses' organizations as bargaining units.

In 1977, the American Nurses' Association published a position paper on reimbursement for nurses. In this paper, the ANA acknowledged collective bargaining as a means for nurses to secure professional recognition in financial and nursing care areas (ANA, 1977).

Unionization of both nonprofessional and professional groups rapidly ensued in the wake of these decisions. Unions had progressed from simply having an economic focus to a point at which they desired a voice in the decision-making process of organizations where they had representation. Decision making had been strictly circumscribed as a management prerogative until a few years ago.

THE NEGOTIATION PROCESS IN HEALTH CARE

The NLRB had many concerns about the impact of organized labor on the provision of health care services. Unlike industry, which can shut down operations for a strike and then continue when an agreement has been reached, a work stoppage in health care could seriously jeopardize the lives and the well-being of many people who are dependent on the system for care. Consequently, strict guidelines about strikes or work stoppages due to the modification or termination of the work agreement were enacted.

The Federal Mediation and Conciliation Service (FMCS), which provides assistance to labor and management for the resolution of differences related to labor arguments, requires a 60-day notice from one or both parties when there is an intent by either party to modify or to terminate an agreement. In those cases in which a new bargaining unit is being certified to represent employees in a negotiated agreement, the FMCS must be notified within 30 days of the date of certification. This procedure then allows the FMCS to assign a mediator in the geographical area in which the health care organization is located. Before a strike can occur, a 10-day strike notice must be given to the employer, and the FMCS must be notified. All precautions are taken to assure that health care clients are not subjected to a cessation of services that could be hazardous to them. When a strike notice is received by the FMCS, the assigned mediator gets in touch with both the labor representative and the employer to investigate the situation. If the mediator finds the strike threat to be imminent and the parties to be at a stalemate, the mediator intervenes to facilitate negotiations. The mediator, seen as an unbiased person with many years of negotiation experience, can make recommendations to both sides for the resolution of conflicts that are impeding the negotiation of an agreement. These recommendations are not mandatory, but often are accepted.

In the event that the mediator is unable to break the stalemate and an agreement cannot be negotiated, the FMCS may appoint a Board of Inquiry, consisting of one or more persons, to begin fact-finding. *Fact-finding* is a method whereby the board gathers all relevant facts in the situation. Hearsay and unsubstantiated information and allegations are excluded. Previously undisclosed information is brought forward in the hope that both parties can come to an agreement through enlightenment of the situation. If this procedure fails again, the conflict goes to arbitration.

In the arbitration process, the arbitrator hears both parties, reviews the fact-finding results of the Board of Inquiry, and makes a decision. The recommendations set forth by an arbitrator, unlike those of a mediator, are binding. Both parties, then, must agree to carry out the arbitrator's decision. If either party feels it cannot abide by the arbitrated agreement, the decision may be taken to court.

Although the sequence of events may seem long and involved, the whole purpose is to provide as much assistance as possible to both parties in a timely manner so that health care services will not be disrupted. It is rare that negotiations go as far as the judiciary system. Most labor agreements are mutually accepted before the threat of a strike occurs.

ASSESSMENT OF ORGANIZED LABOR IN HEALTH CARE

Why Organize?

As the focus of unions changed over time from the economic issues to areas of decision making, a greater impetus arose for professionals to use a collective approach in order to have more control over their areas of practice. Initially, nurses wanted more economic security and better working conditions. As conditions improved, they have seen the use of collective action as a means to control their own practice.

In the psychiatric–mental health care system, as in all health care, nurses often feel impotent in controlling their own practice. Too often, they are not seen by physicians, nurse-administrators, or other disciplines as professionals who have contributions to make on behalf of client care. The bureaucratic nature of the system does little to promote professional autonomy, while it simultaneously increases demands for more nonprofessional work from professional nurses. In many instances, the individual nurse may feel heard only if the voice is loud enough. As a result, nurses join together and collectively seek resolutions to their perceived shared concerns.

Nurses remain divided in their opinions about unionization. Many nurses can see the advantages of unions for such issues as better pay and benefits, improved working conditions, better equipment, and minimal rotation of shifts. They may even see the use of collective bargaining as a vehicle for improving the response of nursing management to their needs.

There are many nurses, however, who believe that the image of unions is detrimental to the profession—an opinion that is difficult to dispute in view of the fact that some nurses have allowed truck drivers' unions to negotiate for such important issues as client safety and nursing practice. Another element of the collective bargaining process that nurses face is the difficulty a person dedicated to providing care and support to clients has in imagining striking and, thus, impeding that care. Many nurses also question why they should pay an outsider to talk with management when they can articulate their needs and concerns directly.

In spite of the mixed feelings of most professional nurses, unions do exist and are a reality in a great many psychiatric–mental health settings. Unionization can also exist among professional or nonprofessional groups within a single psychiatric–mental health environment. Whether collective bargaining agreements exist in either or both groups, the fact remains that the contract formalizes the relationship between the employer and the employee and requires the employer to adhere to it under penalty of law.

Warning Signs of Organizing Activity

It is only natural that the psychiatric–mental health nursing administrator who faces possible unionization should feel threatened and powerless. Certainly, steps should be taken by the nurse-administrator to improve relationships between the staff and management. Such improvement may prevent the need for the staff to resort to an outside group to negotiate for them.

If no collective bargaining unit already exists, recognizable signs may indicate unionization efforts. Any of the following signs should be reported to the personnel department or to the administrator for follow-up:

- Employees cluster together during breaks or lunches with an apparent objective.
- Employees gather around the same few people during breaks or lunches.
- Employees stop their conversations or move away when a supervisor arrives.
- An increased number of questions about benefits and personnel policies are asked.
- Open criticism of the administration becomes increased and intensified.
- Handbills about unions are being distributed, are left in lounges, or are found in wastebaskets.
- Petitions or union authorization cards are being circulated.

Effective Labor Relations

The issues of wages, salaries, benefits, and control over practice are major reasons for collective bargaining. Other problem areas are fairness, equity, and the consistency of treatment of employees. All of these problems can be addressed preventively to promote a work environment that is fair, concerned with employees and client welfare, and competitive in the labor market.

The psychiatric–mental health nursing administrator reviews the wage and salary schedule of all personnel at least annually to determine if pay adjustments are competitive, are within the organization's financial means, and are handled fairly and consistently for all employees. If guidelines for the administration of wage packages do not exist, the nurse-administrator should collaboratively develop these guidelines with the personnel or human resources department. Exceptions to the guidelines must be carefully considered before they are instituted, in as much as unfair treatment can foster negative and hostile feelings. Remember, although wages may be confidential, they are never kept secret. Fair wage decisions, based on written guidelines, can minimize feelings of favoritism and can enhance individual feelings of worth.

After the wage and salary review, recommendations for improved pay and benefits based on the local labor market are made to the personnel department on an annual basis. In some organizations, the personnel department is responsible for reviewing current wage, salary, and benefit programs and recommending changes. If that is the case, the psychiatric–mental health nursing administrator must be kept abreast of existing staff needs and local, regional, and national trends and needs to discuss all recommendations originating from the personnel department before they are submitted to the Board of Trustees for approval. For example, a local trend for a particular benefit may be under consideration for inclusion in the organization's benefit plan. However, if this benefit is not desired by the nursing staff, another benefit should be investigated. Also, if the nurse-administrator is aware of the staff's needs, ideas can be given to the personnel department and a more meaningful benefit package can be arranged. The staff will feel, then, that they have been heard and that the organization is responsive to their needs.

The handling of discipline, promotions, transfers, and grievances also needs to be done in a fair manner. Like wages, guidelines must be constructed and used consistently to maintain an environment of honesty and fair treatment. These guidelines should be developed in conjunction with the personnel department.

Open communication is the key to managing staff in order to reduce conflict and to increase participation. Encouraging nurses to be active participants in departmental and organizational committees can promote creative problem solving and address staff concerns. Nursing practice committees, policy and procedure committees and nurse-physician committees can be used to gain the involvement of the staff and management and nurse-administrators in the day-to-day operations of the organization. When preparing the departmental budget, these committees should hold meetings with the staff and the management to define areas of need and to negotiate items when appropriate. Again, this procedure gives all levels of nursing an opportunity to be heard, and wiser decisions will result. Annual departmental and unit objectives should also be developed with input from the staff—especially at the unit level when the staff members are going to be the instruments for achieving these objectives. Of course, management must always make some decisions without staff participation. However, when possible, staff members should be included in the decision making, as this will improve working relations and promote job satisfaction.

PLANNING FOR NEGOTIATIONS

In spite of all efforts, unionization may still occur. If negotiations are inevitable, the psychiatric–mental health nursing administrator must be prepared for the bargaining table. It is important to remember that the best of relationships between nursing managers and the staff may be strained before and during the negotiating process. It is not uncommon for feelings of suspicion and isolation to ensue. Management and staff become fearful and anxious. Even the most minor concerns can escalate into major issues. In situations in which a union is just being organized, divisive tactics are often used. In general, negotiations can be a most uncomfortable and frustrating time for everyone.

Maintaining Leadership

The nurse-administrator must remain objective and strive to maintain the leadership of the department—a task that is not always easy to do in the face of the anger and fear of both management and staff nurses. Time should be spent with the head nurses and supervisors to discuss the contract and all the issues that are surfacing at the unit level. The nurse-administrator must reassure the management team that the problems are temporary, and must support approaches to be used to alleviate the stress. The nursing managers can also be helpful to the nurse-administrator by providing information that can be used at the bargaining table. The nurse-administrator needs to be proactive in regard to departmental bargaining proposals—not solely reactive to the bargaining unit's demands.

If the organization has a negotiating team, the nurse-administrator may not have much direct involvement in the actual negotiation of the agreement. The team, however, needs information from the nurse-administrator regarding the status of the agreement in the nursing department; the management areas to be addressed at the table; and perceived attitudes, strengths, and vulnerabilities of the bargaining unit. In order to do this, the nurse-administrator must be thoroughly acquainted with the existing contract and all the job responsibilities of all job classifications in the nursing department.

Because the nurse-administrator will be giving a great deal of support to the nursing managers in the department, it is important that the nurse-administrator have a personal means of support as well. This support can be given through the other department heads within the organization as well as through networks outside the organization. Local chapters of the American Nurses' Association Council of Nursing Administration and the American Organization of Nurse Executives of the American Hospital Association (formerly American Society of Nursing Service Administrators of the AHA) can provide information, ideas and support. Never underestimate the importance of a colleague or the need for personal assistance.

Developing a Strike Contingency Plan

Another important aspect of preparing for contract negotiations is the development of a contingency plan in the event of a strike. Meetings of all organizational department heads with top administration can result in everyone knowing the organization's position in the event of a strike. If a nonprofessional group plans to strike, the effects of its plans must be ascertained. Can operations continue as before? Will departments or units or beds need to be closed? Will other personnel walk out in sympathy? All these things must be considered, as well as the security and safety concerns. When a professional group is planning to strike, can operations continue? Can management nurses assume the roles of staff nurses? Will layoffs need to be considered when beds are closed? Will clients have to be moved to another agency for care? Will nurses resign because of the conflict? How long can the organization manage to function under these circumstances? Of course, a strike is not a pleasant situation. In many ways, it threatens feelings of job security and is a frightening prospect for all persons involved. Once plans have been made final, meetings should be held with the staff to inform them of these plans. Support and concern for both staff and clients must be shown. In the interim, negotiations should continue, using a mediator if necessary.

IMPLEMENTING THE CONTRACT

Elements of the Agreement

Once an agreement has been reached, operations should return to normal as quickly as possible. Even if the threat of a strike has not been present, the atmosphere will still show marked improvement after the ratification of a new agreement. Both management and labor want to ensure the continuation of services and employment, and the ratification of an agreement brings relief to both sides.

The agreement, or contract as it is also called, contains several elements (Exhibit 6–1). Not all agreements contain all of these elements, but most of the issues included in each element are addressed somewhere in the contract. The contract is signed and dated by representatives of both parties. Once the contract is signed, it becomes a legal document binding both parties.

It is essential that all nursing managers understand the contract so they can administer it appropriately. The head nurse is usually the closest manager to the staff members covered by the union contract. If the head nurse is not aware of the contract provisions, practices that violate the contract may occur. It is the responsibility of the psychiatric–mental health nursing administrator to educate the head nurse and all the nursing managers about the contract. Although a contract may give a manager a feeling of loss of power, it can be used to channel the energies of the staff to achieve improved practice.

The contract should make nursing managers more aware of the need to be fair and consistent in dealing with staff, especially in disciplinary matters. Discipline

Exhibit 6-1 Elements of a Contract Negotiation Agreement

- *Preamble*—opening remarks about the agreement and the relationship of labor and management
- *Union recognition*—statements about the right of the labor representative to be the official representative of certain names, groups, or job classifications
- *Union security*—remarks about how employees become union members
- *Financial aspects of employment*—includes the wages or salaries, holiday pay, and shift differentials agreed upon for each job classification
- *Nonfinancial aspects*—includes fringe benefits, such as hospitalization, sick pay, vacation time, and lunch and coffee breaks
- *Seniority*—the process by which promotions, transfers, and lay-offs are handled
- *Discipline*—description of the discipline procedure to be used
- *Grievance procedure*—establishment of a step-by-step procedure to be used when a violation of the agreement is suspected
- *Management rights*—including management prerogatives for hiring, firing, promoting, disciplining, laying off, adding jobs, changing jobs, setting work hours, assigning tasks, eliminating jobs, and so forth
- *Professional standards* (professional groups only)—includes such things as the right of a professional to refuse to perform tasks viewed as unsafe for clients, the performance expectations to be adhered to by the employees, and the role of the professional group in decision making related to practice in the organization
- *Other elements*—could include a no-strike or no-lockout clause, safety issues, leaves of absence policies, and so forth
- *Duration of the contract*

Source: Adapted from *Labor relations in the health professions* (p. 93) by W.B. Werther & C.A. Lockhart, 1976, Boston: Little, Brown & Co. © 1976 by Little, Brown & Co. Adapted by permission.

---

and discharge must be for "just cause" and not at the whim of the supervisor. This approach is sound management practice, whether an agreement exists or not. The steps of the disciplinary process must be followed, with management retaining the right to alter those steps when the seriousness of the situation warrants.

Handling Grievances

A *grievance* is a complaint about a violation of fair labor practice, whether spelled out specifically in a bargaining unit contract or by organizational policy. Employee complaints may, however, be only complaints and not actual violations of the contract, even when presented as grievances. It is only through time and a testing of both sides that labor and management confine grievances strictly to contract violations. If employees have other avenues available to handle complaints and concerns, formal grievances should be minimal.

In some cases, harassment grievances may occur. Werther and Lockhart (1976) define a *harassment grievance* as a method employed "in the hope that a flood of grievances will cause management to remove an obnoxious supervisor" (p. 132). When nursing managers apply consistent management techniques with a staff who had, previously, been free to do whatever they wished, friction is bound to occur. Even with explanations and staff participation in the forthcoming changes, some staff members resent being managed and rebel by resorting to harassment grievances. The psychiatric–mental health nursing administrator should be supportive of both the nursing manager and the staff while maintaining the manager in the management position. The grievance procedure should not be abused, nor should it be used as a means to attack anyone on a personal basis.

The grievance procedure usually follows a formal process that begins with an informal discussion between the grievant (or the grievant's representative) and the immediate supervisor. If both parties are not satisfied, a written notice may go to the nursing supervisor with a written formal response to be given by the nursing supervisor within a specified period of time. Should difficulties still exist, the grievant may appeal the supervisor's decision to the psychiatric–mental health nursing administrator with a written formal response to be given, again, within a specified period of time. That response may then be appealed in writing to upper administration, requesting a meeting with the administration and the union representation. If that decision is not accepted, the grievance may go to arbitration for a settlement.

If a grievance is presented to the nursing administrator, it should be handled in the following manner:

1. Be objective.
2. Obtain the facts.
3. Share the facts with the grievant or the grievant's representative.
4. Maintain a united front as a management team; if you disagree, do it in private.
5. Be calm.
6. Respond in a timely manner as established in the contract.
7. Consider how the other side will respond.
8. If emotions get out of control during a meeting, adjourn the meeting and reschedule it for another time.
9. Be prepared to compromise.
10. Again, respond in a timely manner.
11. Document everything.

Arbitration is a process that resembles an informal court. Both parties agree upon a third party arbitrator from the American Arbitration Association or the FMCS. Because arbitration is costly, both parties share the expense. The burden of proof is on the bargaining unit, except in cases of the discharge of an employee. Witnesses for both parties are sworn in, and testimony is given. The bargaining unit speaks first. Witnesses are examined and cross-examined. The arbitrator may also examine the witnesses. There is no jury, and the arbitrator alone compares the facts presented with the language of the contract. Briefs are sometimes prepared and submitted after testimony is given. The arbitrator makes a decision in favor of management or the grievant. A written response is given to both parties, and the decision of the arbitrator is usually final. In rare instances, the decision may be appealed to the courts for a final settlement.

Being involved in the arbitration process can cause the nurse-administrator and all witnesses some anxiety. The point of arbitration is to arrive at an impartial judgment as to the appropriateness of the application of the union contract. If the nurse-administrator performs the job well at lower levels of the grievance procedure, the stand taken during arbitration will be a confirmation of the appropriate action of management.

EVALUATION

Unionization is relatively new in the health care industry, and professional feelings reflect ambivalence; nevertheless, more nurses are organizing for pay, benefits, and control over practice. In spite of the mixed reception, unions should not be viewed as inherently evil; they serve as a voice for those who would not be heard individually. If the psychiatric–mental health nursing administrator strives to provide a work environment that is fair and consistent and encourages participative management, the likelihood of a union effort is diminished. Even with the presence of a union, fairness, consistency, and participative management can channel staff energies to improve the psychiatric–mental health nursing staff and staff morale.

When preparing for contract negotiations, the nurse-administrator must look at the work climate, current practices, and competitiveness with other psychiatric–mental health organizations. Contingency plans must be made in the event of a strike. The nurse-administrator should also develop demands for the department to be taken to the bargaining table.

In administering the contract on a day-to-day basis, all nursing managers must be thoroughly aware of the contract provisions. Discipline, in particular, must be carefully planned and applied. In the event of a grievance, the nurse-administrator must investigate the situation carefully and be prepared to respond in a timely manner. Compromise may be necessary and could improve relationships if done appropriately and without destroying management's credibility and effectiveness. If a grievance goes to arbitration, the nurse administrator must prepare witnesses to testify in a manner similar to a courtroom. Arbitration is used to obtain a neutral third party judgment in those cases in which labor and management cannot agree. In rare situations, arbitrated decisions can be appealed to the judicial system for a final opinion.

REFERENCES

American Nurses' Association. (1977). Reimbursement for nursing services: A position statement of the commission on economic and general welfare. Kansas City, Mo: Author.

Werther, W.B., & Lockhart, C.A. (1976). *Labor relations in the health professions*. Boston: Little, Brown & Company.

SUGGESTED READINGS

Belitz, E.E. (1982). Nurses' participation in bargaining units. *Journal of Nursing Management, 13*(10), 48–57.

Cannon, P. (1980). Administering the contract. *Journal of Nursing Administration, 10*(10), 13–19.

Castrey, B.G., & Castrey, R.T. (1980). Mediation—what it is, what it does. *Journal of Nursing Administration, 10*(11), 24–28.

Johnson, L.M., Roy, K., & Shippey, S. (1983). Union–yes or no? *Journal of Nursing Management, 14*(4), 45–48.

Rowland, H.S., & Rowland, B.L. (1980). *Nursing administration handbook*. Rockville, Md: Aspen Systems.

Stevens, W.F. (1978). *Management and leadership in nursing*. New York: McGraw-Hill.

Chapter 7

Budgetary Planning in Psychiatric–Mental Health Nursing

OVERVIEW

Faced with the challenge of providing the highest possible quality of care while maintaining costs at an acceptable level, the psychiatric–mental health nursing administrator is keenly aware that one of the most important aspects of management is the budgetary process. In order to meet this challenge, the nurse-administrator needs a working knowledge of the budgetary process employed by the organization, must have ready access to the data, and must be familiar with the economic trends of the health care industry.

The budgetary process, like the nursing process, requires an assessment of the existing economic position of the department; careful planning for the financial needs of the department; implementation of the approved, finalized budget; and evaluation of the effectiveness of the budget through a budget reporting mechanism. Guenther (1979) defines the *budget* as "1) the annual operating plan, 2) a financial road map, and 3) a financial plan which serves as an estimate of and control over future operations through an estimate of future costs and a plan for utilization of manpower, material, and other resources to cover capital projects in the operating program" (p. 127).

Budget Components

The overall departmental budget is separated into three components: the salary and wage budget, the operational budget and the capital budget. The *salary and wage budget* comprises the largest element of the psychiatric–mental health nursing departmental budget. In addition to wages, this budget includes employees' earned benefits, such as vacations, personal or sick leave, and holidays.

Premium pay, such as shift differentials, on-call pay and educational differentials for advanced educational preparation, as well as step- and merit-pay raises, are also incorporated into the wage and salary budget (Schmeid, 1979).

The *operational* budget contains funds for needed supplies required by the day-to-day operations of the department. Paper supplies, small equipment, table games, stock medical or surgical supplies (not charged to the client), tongue blades, cotton-tipped applicators, bandaids, alcohol sponges, and syringes are a few of these operational expenses. Each setting has its own defined operational budget. In some instances, however, there may be separate budgets for education, travel, recruitment, or administration.

Anticipated purchases of new equipment or the replacement of major items that amount to over $500 are components of a *capital* budget. Furniture for client bedrooms, lounges, and unit or departmental offices; audiovisual equipment; office equipment, such as word processors, typewriters, and dictation machines; carpeting; and draperies are a few of the items that would be incorporated into the capital budget. However, some organizations maintain separate budgets for furnishings in order to provide greater overall control of furniture needs and costs. By coordinating large capital purchases in this way, price breaks can be used effectively.

Budget Development

Development of the psychiatric–mental health nursing budget requires a systematic approach with an associated timetable of activities to ensure the approval and implementation of the budget in a timely fashion. The budgetary process is a series of activities. When completed, they lead to negotiation with the administrator or between department heads for monies and result in an approved budget. Ganong and Ganong (1980) outline the sequence of activities in the annual budgetary process.

1. Formulate departmental or unit objectives for the fiscal year.
2. Develop strategies and plans for the implementation of objectives, anticipated projects, or program changes.
3. Determine a projected cost for each objective, project, or program change.
4. Review the previous budget record, giving special attention to areas that are over or under the budget.
5. Forecast income.
6. Review wage and salary costs, and determine costs for the future.
7. Prepare budget recommendations.
8. Submit budget proposal.
9. Negotiate, make revision, and secure approval.

Although the proposed budget should include all items being considered for funding, each item needs to be given its proper priority. When negotiations result in less money than is anticipated, these funds can be allocated to those items of highest priority.

Before the proposed budget is formulated, an assessment of the department's needs must occur. Several factors make this procedure necessary. In many facilities, the budgets are dependent on government grants. In these situations there is less possibility to negotiate for funds. In addition, the health care industry is seeing greater fiscal control due to diagnosis-related groups (DRGs), cost containment programs, and similar belt-tightening efforts by federal, state, and third party payers. As a result, the nurse-administrator has a greater responsibility to evaluate nursing department objectives carefully in order to provide care within a feasible framework. Because greater justification for approval of budget increases continues to be required, nursing programs may need to be deleted, postponed, or modified from their original proposed methods.

ASSESSING DEPARTMENTAL NEEDS AND PLANNING THE BUDGET

In order to obtain adequate information about the budgetary needs of the psychiatric–mental health nursing department, service, or unit, the psychiatric–mental health nursing administrator must work cooperatively with the nursing management team to establish departmental objectives. This occasion is also an opportune time to teach and to enforce cost containment measures. The formulation of objectives and the subsequent tasks associated with the objectives provide an overall direction for the program and determine the amount of funding necessary to implement the objectives. When developing objectives, associate a cost with each objective, and give each objective a priority.

Long-range planning is necessary for the implementation of involved, large-scale goals. These long-range goals (3–5 years) can be achieved through a series of short-term objectives (annual), which distribute the cost over a period of years. For example, implementation of a primary nursing model may be planned over a two- to three-year period. The first-year objective may be to upgrade lower paraprofessional positions to higher paraprofessional positions (aides, to mental health technicians). The second-year objective may include the addition of a certain number of full-time equivalent RN positions and the beginning of educational preparation for primary nursing. The third-year objective may be the addition of the remainder of the desired RN positions, renovation of the nursing unit, and the implementation of the primary nursing model.

Whatever the goals of psychiatric–mental health nursing, departmental objectives play a major role in the budgeting process—not only for the salary and wage budget but also for the capital and the operational budgets. A major change, such as primary nursing, may have a positive or a negative impact on the capital and operational requirements. This kind of change may require additional staff positions, equipment, and day-to-day expense. In some cases, the impact of the proposed objective may increase one budget and reduce funds needed in another budget category. All of these factors must be taken into careful consideration if the proposed budgets and programs are to be successful.

The nurse-administrator needs to receive input from the nursing staff directly, through a nursing budget committee, or through the nursing managers to determine the needs of each nursing unit. The uniqueness of each psychiatric–mental health nursing area within the same department or service necessitates different budgetary needs. For example, the costs of a psychiatric–mental health walk-in clinic that is open 12 hours a day, 5 days a week, are far less than that of a 30-bed acute-care inpatient unit staffed 24 hours per day and 7 days per week. Therefore, meetings with the persons directly involved in administering each psychiatric–mental health area are necessary because the nurse-administrator cannot know all of the needs of all of the areas all of the time. During this assessment process, the nurse-administrator reviews staffing costs, anticipated equipment replacement, and future purchases of new equipment. Budgets are usually projected for a three-to five-year period. Consequently, it is necessary to make a careful evaluation of unit or departmental objectives, the anticipated impact on personnel, and the supplies and equipment needed over the time frame of the objectives. If the evaluation is done with foresight, unanticipated needs will be minimal, and costs can be kept within the budgeted amount. Failure to consider all possible needs can result in an unbudgeted expense becoming a priority and no funds being allocated for that purpose.

An audit of supply usage and an inventory of all equipment are essential. Trends in supply usage should be examined. For example, implementation of a new activity within the overall program may require a considerable unanticipated increase in paper supplies. Seclusion-room television monitoring equipment may need continual repairs, indicating an unexpected need for replacement. Replacement of such items as television monitoring cameras can lead to several thousands of dollars in expenses that were not included in the budget. Such a reallocation of funds could necessitate a rebudgeting process and cause a delay in the acquisition of these needed items.

The personnel costs (included in the salary and wage budget) must be carefully determined, and accurate projections must be made. Determining the cost of nursing care is a new process for the psychiatric–mental health nursing administrator. Historically, inpatient nursing care has been viewed as an expense included in room rates. Per diem payment, based on client days and including the hospital's actual costs, is being abandoned. Inflationary spending and health care costs have forced a change in the reimbursement system.

Prospective Reimbursement—DRGs

Witalis (1979) defines *prospective reimbursement* as "payment at a predetermined, anticipated rate [which] . . . requires that the payment rate between a third party and an institution be determined prior to the beginning of the service period" (pp. 12–13). Instead of using client days as the payment unit, DRGs are used to assign a dollar amount to a diagnosed condition. This system is based on the average cost of care for all clients with that diagnosis. Client stays in excess of the DRG-assigned length of stay (LOS) mean a loss of income for the facility because days beyond the assigned LOS are not reimbursed. Conversely, client stays of less than the assigned LOS are reimbursed at the assigned rate, which means an increase in revenue for the facility.

Currently, the DRG prospective reimbursement system has been implemented in hospitals for all services except psychiatric–mental health. It is anticipated that, ultimately, psychiatric–mental health services will also be reimbursed on the basis of DRGs. Payment based upon DRGs does include nursing care. However, nursing care must be clearly defined and a dollar amount must be attached to it. This goal can be accomplished by establishing costs related to a client classification system. In this way, nursing can begin to identify the actual costs involved in providing care. In the billing based upon a client classification system, nursing acknowledges that there is more than one level of care and that clients who do not require the highest level of care should not subsidize those who do.

This type of billing is known as variable billing (Exhibit 7–1). Higgerson and Van Slyck (1982) define it as "billing for specific aspects or levels of nursing care, which vary from [client] to [client]" (p. 20). They further add that "for each level [of care,] the required staffing [in full-time equivalents] and supplies serve as the cost basis for the changes" (p. 20). Because the prospective reimbursement system is concerned with reasonable costs, qualification and quantification of the nursing care given to psychiatric–mental health clients establish actual costs for those services separate from room and board costs.

With the full impact of prospective reimbursement as yet unknown, it is important that the psychiatric–mental health nursing administrator be aware of the possibility of future revenue constraints. As a result of the close scrutiny being given to health care costs, the nurse-administrator needs to base staffing requirements on predetermined, objective criteria. The development of staffing patterns based on actual client care requirements can provide justification for staffing patterns and can keep costs within acceptable limits. The use of client classification systems in conjunction with variable billing can provide concrete data for the validation of costs in psychiatric–mental health nursing care and can support budget recommendations. Witalis (1979) warns that, "until professional nurses make a convincing case for their services to the [client], hospital budget cuts will be levied primarily on the nursing department" (p. 17).

Exhibit 7–1 Variable Billing

What is variable billing? The term means billing for specific aspects or levels of nursing care, which vary from patient to patient. For variable billing to be successful, the corporation must accept certain assumptions:

- Revenue and expenses are defined and assigned to appropriate cost centers.
- The cost of providing each individual service is identified.
- Patients' bills are based on that cost plus a contribution toward profit.
- Each patient pays only for services received and does not subsidize services received by other patients.

Assumptions specific to nursing should include the following:

- Nursing care is an identifiable entity that can be defined, measured, and costed.
- Nursing care varies with the patient's diagnosis, level of illness, age, and so forth.
- A direct relationship exists between nursing care provided and costs (staff and supplies).

Source: From "Variable billing for services: New fiscal direction for nursing" by N.J. Higgerson & A. Van Slyck, 1982, *Journal of Nursing Administration, 12*(6), p. 20. © 1982 by the J.B. Lippincott Co. Reprinted by permission.

The Master Staffing Plan

Appropriate staffing levels based on a client classification system need to be established. (See Chapter 14) Because allocation of staff in this manner is based on a scientific method rather than on estimates, the nurse-administrator needs to review the past year's census and acuity information to determine the average client acuteness level for the year. If the census reveals great fluctuation, the trends should be monitored. Monitoring can indicate the periods of high and low acuity so that staffing schedules can be modified accordingly and maintenance and repair work can be projected.

The cost of employing RNs can seem staggering when compared with paraprofessional (mental health workers, etc.) and nonprofessional (clerks, etc.) staff costs. The use of RNs and mental health workers or nurses aides is determined by the organization's philosophy of treatment, the financial resources, and the availability of human resources. Each setting requires a unique staffing pattern. An all-RN staff may be appropriate and may be required for a walk-in clinic. An acute-care inpatient unit may desire all RNs, but it may require such a large number of RNs that the supply and the budget cannot permit such a staffing pattern. In some instances, the level of care required by the client population may actually dictate the need for RNs and paraprofessional staff. Although the cost for RNs is high, many benefits to the client and the organization can be gained through their effective and efficient use. RNs used in a primary nursing model would be providing a greater amount of direct nursing care than RNs engaged in the team nursing model. Client and nurse satisfaction can be higher in the case of the primary nursing model, with a shortened client stay in some instances.

The New England Deaconess Hospital in Boston conducted a comparative study of two nursing units in 1974 and 1975. One unit used a primary nursing approach; the other unit, a team nursing model. Each unit used the same master staffing pattern. The team unit had three fewer clients. The results of the study revealed that the cost per bed for the primary unit was $141.67 less per month (Marram, Flynn, Abaravich, & Carey, 1976). In addition, Marram et al. noted a difference in the quality of the care provided by the two units.

> There is data to suggest that the primary unit not only cost less to operate, but also had higher quality care outcomes. The results of this entire endeavor indicated that even though these modes were both regarded as very good units, on the primary unit:
>
> 1. Nursing staff and clients were more satisfied;
> 2. Nursing staff reported that they more often got highly involved with their clients;
> 3. Clients perceived the nursing care to be more individualized, and personalized;
> 4. Nurses were found to perform greater numbers of tasks more frequently for all or most of their clients and to spend more time on more professional tasks; and
> 5. Nursing assessments more often incorporated the client's perception of his illness, nursing needs were more often recorded and included a wider variety of needs and nursing care plans were more frequently completed. (p. 84)

The data, then, seem to suggest that it may be fallacious to discount the possibility of implementing primary nursing because of anticipated higher costs. Although there has been little written about the financial impact of primary nursing in psychiatric–mental health organizations, the administrator should still weigh carefully the cost of the current modality and should project the costs of a primary model. Furthermore, the use of primary nursing as a pilot project can be helpful in determining the costs and benefits of such a change. With preparation, mental health workers can be used as associates to an RN who would serve as primary nurse. This arrangement can assist in keeping costs down, in comparison to the costs for an all-RN staff.

Whatever the staffing pattern or mode of nursing, costs for salaries and wages need to be projected for the budget. Meetings with the financial officer can assist the nurse-administrator in determining a sufficient amount for anticipated salary needs. The financial officer has an established computation formula that accounts for each full-time equivalent position in each job classification, the benefits to be accrued for each position, anticipated vacancies, approximate length of time until current vacancies are filled, and planned reduction or increase of positions. In addition, an overview of the client census and a projection of income can be made. Comparisons between the current and the projected budget can be assessed, and further adjustments can be made before the salary and wage budget is ready for review by the administration. Any changes in staffing that require the deletion or the addition of positions need to be carefully and thoroughly documented by the associated rationale for projected costs. The rationale for additional positions should include supportive data, such as acuity information and any change in program direction. When reducing positions, remember that once a position is deleted, the nurse-administrator must rejustify it before adding it in the future. In some instances, lower level positions, such as nursing aides or mental health workers, can be deleted and then combined and upgraded to an RN position, if desired—e.g., delete two full-time equivalent mental health worker positions and change them to one full-time equivalent RN position. Combining and redistributing positions can provide a relatively easy alternative for meeting staffing needs in the most cost-efficient way.

When the salary and wage budget, the capital budget, and the operational budget have each been prepared, the total budget package is ready for presentation to the administrator for approval. (In some organizations, each department is responsible for developing its own budget, which is then shared with all departments.) The financial officer then presents the acceptable overall organizational budget. Next, each department must negotiate with other departments until the organizational budget is equal to the combined departmental budgets. Through this process, the department heads become aware of the combined organizational operation and their own departments' relationship to that whole. Through discussion of the goals, objectives, and needs of each department and the goals and objectives of the organization, the participants rank their budget needs in relation to the overall organizational needs. Ultimately, compromises are made that balance the projected budget of each department with that of the overall organization. This process is an arduous one and requires the nurse-administrator to be knowledgeable about all aspects of the psychiatric–mental health nursing budget. Concessions and support can be obtained informally through networks with other department heads before the final budget negotiations. In this way, the psychiatric–mental health nursing administrator can support another department's efforts in one area for their return support to the nursing budget. Finally, the proposed budget with all necessary revisions is approved and ready for implementation.

IMPLEMENTING THE BUDGET

In order to provide a systematic and an orderly implementation of the budget, time frames are established for the addition of staff positions, for the purchase of equipment, and for capital improvements. Discussion with the financial officer, the purchasing agent, and the maintenance director provides the psychiatric–mental health nursing administrator with the assurance of adequate cash flow for the purchase of large items, the scheduling of improvements at the best possible time for the area involved, and the receipt of purchases in a timely fashion. This timetable, which can be documented on the budget itself, reduces the tendency to request staff, equipment, and improvements at the same time, thereby causing financial hardship to the organization and chaos to the purchasing and maintenance departments. Pay increases are implemented as scheduled, and new programs are instituted within the time frames established during the planning phase.

EVALUATING THE BUDGET PROCESS

Evaluation of the budget process is ongoing. Several aspects of the budget are reviewed and evaluated on a routine basis. These aspects include biweekly (or weekly or monthly) payroll summaries, monthly department performance reports, quarterly financial reports, and labor productivity reports. Each of these mechanisms provides information to the psychiatric–mental health nursing administrator about the projected, actual, and year-to-date performance of the department in relation to its budget.

Biweekly payroll summaries indicate for each position the amount of regular and overtime hours worked in each cost center (nursing unit, department, service) along with the dollar amount paid in regular, overtime, and other pay (such as holiday, vacation, and sick leave). The number of authorized hours is indicated as well as the budgeted and actual figures. This summary tells the nurse-administrator how many hours under or over the authorized hours (based on FTEs) have been worked, and it compares the hours worked and the cost for the period with what was budgeted. If there is a large variance in either costs or savings, the nurse-administrator should ascertain the reasons as soon as possible and should monitor this activity for trends. Adjustments in staffing may be warranted, such as calling in additional help during a busy period (instead of having the staff work overtime) or allowing the staff to take time off during low periods.

Monthly department performance reports compare the monthly payroll information, other expenses, and revenues with monthly budgeted amounts, year-to-date budgeted amounts, and actual figures. This information tells the nurse-administrator exactly how the revenues and the expenses of that period compare with projected revenues and expenses for the period and with past revenues and expenses from the previous fiscal year. This report presents a more comprehensive picture of the entire psychiatric–mental health nursing budgets because it involves salary and wages, operational expenses, and capital items. Variances noted in this report require investigation by the nurse-administrator to determine causes and needed modifications. Is the variance an emergency, one-time-only problem, or has something occurred that will continue to have an impact on the budget? These questions need to be answered. The quarterly and annual financial reports give comparative information in the same manner as do the monthly reports. All of these reports are designed to assist the nurse-administrator in evaluating the effectiveness of the budget.

Labor productivity reports are new to psychiatric–mental health nursing. Similar to the biweekly payroll summary, the labor productivity report should be prepared and sent to the nurse-administrator promptly after the reporting period. The administrator then has sufficient time to investigate any apparent difficulties and to make changes in the staffing, if necessary. Productivity is the amount of client days for a specific period divided by the total number of hours worked during that time (P = client days/hours worked).

Productivity reports are intended to provide meaningful information to the nurse-administrator for a more finite determination of the direct-care hours provided. By this process, the average amount of time of nursing care given by each job classification can be divided. The number of nursing-care hours provided during each client day can be calculated by dividing the number *one* by the productivity ratio (nursing care hours = $1/P$). Monitoring the nursing-care hours can prove to be enlightening. For example, when RN staff members are assisted by para- or nonprofessionals, the amount of RN time per client may prove in some instances to be extremely low and may be an indication of the type of care being rendered. Further investigation may show an extreme amount of time being used by the RN in paperwork, which has taken the RN from direct client care. When nursing hours worked are adjusted by client acuity, the nurse-administrator can see the actual amount of psychiatric–mental health nursing time devoted to direct client care. Productivity ratios, nursing-care hours worked, and nursing-care hours worked but adjusted by client acuity all provide valuable information to the nurse-administrator. These data regarding the workload of staff on a given unit during a given period can then be compared with past performance and can provide an average of the performance for the fiscal year-to-date.

Changes in the client population or the services being provided also affect the productivity ratio. For example, a modification in the screening procedure in an outpatient service may allow more timely referrals and, subsequently, may give the staff additional time to see more clients during the course of the day. In this case, the output is the number of client visits rather than client days. If this situation occurred and staffing remained the same, productivity would increase. Trends in the workload and labor productivity can be seen graphically when monthly productivity information is plotted on a graphic chart. This information, along with other budget information, can assist the psychiatric–mental health nursing administrator in the identification of trends that will be useful in future budgetary planning.

REFERENCES

Ganong, J.M., & Ganong, W.L. (1980). *Nursing management*. Rockville, Md: Aspen Systems.

Grimaldi, P.L. (1982). DRGs and nursing administration. *Journal of Nursing Management, 13*(1), 30–34.

Guenther, H.H. (1979). Frequently asked questions about budgeting. In E. Schmeid (Ed.), *Maintaining cost effectiveness*. Rockville, Md: Aspen Systems, 127–130.

Higgerson, N.J., & Van Slyck, A. (1982). Variable billing for services: New fiscal direction for nursing. *Journal of Nursing Administration, 12*(6), 20–27.

Marram, G., Flynn, K., Abaravich, W., & Carey, S. (1976). *Cost effectiveness of primary and team nursing*. Rockville, Md: Aspen Systems.

Schmeid, E. (1979). Allocation of resources: Preparation of the nursing department budget. In E. Schmeid (Ed.), *Maintaining cost effectiveness*. Rockville, Md: Aspen Systems, 143–150.

Witalis, R. (1979). The state of the budgetary art: Survey shows many hospitals are not prepared to comply with new law. In E. Schmeid (Ed.). *Maintaining cost effectiveness*. Rockville, Md: Aspen Systems, 10–12.

SUGGESTED READINGS

Althaus, J.N., Hardyck, N.M., Pierce, P.B., & Rodgers, M.S. (1982). Decentralized budgeting: Holding the purse strings, part 1. *Journal of Nursing Administration, 12*(5), 15–20.

Grimaldi, P.L., & Micheletti, J.A. (1982). RIMs and the cost of nursing care. *Journal of Nursing Management, 13*(12), 12–22.

Henninger, D., & Dailey, C. (1983). Measuring nursing workload in an outpatient department. *Journal of Nursing Administration, 13*(9), 20–23.

Rowland, H.S., & Rowland, B.L. (1980). *Nursing administration handbook*. Rockville, Md: Aspen Systems.

Shaffer, F.A. (1983). DRGs: History and overview. *Nursing & Health Care, 4*(7), 388–396.

Chapter 8

Supervision in Psychiatric–Mental Health Organizations

Supervision is often viewed as a negative component of nursing administration. However, supervision can exert a positive influence on the nursing department's overall program to develop the staff's competencies—particularly within psychiatric–mental health nursing. Those who provide supervision at all levels within the department are role models (refer to Chapter 11) for all nursing staff and continually facilitate the department's ability to deliver quality client care. In order to provide quality care, the supervision provided must be appropriate to the specific psychiatric–mental health organization. "In a health care organization, knowledge of the specific functions performed is of primary importance and one cannot bring so-called generic management methods into health care and expect them to work" (McConnell, 1982, p. 1).

ASSESSING SUPERVISORY COMPONENTS

Organizational Structures

The organizational structure of the psychiatric–mental health nursing department should be examined to determine the type of supervision needed or to assess whether the supervision in place is appropriate. There are two basic organizational structures in nursing departments: centralized (the traditional structure) or decentralized (Calkin, 1982). Within the centralized structure, decision making is usually retained at the higher levels of management; little input is sought from the staff nurse level. Traditional positions include the director of nursing, associate and/or assistant directors of nursing, shift supervisors, head nurses, and charge nurses on the off-shifts.

Decentralized organizational patterns, in contrast, delegate the primary managerial accountability and authority to the unit, the director of nursing retaining ultimate authority (Calkin, 1982). Through this system, the decision-making process is moved closer to the staff nurse level and, it is hoped, incorporates direct input from the staff nurse. This arrangement serves to retain "the [client as] the center of the nursing care system" (Munschauer, 1983, p. 21). In these patterns, supervisory positions would be the director of nursing, head nurses, and charge nurses with shift supervisors who serve as resources rather than as line staff.

Participative Management

In either system, a process called participative management can do much to increase the staff's job satisfaction and commitment (Calkin, 1982). It has also been determined that shared decision making decreases turnover and resistance to change (Deines, 1981). Through involving all levels of psychiatric–mental health nursing personnel in the department's decision-making process, nurses are involved who are often the most resistant to change. Their involvement can decrease resistance because of their greater commitment to the achievement of specific goals. By integrating this process throughout the department, the nurse-administrator could also use management-by-objective techniques with the staff.

Clinical Specialist

Another organizational issue that often needs to be resolved is the position of the psychiatric–mental health clinical nurse specialist. The clinical nurse specialist may be a staff or a line position. Nursing's problems often arise as a result of responsibility without authority; yet the position of the clinical nurse specialist often has little authority. Of course, the resolution of this problem depends on the organization's role expectations of the clinical nurse specialist. Should the position be solely advisory, authority may not be needed; however, if the clinical nurse specialist is to serve as a change agent within the organization, the position should be granted the authority (through a line position) to facilitate change. Moreover, if the role is to be designated as a combination of a direct care giver and supervisor, time must also be allotted for both aspects of this role. Otherwise, neither role will be carried out to the satisfaction of the department.

Supervision

Once the organizational structure has been assessed, the meaning of supervision within the department should be clarified. *Supervision* can be viewed as "a dynamic process in which the supervising person encourages or participates in the development of subordinates . . . [through] planning, communicating, direction, instruction, technical assistance, support and evaluation" (Yura, Ozimek, & Walsh, 1981, p. 76). The supervisor accomplishes these activities through the assumption of five subroles: "1) role model with [clients] and personnel, 2) participant-observer, 3) informal teacher, 4) instigator and innovator, and 5) over-seer, assessor, evaluator" (Fagin, 1967, p. 34).

As participative management becomes more prevalent within psychiatric–mental health nursing departments, supervisory personnel should also recognize the role supervision plays within this process. "A positive attitude about the staff, the use of positive rewards, a willingness to become involved, and a belief in the nurses' ability to function effectively are vital perspectives for the . . . supervisor to develop" (Hayes, 1979, p. 30). Through the implementation of these behaviors, the staff become increasingly involved in the decision-making processes, and also increases their self-esteem within the work environment. This increase in self-esteem generally results in a subsequent improvement in client care.

In addition, through using knowledge of group dynamics and group process, the supervisor works with the nursing staff to improve the quality of care. This knowledge of groups enables the supervisor to recognize potential staff difficulties resulting from group interactions. Skillful facilitation of the group process enables the supervisor to encourage and to support the positive development of groups of nursing staff. Particularly in in-patient settings, the nursing staff must work within a group—even if involved in primary nursing. Recognition of this aspect of the work environment enables the supervisor to develop a holistic approach to the supervision of personnel. Such a people-centered approach to management is more appropriate for a health care setting than is production-centered management (McConnell, 1982).

Leadership

Supervisory personnel should also be encouraged to function as leaders, rather than solely as managers. "Effective leadership is vital to a group's success" (McConnell, 1980, p. 106) and is defined "as a set of actions that influence members of a group to move toward goal setting and goal attainment" (Diers, 1979, p. 67). Rather than focusing on the day-to-day activities of a manager, a leader looks toward an improved tomorrow and the strategies to facilitate the group in reaching that tomorrow. "There [can] not be an environment supportive of quality bedside nursing without strong nursing leadership" (Wilsea, 1980, p. 48).

By creating the appropriate combination of "leadership style and group environment" (Bassford & White, 1977, p. 83) in the psychiatric–mental health nursing department, the supervisor can promote the effectiveness of the department. The department should be assessed to determine the type of leader needed, particularly when filling open leadership positions. Should a discrepancy be discovered between the group environment and the leadership style, steps should be taken to work with nursing leaders to increase their awareness and to decrease the discrepancy.

Further assessment of supervisory personnel can also aid them in becoming more leadership oriented. This objective can be accomplished through a variety of approaches. Attitudes toward goals should focus on a personal and active approach rather than on a passive, impersonal one. Furthermore, supervisory staff should be involved in goal formation rather than simply being instruments for its implementation. "Collaborative . . . leadership places personnel in a position which they do not feel a need to defend" (Kepler, 1980, p. 18), and this diminished need for defensiveness can then be passed on to the staff being supervised.

Work should be viewed as the opportunity to develop new solutions to previous problems and to expand options rather than as a process that results only in decision making. The staff should be encouraged to relate with others in more empathetic ways but also to allow themselves time alone to foster creativity (Zaleznik, 1981). Through the fostering of leadership qualities, the growth of leadership in the supervisory staff can be facilitated.

PLANNING FOR IMPLEMENTATION OF RELEVANT SUPERVISORY ROLES

Policy Review

Once the review of the supervisory component of the department has been completed, the planning phase begins. In this phase, the decision is made as to how supervisory roles within the department are to be implemented according to the current needs of the department, the staff, and the client population. Of course, this plan may change periodically as needs change.

After the basic roles of supervision have been delineated, department policies and job descriptions should be created that support the predetermined roles. All policies related to supervisory behavior should be reviewed to ensure that they support current behavior and facilitate future growth. For example, policies concerning evaluations should reflect current practices rather than dictate an outmoded, nonpracticed evaluation method. Outmoded policies should be rewritten with the future in mind so that annual revision is not necessary. As in the case of other administrative actions, these revisions should be delegated to a committee of the staff involved in policy implementation. The nurse-administrator should review the final revisions.

Job Descriptions

Crucial to the development of a clearly delineated behaviorally-based evaluation format is the existence of equally clear behaviorally-oriented job descriptions.

Unless the two are consistent, ambiguities result and the evaluations do not reflect actual performance. Job descriptions must "reinforce the objectives of the department and the expected standards of care" (Lerch, 1982, p. 28). Associated with each job description should be "standards of performance specific to each classification with given criteria relative to and supportive of each standard" (Lerch, p. 28). These standards should be based upon the professional organization's standards for psychiatric–mental health nursing practice and, when applicable, the standards for nursing service administration.

Guidelines for the review of current job descriptions ensure that a sound basis is provided for the evaluation process. The job description, as stated above, should be specific and clearly defined. It should be realistic and current (Cook, 1979). If the job description is outdated, then the evaluation also is measuring standards that no longer apply.

If total revision of the department's job descriptions is warranted, job analysis might be done. "Job analysis is the process of identifying, specifying, organizing, and displaying the duties, tasks, and responsibilities . . . actually performed in a given job" (Ignatavicius & Griffith, 1982, p. 37). Through this process, a job description is developed that describes a specific job. Job analysis is also an effective method for dispelling the myth that a nurse is a nurse is a nurse. A job description developed through job analysis behaviorally describes a job in a way that clearly lends itself to evaluating a specific type of nursing staff. As a result, the staff members know exactly how they will be evaluated.

Communication and Supervision

The roles that the supervisory staff of psychiatric–mental health nursing should assume vary according to each setting. However, in planning for their initial or continuing implementation, certain universal components of supervision should be facilitated. The administration "sets the working environment's tone—the style of human relations and communication basic to it" (Foster, 1981, p. 18). The tone of the working environment is particularly crucial in psychiatric–mental health nursing, because interpersonal communication and self-awareness skills are basic to the provision of quality care. If the nursing administration does not emphasize the importance of these two areas, the quality of care suffers.

Personal Assessment

Hence, the level of communication within a department depends upon the administrator's skills. As in any interaction within psychiatric–mental health nursing, a communication problem between two persons may exist because of a personality conflict. Should miscommunication exist, a personal assessment should be made to determine whether the source of the difficulty lies within the individuals. "If [one] can deal objectively with [one's] own strengths and weaknesses in a constructive way, it is much easier to adapt to powers and defenses in others" (Kepler, 1980, p. 17). By assuming responsibility for one-half of the communication difficulties in which they are involved, the nurse-administrators serve as role models for other staff members, encouraging each to assume responsibility for a role in communication successes and problems. This sharing of responsibilities also establishes an environment in which the staff can communicate in an open fashion, rather than defensively.

In assessing one's ability to communicate effectively, the psychiatric–mental health nursing administrator should recognize that communication techniques, like leadership styles, may vary according to the situation. "The truly expert manager or supervisor can create a climate in which subordinates *want* to assume responsibility and further their personal development" (Wilkinson, 1981, p. 44). One primary method for facilitating this change is by remembering the perspective of the subordinate when involved in discussion. This perspective allows the administrator to anticipate difficulties that may arise during the communication session.

Informal Organization

Once effective communication techniques have been developed within the department, the informal organization should be considered by the supervisory staff. If the staff practice effective communication skills with noneffective results, the informal organization may be a factor. The *informal organization* can be defined as "that network of personal and social relations which is not established or required by formal organization" (Schuldt, 1978, p. 21). This group, with its own leader and norms, can do much to encourage or to hinder the organization's progress towards identified goals. By recognizing that this group exists, the supervisory staff can use their knowledge of group culture and dynamics to facilitate positive growth. If an organization's communication system is open and direct and the supervisory staff are able to work with and be empathetic to those being supervised, a collaborative team approach to the delivery of psychiatric–mental health care can develop.

Counselling Staff Members

Another communication technique that can serve to improve the quality of care is the counselling of staff. *Counselling*—"face to face meetings between supervisor and subordinate" (Walker, 1976, p. 10)—is used for multiple reasons. A basic goal is the identification of staff performance deficits that hinder that staff's ability to develop professionally and, possibly, to maintain the position. Counselling differs from discipline in that it is an attempt to increase the employee's awareness of a problem area, so that corrective action can be taken before the need for discipline arises. This identification should enable the staff to change specific behaviors and so alleviate deficits and improve job performance. In this communication technique, the supervisor attempts to facilitate the staff's own corrective actions rather than resorting to discipline. Counselling should focus on the employee's ability to be accountable for personal behavior. Without this accountability, changes in behaviors are unlikely (Murphy, 1983).

The actual counselling process can be fostered through a variety of techniques. A relaxed environment should be created, but the counsellor should be verbally direct during the discussion. Through the use of active listening, the staff's goals are identified while gaining the individual employee's confidence. During open discussions, the staff's awareness of how the identified behavior is hindering the achievement of certain goals is increased.

The staff should fully understand the content of the discussion. Asking the staff to rephrase or to summarize the discussion may help to clarify any confusion before the close of the meeting. By maintaining the staff's active role in this communication process, the staff's assumption of responsibility for actions and their consequences is encouraged.

After the discussion, the content of the meeting should be recorded. Through this process, the data for future directions are provided if the staff's problem behavior continues. It is difficult to recall the content of a discussion several months later, and a written summary not only refreshes memories but may serve to alleviate future problems. Because the discussion did not include disciplinary action, this documentation is solely for the use of the counsellor and need not be signed by the employee.

Staff Development

Throughout all supervisory communication and activities, the focus is on staff development—i.e., aiding the supervisors and staff in their progress toward increasing competency and improved client care. The psychiatric–mental health nursing administrator does this by serving as a role model (see Chapter 11) to facilitate the supervisory staff's professional growth.

Administrative responsibility further includes the assessment of the strengths and weaknesses of each supervisory staff member, and the communication of this assessment to the relevant persons in a manner the staff is able to receive and use. The nurse-administrator should ensure this reception through skillful communication techniques. Strengths should be supported and developed and weaknesses minimized or eliminated through collaborative educational efforts with the individual staff members. It is then expected that the supervisory staff would treat their subordinates in a similar fashion. Any of these efforts may use standardized materials, but they should be individualized in order to ensure the staff's receptivity.

One of the largest challenges is the development of initiative and the independent assumption of accountability by all staff members—particularly those who are no longer challenged by their positions. A basic technique is communication that focuses on the staff's accountability for the care delivered. If staff members do not routinely assume another's accountability—except temporarily—all staff can progress. Communication should indicate that each person is capable and is competent to fulfill the designated position requirements, with support being given if needed (Worthington, 1982). These mechanisms encourage the growth of the staff's self-esteem and should result in an improvement in the delivery of care.

Another mechanism for fostering staff growth is the encouragement of staff involvement in problem solving and decision making according to participative management techniques. Decisions should be made at the lowest level possible. Not only does this approach encourage the staff's involvement in the management of the department, but it also frees the supervisory staff from unnecessary work.

Staff variances in the completion of assignments should also be respected. There is seldom only one right way to deliver client care. Forcing standardization fails to recognize the uniqueness of the individual staff member and the client; rather, it results in a lower quality of care. Recognition of this uniqueness also fosters creative problem solving by the staff, which, in turn, facilitates the delivery of individualized client care and increased staff morale.

Clinical Supervision

An important aspect of psychiatric–mental health nursing supervision not always included within other nursing areas is *clinical supervision.* "Clinical supervision is having someone who will assist . . . in studying what [is occurring] in an investigative, teaching-learning environment. . . . It is one of the major differences between professional and technical practice" (Benfer, 1979, p. 14). Trainor (1978) further points out that "the goal of [this] helping relationship is to facilitate growth and assist persons to develop and use their inner resources in order to improve their functioning" (p. 30).

Within psychiatric–mental health nursing, all professional nursing staff should have access to regular clinical supervision by qualified supervisory staff. As stated elsewhere, these clinical supervisors should have a master's degree in nursing, specializing in the particular aspect of psychiatric–mental health nursing being supervised. It is important that the staff develop a trusting and respectful relationship with the person providing the supervision. Often, the first thing that should be done is to "change the attitude of staff toward authority figures" (Fagin, 1967, p. 36)—particularly if the attitude has been an antagonistic one. Through the development of a collaborative atmosphere, the two persons can work together to improve the quality of the care provided.

The content covered during clinical supervision is also important. It should be selected carefully and with a focus on the improvement of the staff's therapeutic abilities. "It is important to include only present material in confronting both the basic personality of the [staff], and his/her ego strength and nature of defenses, so that the discussion will focus on the therapeutic process and its meaning" (Feather & Bissell, 1979, p. 268). During the meeting, the impact the staff's behavior has on the client should also be carefully reviewed. This self-awareness on the part of the staff should extend also to the supervisory staff.

Conflicts between the supervisor and the staff may result from various sources: for example, a differing view of the treatment given to the client, countertransference, or the differing philosophies of the staff. These conflicts should be recognized when they occur and should be resolved, either with the staff or during the clinical supervisor's own supervision time (Feather & Bissell).

Trainor (1978) has found that, in order to establish a helping relationship with the staff, certain characteristics have a positive influence: "genuineness, positive regard, empathy, . . . positive view of the person being helped, a willingness to become involved, and a belief in the person's ability to act on his [/her] own" (pp. 32–33). These factors have been found to cause a positive change in the staff receiving supervision. How the clinical supervisor conducts the meeting and behaves during it can also greatly affect the staff's behavior after the meeting. "In order to establish a helping relationship, the . . . supervisor and the [staff] must clarify mutual expectations, establish common goals, and initiate cooperative action" (Trainor, p. 33).

Certain techniques may be used to foster these characteristics. Trainor (1978) lists ten:

> 1) providing positive feedback on an informal basis, 2) minimizing defensiveness in confrontation interviews, 3) promoting the involvement of nursing in decision making, 4) focusing on what is not being expressed as well as on what is being expressed, 5) refraining from acting on the evaluation of others, 6) increasing attention to listening, 7) responding non-defensively, 8) minimizing playing a role and hiding behind a mask, 9) creating an environment in which other persons feel free to disagree and express their own ideas, [and] 10) expressing feelings appropriately. (pp. 34–36)

Many of these actions have been discussed elsewhere in this text in relation to other activities. They are mentioned here to demonstrate the importance of interpersonal skills in psychiatric–mental health nursing not only with clients but also in clinical supervision in order to foster the development of the entire department.

Management Development

In addition to the development of the clinical staff, the supervisory staff should also be fostered. Efforts should be directed not only at current supervisors but also at those staff members who demonstrate the potential for future supervisory positions. Through this mechanism, the department can continue to have strong leaders despite unavoidable turnover.

One basic method for providing developmental support to supervisors is the provision of position descriptions and departmental policies that are clearly worded (Stevens, 1979). A sound basis is thus provided for consistent behavior by all supervisors. Policies that are clearly stated are much easier to implement, and they provide a support for future policy-consistent programs. This clarity enables supervisors to maintain the standards established by the department. Furthermore, such clearly defined expectations help to ensure that supervisors assume the accountability related to their respective positions (Stevens, 1979).

Management Focus

The supervisor should also have a realistic approach to management, which includes the blending of a future orientation with current personnel practices (Stevens, 1979). To be an effective leader, a supervisor should be goal-oriented and directed. The focus should be upon the future and how to reach future goals efficiently and effectively. To not do so is to become bound up in a crisis mentality of simply surviving day-to-day problems.

Of course, the supervisor should be well versed in current personnel policies and procedures. If any staff members belong to a bargaining unit, the bargaining agreement should be thoroughly understood. It is imperative that the supervisor be extremely knowledgeable in these matters in order to be able to apply them consistently to all the staff.

Developmental Supports

The development of management staff requires personnel and financial support. The departmental budget should, of course, designate funds for staff development. At the same time, within those staff development funds, a cost item should be management development. Seminars, workshops, and self-directed learning experiences require financial resources. Supervisory coverage for those activities, as well as for clerical support and supplies, requires financial outlays. These costs should be included in the budget as a demonstration of the commitment of the psychiatric–mental health nursing administrator to this aspect of the development program.

Content of Management Development

If a nurse-administrator wishes to facilitate the growth of the department, the supervisory staff should be recognized as key resources for that growth. If they are allowed to stagnate and become outdated, the entire department suffers. Not only should there be a management orientation program; there should also be continuing educational efforts to improve a person's level of functioning. In one study, Stetler, Garity, Macdonald, and Smith (1980) identified basic educational topics relevant to nursing management: "change, conflict management, evaluation, group dynamics, interpersonal relations, interviewing, professionalism, implications for management, leadership, motivation, organizational systems, problem solving, theories of management" (p. 21). Other topics found by Wilsea (1980) to be useful include "assertiveness, . . . personnel management, cost-containment, staffing and scheduling, labor relations, . . . accountability, fiscal management, politics, power, quality assurance, organizational theory, communication theory, . . . human relations theory, . . . management by objectives, nursing audit, [and client] classification" (p. 48). These topics are not exclusive or necessarily relevant to all organizations; they can be arranged, however, to fit the individual needs of the psychiatric–mental health nursing department.

Methods for the presentation of these topics should be based on individual, organizational, and staff needs. Seminars could be held regularly, or much of the work could be done through self-study modules. Investigation could also determine whether such educational efforts could be approved for continuing education credits. Such credits serve to reinforce the staff's efforts and are useful for certification purposes.

Management Career Ladders

As in the case of clinical career ladders, an administrative career ladder can be developed. To do so, a similar process would be utilized, but with a different career focus. The development would include a job analysis of each supervisory position, identification of the standards incorporated into each position, and identification of the requirements needed to comply with these standards. One such ladder utilized the decision-making process as its focus, dividing the areas of decision making into those involved with the "interface of the organization with the environment, organizational design, and managerial strategies" (Fralic & O'Connor, 1983, p. 10). In this situation, the differences between levels of decision making involved the "amount of information needed to make those decisions and the perception or knowledge of the organization each manager has at each administrative level" (Fralic & O'Connor, p. 13). Through this process of identifying competencies, staff members who demonstrate the capabilities important to the organization can be identified and supported if they wish to become managers in the future.

IMPLEMENTING SUPERVISORY PROCESS

Once competent, confident supervisory staff have been developed, it is up to these persons to implement the supervisory process. Furthermore, this process should be implemented in a fair and consistent manner by all supervisory staff on all the shifts. Inconsistencies between shifts can result in discrimination, poor morale, and, ultimately, a lowered quality of care. By expecting accountable behavior from all supervisory staff, the nurse-administrator is likely to receive it (Sherwood, 1982)

Again, communication is extremely important. In order to facilitate open and honest communication, a variety of techniques can be utilized. One author, Mlynczak (1982), suggests using a communication book, which aids in the sharing of written information by all shifts. In addition, the communication letter can serve as an updating newsletter to keep staff informed of "remedies, new procedures, and upcoming events" (p. 45). Finally, staff meetings can be held on a regular basis on all shifts to provide for face-to-face discussions.

Orientation to changes in procedures can be done through a teaching-learning tree in which all staff are responsible for passing on the new information. The head nurse then meets with the last staff member, receiving the information to ensure that no details were lost in the process. This technique involves all of the staff and holds them accountable for communicating changes to others accurately. Whatever communication techniques are utilized, it is important that the process be done consistently on all shifts by all supervisors.

Positive Reinforcement

Another factor that is crucial for successful supervision is the use of positive reinforcement or praise. It has been stated that all staff should be encouraged to use self-awareness and evaluation to improve themselves. However, without praise, such behavior is likely to be extinguished. Leaders who use positive reinforcement on a frequent and appropriate basis do much to improve staff motivation. Through this dynamic approach, these leaders provide a working environment in which all of the staff are able to function at their highest level of competency.

Conflict Management

Naturally, conflict exists. Any situation that involves differing opinions has some degree of conflict. Techniques for handling conflict include "competing, collaborating, compromising, avoiding and accommodating" (Marriner, 1982, p. 29). Collaborating is the most productive of these mechanisms because it results in each party experiencing a satisfactory conclusion to the conflict. This mechanism requires, however, a substantial amount of time.

Oermann (1977) has suggested a form of collaborative supervision that is useful not only in times of conflict but as a problem solving approach (diagnostic supervision). Although the author discusses it in relation to staff development, this mechanism can be used at any time to aid the supervision process. Basically, it is a technique similar to the nursing process and is composed of these steps: "recognition, determination of objectives, assessment, plan development, implementation and evaluation" (p. 10). This model supports the basic concept of this text—that the nursing process and the administration of a psychiatric–mental health nursing department are complementary. Through this mechanism, investigation occurs before action is taken, so that much unnecessary or reactive behavior is eliminated.

Because conflict is often a daily occurrence, the supervisory staff must be capable and confident in working with it. Resolving conflict is much the same as solving a problem, and so it should be approached in a similar fashion. There are, however, some basic techniques suggested by Cooper (1979) that can be used to minimize the amount of conflict (Exhibit 8–1). All of them use good communication skills and common sense.

Exhibit 8–1 Minimizing Conflict

- Keep a positive approach; it can often decrease the possibility of confrontation.
- All communication should be clearly understood by both parties; missed communications are a frequent source of conflict.
- Communicate to the staff with respect.
- Be as involved in client care as possible. Conflict is less likely to develop over client care activities when the staff recognize supervision's willingness to become involved.
- Give positive feedback as much as possible.
- Avoid making quick judgments and discuss the issues. Listen and ask questions in order to obtain as much information as possible before making decisions.
- Avoid gossip; it is unproductive and a waste of time.
- Attempt to exclude personal problems from the work environment. Resolve feelings as much as possible before becoming involved with staff.
- Leave a situation if it cannot be objectively handled; unless it is an emergency, there is no reason to remain in a situation in which feelings are explosive. Before leaving, however, make a commitment to work with the issues at a later date, and keep it.
- Do not hold grudges; residual resentment has no place in supervision.
- Recognize and accept your own mistakes. Examine them to determine how they might have been prevented and to learn from them. Do not ruminate on past mistakes. (This behavior serves as a role model for the staff.)
- Confer with a superior. If the conflict cannot be resolved by the two parties, they should agree on a third person who can assist them in working through the issues.

Source: Adapted from "Conflict: How to avoid it and what to do when you can't" by J. Cooper, 1979, *Nursing 79*, 9(1).

Lamp (1982) adds a final suggestion. Do not censure staff in public. Nothing is gained and much could be lost by publicly embarrassing a staff member. This type of conference should take place in private with only the persons involved present. This policy applies to all levels of the staff.

Conflict cannot be avoided. However, if supervisory staff members recognize it as a problem that needs solving and attempt to do so, it will no longer serve as a stumbling block. Communication used to resolve conflict can also serve to open and to improve channels of communication between supervisors and staff.

Counselling versus Therapy

An issue pertinent to psychiatric–mental health nursing supervision is counselling versus therapy. In attempting to improve a staff's nursing care or work behavior, personal issues arise that are related to the problem areas. The supervisor should recognize this occurrence and continue to focus on the resolution of the current work-related issues. Should the supervisor recognize that therapy would be beneficial, this possibility could be explored with the staff. By demonstrating this recognition and associated concerns for the best interests and confidentiality of the staff, the supervisor can assist the staff in receiving the assistance needed from the appropriate people (e.g., employee assistance programs).

Documentation

Throughout all supervisory activity, documentation is crucial because it provides the basis for evaluations and, should it be necessary, disciplinary action. Without documentation, the supervisor cannot accurately evaluate a staff and is subject to all the evaluative flaws—e.g., the halo effect. With it, an accurate portrayal of the staff's strengths, weaknesses, and progress can be drawn. Furthermore, the supervisor who has documentation has a firm basis and rationale for continued disciplinary action if necessary. Whether documentation is in the format of informal anecdotal notes or on a form supplied by the department, it is crucial for the equitable and consistent functioning of the supervisor. Any documentation should include the date, the name of the employee, the facts of the situation, the content of the discussion between the supervisor and the subordinate, the staff's understanding of the problem, the expected results of the meeting, and the related deadlines.

EVALUATION

Evaluations are generally stressful for both supervisor and staff. Whether it is due to the ambiguity of the evaluation form, the infrequency of its occurrence, or the communication styles of those involved, an evaluation seldom seems to result in a staff member's development. Evaluation problems that have been identified include the subjective nature of the process, the one-way communication pattern, and the annual occurrence, which does not lend itself to learning (Breeden, 1978).

Also, when reviewing a staff's problem behaviors after an evaluation conference, one may find—

- that the staff do not receive reinforcement from supervision for the occurrence or the lack of occurrence of expected behaviors;
- that the staff are rewarded for not complying with expected behaviors;
- that the staff are sanctioned by peers for positive performances;
- that impediments may exist that are beyond the control of the staff but that hinder the attainment of desired behaviors. (Milnar, 1981)

Hence, negative evaluations may have resulted because of system impediments rather than staff's deficiencies.

Evaluation can be defined "as the process of measuring an object, an activity (such as performance), or an abstraction to determine the extent to which it meets established criteria" (Breeden, 1978, p. 14). Reasons for the existence of evaluations are many. They exist—

- to affect performance by measuring it or improving it,
- to increase staff's motivation,
- to determine merit raises,
- to facilitate promotions and transfers,
- to identify educational needs of the staff,
- to validate the need to terminate unsatisfactory staff. (Clark, 1982; Stevens, 1976)

Because of the problems outlined previously (which are often inherent in the evaluation process) the goals stated above—although attained—may result from a stressful experience.

Guidelines that Facilitate Process

In order to facilitate the evaluation process within an existing system, the program can be reviewed to determine if the following guidelines are being met. Communication during an evaluation should be a two-way process, not just the superior speaking and the subordinate listening. "It is important [and valuable to the department] that individuals feel free to express their opinions without fear of exposure'' (DeGiovanni, Gordon, & Schlesinger, 1978, p. 29). The behaviors evaluated should be clearly delineated for subordinates and superiors. Any ambiguity leads to conflicts and stress. Hence, job descriptions should be clearly and behaviorally stated. All superiors should consistently expect the same levels of practice, and common disciplinary practice should be consistent with what is expected by the department. If there are discrepancies in either area, evaluation problems will continue to exist.

The effective receipt of communication is related to its relevance to the staff. If the staff believe that the communication does not apply to them, they do not accurately receive it. The superior should ensure that the staff hears what is actually being discussed. There will be no carry-over or progress if the staff did not comprehend the specific nature of the needed change or recognize that the communication was directed toward them.

The staff must be informed in advance when the evaluation is to occur (Cook, 1979). This is crucial when participative evaluations are expected. The staff members must have time to complete their self-evaluations in order to discuss discrepancies that arise during the evaluation conference.

An evaluation should review both the staff's strengths and weaknesses. Praise and positive reinforcement are crucial to maintain a staff's motivation and to provide energy for the improvement of deficits. The goal of the evaluation is a holistic view of the staff's abilities and competencies. By focusing only on strengths, the staff may never change problem areas.

The annual evaluation should be documented with copies for the employee and the personnel file, but the evaluation process should be an ongoing one, not just the annual meeting. The staff should receive frequent feedback about their progress in identified deficit areas. Positive reinforcement and praise should be given when appropriate to reinforce strengths and to give recognition to the individual staff member.

Development of an Evaluation Format

If the department's evaluation format is not satisfactory, a new format that more adequately meets the department's needs can be developed. According to Brief (1979), two important points must be considered when assessing the current evaluation program: (1) Is the current system valid? Does it measure what it purports to measure? and (2) Is the evaluation tool trusted by those involved? If the answer to these two questions is yes, there is no need for a revision of the system. If, however, the answer is no, the department should review and revise current practices.

There are "four basic steps for developing a workable performance appraisal system: 1) determination of employee behavior to be evaluated, 2) establishment of methods for measuring the performance dimension, 3) documentation of procedures for using the appraisal instruments, [and] 4) ongoing evaluation of the system" (Brief, 1979, p. 8). This process would, of course, follow other such developmental processes examined in this text and would involve the appropriate staff at all levels of the department.

Content

General guidelines already exist for the content of the evaluation format for psychiatric–mental health nursing. In determining important performance factors, Bernhardt and Schuette (1975) identified those factors generally relevant for the registered nurse: "teaching, observational ability, organizational ability, professional growth, responsibility, interpersonal skills, management skills, appearance, attendance, clinical skills, reaction under pressure, nursing process, and length of service" (p. 19). Similar factors have been cited by Marshall and Schau (1976) as being relevant for nursing assistants in general hospitals: "emergency responsiveness, interpersonal relations, attitude toward job, judgment, observation and reporting, skills, initiative, emotional stability, dependability, knowledge, acceptance—work changes, . . . safety, learning ability, charting, integrity, attendance pattern, [and] appearance" (p. 39). Although these have relevance for a general hospital setting, they lend themselves to a psychiatric–mental health setting as well.

Not all factors need to be evaluated. Each department needs to identify only those factors crucial to the delivery of quality client care within the specific organization and that reflect the organization's or department's standards of care. Each factor should then be examined to identify significant behaviors that are indicative of satisfactory job performance. If staff members are evaluated on nonimportant behaviors, they find it difficult to recognize and to emphasize the important ones (Cook, 1979). Hence, the committee should focus upon identifying the competencies required for job performance. The behaviors being evaluated should occur on a regular basis in order to receive satisfactory ratings. Isolated incidences do not demonstrate that the person is capable of performing in a similar manner on a consistent basis (Bernhardt & Schuette, 1975).

Staff Involvement

The staff being evaluated should be involved in the development process for the tool. This involvement should not only decrease resistance to the final tool, but it should also demonstrate to the staff the administration's commitment to the use of staff input. In many instances, the involved staff can assist management in realistically evaluating a position that has changed in subtle, but important, ways over a period of time. The staff can identify what they do, and management can determine whether this process is the way in which care should be given.

Types of Evaluations

There are many types of evaluative processes. All of the processes detailed by the authors focus upon the involvement of the staff in an effort to decrease the stress involved in the experience and to promote the development of an involved staff. Through these processes, staff members are continually encouraged to assume the responsibility and accountability commensurate with their nursing practice.

Self-Evaluation

An important element in all evaluation processes in psychiatric–mental health nursing is self-evaluation. Consistent with nursing's commitment to involve the client in the health care process is nursing administration's commitment to involve the staff in the evaluation process. This involvement also serves to provide motivation for the involved staff (Edwards & Powers, 1982). As is the case with other new policies, the involved staff members need sufficient orientation in order to feel comfortable with what, for many of the staff, may be a foreign and uncomfortable experience. They should be advised that the self-evaluation should include a summation of past performance, current functioning, and future goals (Colerick, Mason & Proulx, 1980). Supervisors should realize, however, that certain staff members may be hesitant or noncompliant with the request for a self-evaluation. In those instances, the supervisor needs to work with the staff to resolve this problem. Should noncompliance continue, it is up to the nursing administration to determine the responsive reaction, whether educational or disciplinary.

Participative Evaluation

Another example of staff involvement is participative staff evaluations. In this process, both the staff and the supervisor come to an evaluation conference with a completed evaluation. During the conference, both evaluations are discussed, and a composite emerges. Through discussion and elaboration, facts of which both parties may have been unaware come to light, and the resulting evaluation is a more accurate picture of the staff's performance than is created from one person's viewpoint. This process, according to Breeden (1978),

> decreases threat, improves understanding of performance requirements, fosters early problem recognition, and increases creativity, self-actualization, and job satisfaction for the supervisor and [staff]. [It] provides recognition for quality work, advises [staff] of performance adequacies and inadequacies, . . . identifies training and development needs, . . . can be used to improve communication between the supervisor and the [staff], and [the sharing of] ideas relevant to the work situation. (p. 14)

Several points are crucial to the success of this process. All staff members should be involved in and oriented to the process, the forms, and the terminology. Should there be ambiguity in any of these, unnecessary conflicts can result, which would need to be resolved during the evaluation conference. This ambiguity adds, rather than decreases, stress and should be avoided through the clear delineation of the content of the form during a well-defined evaluation. These evaluation conferences would also be held on a regular basis, rather than annually. Through this mechanism, progress can be ascertained, and changes that reflect such progress can be made in plans, with modification of earlier established needs (Breeden, 1978).

Benefits resulting from a participative evaluation program have been identified by Clark (1982).

> Participatory goal setting and objective appraisal develop the leader's authority and skill. The communication network—upward, downward, and horizontal—strengthens. The organization moves toward unity through its common goals and objectives. Since the basis of the performance is explicit and objective, validity and realiability increase. Appraiser and appraisee understand their responsibilities better. The collection of data regarding training and development improves. Human resources and career assessment and planning receive systematic recognition of their importance. The [staff] is increasingly motivated to control herself[/himself] and to direct her[/his] work more objectively. The [staff] is less defensive. The active [staff member], who set her[/his] goals, determines the method of measurement and self-evaluates is more likely to feel she[/he] has been fairly appraised. (p. 28)

Management by Objectives

A further refinement of the participative evaluation process involves the use of a modified form of management by objectives. In this evaluative process, the superior and the subordinate meet to choose work goals, to identify measurable objectives and time frames for each goal, to determine progress, and to identify necessary corrective actions that must be taken in order to facilitate goal or objective attainment. This mechanism, as with all revisions of evaluative programs, cannot be accomplished quickly. *All* aspects of the planning process defined previously should occur. This mechanism may require several years, however, before it is operational and functioning to the satisfaction of all those involved (Council & Plachy, 1980).

Guidelines are also associated with this process in order to facilitate its successful implementation. In addition to being patient, all persons involved should be sure that defined goals and objectives are consistent with those of the department and organization.

These goals and objectives must also be stated in behavioral terms, and must be measurable. Without this specificity, ambiguity recurs and produces unnecessary conflict and resistance. Furthermore, superiors need to identify crucial behaviors that need changing in order to provide quality care. The standard expectations of performance should be clearly delineated in order to identify the level at which each staff member should be functioning so that the predetermined quality of client care is provided. During this process of goal and objective setting, review dates should be established to continue the evaluation process. Through this mechanism, both parties know when the goals and objectives will be evaluated and can plan for a review conference on that date. Thus, staff members are not taken by surprise; instead, they have control over the time frame by knowing what is expected and when (Council & Plachy, 1980).

Performance Profile

The performance profile system is "designed to reduce the dominance of the evaluation theme on both supervisor and subordinate and, at the same time, to facilitate counselling [and] development efforts" (South, 1978, p. 27). The profile is developed through a three step process:

1. Select the performance components—usually four to eight.
2. Convert the ratings of these components (when necessary) to numbers by giving numerical values to qualitative terms.
3. Plot the sums on the profile to identify the staff's strengths and weaknesses. (South, p. 29)

Because this process identifies areas of strengths and weaknesses for specific staff members and focuses on performance patterns, it lends itself to staff development. Furthermore, it emphasizes to the staff that the nursing administration is attempting to review the overall performance and to determine areas in which staff members may need assistance. This process can also be combined with a self-evaluation that is compared and contrasted with the supervisor's evaluation (South, 1978).

Furthermore, this system serves to identify those staff members with strengths who may benefit from involvement in special projects or educational programs or, perhaps, promotions. It serves to identify common educational or training needs and can identify supervisors who tend to evaluate the staff on a general basis rather than on an individualized basis. As a rule, this process "lessens the overall evaluative tone of the performance review, facilitates the diagnostic thinking, and reduces the resistance of the subordinates by shifting the discussion toward understanding one's performance rather than comparing it to that of others" (South, 1978, p. 31).

Supervisor-Staff Conference

In all of the evaluative processes, the supervisor-staff conference plays a crucial part. The purpose of most of these conferences "is to compare objectives, set priorities, establish approximate timetables for achieving objectives, and discuss follow-up procedures" (Cook, 1979, p. 84). In order to achieve this goal, there must be a two-way communication process. Both parties should send and receive clear messages.

In this situation, the main responsibility for the clarification of communication lies with the supervisor. "The skill with which a supervisor conducts an evaluation conference appears to be a key factor in determining whether the procedure will be effective in motivating behavioral change" (Breeden, 1978, p. 15). Breeden further identifies important skills the supervisor should cultivate: "listening, participating, structuring the interview situation, asking for elaboration, and reflecting" (p. 18).

Two types of conferences are also identified—the work conference, which occurs at predetermined times throughout the year, and the formal evaluation conference, which occurs annually. The work conference focuses "largely on discussing progress toward goals set in the previous conference, sharing ideas about the work situation, receiving comments on [the supervisor's performance], and talking about factors influencing [the staff's] job satisfaction and self-development" (Breeden, 1978, p. 18). The annual conference, similar to the work conference, is used, additionally, to review salaries and positions.

Because these conferences are extremely important for supervisor-staff relationships, the supervisor must establish the conference's goals when contracting with the staff member to arrange the date, the time, and so forth. The place of the conference should be one in which both persons feel comfortable. The supervisor reviews the job description and performance standards, applying the content of the staff member's actual performance. During the conference, both persons review these while comparing the two evaluations. From this discussion, the two develop goals and related time frames for their accomplishment. Finally, it is crucial to recognize the staff member's strengths, as well as weaknesses, and to give the staff member support in maintaining the strengths and overcoming the weaknesses. This type of focus presents a holistic view of the staff and alleviates the feeling that the conference was only a fault-finding experience.

A summation of the conference is important and occurs at two points. At the conclusion of the conference, the supervisor should verbally summarize the content for validation with the staff. "Following the annual evaluation, record the conference outcomes, translating performance standard levels into behavioral descriptions. Summarize areas of agreement and difference from the . . . conference, and list the agreed-upon goals for improving work performance" (Breeden, 1978, p. 18). After this is typed, the staff member should read and sign it, and it should be filed in the staff member's personnel file.

Peer Review

"Peer review can be defined as a process by which practitioners of the same rank, profession, or setting critically appraise each other's work performance against established standards" (O'Laughlin & Kaulbach, 1981, p. 2). It is a "method for monitoring nursing practice [which] addresses the norms required by bureaucracy and also provides professional assessment of practice which promotes the nurse's accountability" (Mullins, Colavecchio & Tescher, 1979, p. 25). The purposes of peer review are much the same as other evaluative processes. The documentation, however, may differ substantially from that used in the more traditional approaches.

The information provided must identify "technical competency; whether the [client] care outcomes reflect the nurse's technical competency; what the professional nurse does, as primary nurse, that is unique; superior work worthy of recognition and commendation, and areas for growth development" (O'Laughlin & Kaulbach, 1981, p. 23). Mullins et al. (1979) recommend the following documentation format: "two behavioral performance evaluations, two reference letters, self-evaluation, two nursing histories or assessments, and one example of current, original work" (p. 26). The material is reviewed by a committee selected by the psychiatric–mental health nursing department. The nurse is also interviewed, and the results of the process are shared with the nurse and other persons as necessary. The actual committee selected and the details of the review process vary among organizations.

Before beginning the planning process for the implementation of peer review, five questions can be asked to determine if peer review is appropriate for the organization and the department.

1) What are the risks associated with implementing a process for which the outcomes are largely unknown? 2) Once the organization is committed to the implementation of peer review, what alternatives are available if the review process is not suitable? 3) Given that confidentiality is an issue, what, if any, should be the feedback mechanism between peer review committees and the various departments in the institutions? 4) What responses can be anticipated from other disciplines within the institution? 5) Can the expense of initiating such a process be justified? (Mullins et al, 1979, p. 30)

If the answers to these questions are affirmative, the nurse-administrator can then initiate the planning process. If these questions raise additional questions or are answered in the negative, other alternative evaluation processes should be examined.

As with any new program, there will be problems and resistance. Much can be done, however, to decrease the potential for both. Sufficient time should be allowed for personnel to institute the program. The development of the mechanism, and the initial orientation of the department to this process, require an extended period of time. A reasonable amount of time is also required for the actual review process, although this time decreases as individuals become more adept at reviewing. Support services must also be available in order to facilitate the documentation aspects of the process. Without such support, the persons involved in the process may become discouraged and may be unable to concentrate on the actual review (Mullins et al, 1979).

The insecurity inherent in the institution of a new process should also be considered. Not only do those nurses being reviewed feel threatened by the unknown of the new process, but those doing the reviewing often do not feel qualified to review other nurses (O'Laughlin & Kaulbach, 1981). Some of this insecurity decreases as those involved become more familiar with the process. By having the program clearly delineated and defined, and based upon observable behaviors, much of the ambiguity that often leads to this insecurity can be eliminated. However, these feelings should be recognized and handled through discussions and an exploration of causes as part of instituting the actual process.

Peer review is a professional process for use in a profession's monitoring of its members. By determining whether such a program is appropriate for a particular department, the stage can be set for future reimbursement for the nurses within the organization. The process also serves to demonstrate that the nursing profession can be self-monitoring without the direction of outside disciplines or agencies.

Merit Increases

Many organizations use the annual evaluation to substantiate merit increases. In order to make such a program valid, the evaluation program should be behaviorally based and clearly defined. If it is not, every staff member, generally, receives the same merit raise, regardless of variances in performance. However, when "tied to known performance expectations within the control of the [staff], a desired merit increase becomes a direct motivator of performance" (Lerch, 1982, p. 31). Through this technique, staff members are able to earn merit raises dependent solely upon demonstrated behaviors, not in response to a supervisor's subjective opinion. By locating the control with the staff, the staff members become accountable for the existence or the absence of a raise, not the supervisor.

Evaluation of Nursing Leaders

The type of quality evaluative process discussed above is not confined to the staff alone but also to nursing leaders. The rationale for this is the same as for the staff—to improve the quality of performance. Writing about management, Holland (1981) has defined "six specific role prescriptions . . . identified as essential for managing within a hierarchical organizational setting" (p. 17). Inasmuch as this description is applicable to psychiatric–mental health nursing leaders, these traits should also be considered when developing job descriptions or evaluation forms for this group. According to Holland, these are the six essential role prescriptions:

1) Managers are expected to deal effectively with their superiors and to obtain support for actions at high levels. Thus, managers should have positive feelings towards those holding positions of authority over them.
2) Because of the competitive nature of managerial work, managers are expected to accept the challenge of the job and achieve results for themselves and their subordinates.
3) A manager is expected to take charge and behave in an active and assertive manner.
4) A manager must exercise power over subordinates.
5) The manager is expected to be willing to be unique and assume a position of high visibility.
6) Because of the realities of the managerial job, a manager must be willing to face the routine administrative tasks which accompany the job. (pp. 17–18)

The general evaluative process for a nurse-manager should be similar to that of the staff: e.g., self-evaluation, participative evaluation, focusing on strengths as well as weaknesses. An additional consideration in the evaluation of nurse-managers is the use of staff evaluation. Hamric, Gresham & Eccard (1978) identified several advantages for this aspect of managerial evaluation. According to them, it

1) provides a written index of overall performance; 2) demonstrates general trends in performance (general areas of strength and weakness); 3) validates or invalidates the leader's beliefs as to the scope, appropriateness, and effectiveness of her[/his] practice by comparing them to the staff's perception; 4) facilitates diagnosis of overall staff problems, pointing out problem areas of which the leader may have previously been unaware; 5) produces data for a concrete baseline definition of the quality of performance that can be used in future evaluations; 6) enables the staff to participate in a constructive professional evaluation of the leader; . . . [and] 7) for staff to feel that their opinions are valued can certainly enhance the total effectiveness of the clinical leadership. (p. 25)

Of course, problems associated with this process may be anticipated. An initial threat exists that is involved in any innovative evaluation. The staff may be less than honest if they question whether the confidentiality of their responses will be honored. Their responses may also be unfairly hostile as they use this program to vent anger that may be unrelated to the particular superior. It is, therefore, important that this program be introduced in a fashion similar to any long term departmental project. Crucial to its success, as mentioned previously, is the maintenance of confidentiality so that the involved staff may be assured of anonymity, and may be able to express their perceptions honestly.

As in the case of client care, it is essential in psychiatric–mental health nursing for a nurse leader to be aware of the perceptions of others. Staff evaluations provide the leaders with a unique perspective that can be achieved in no other way. This additional input enables the leader to further validate previously developed self-perceptions and to make corrections as needed.

Discipline

Realistically, the evaluation process does not always involve only the positive aspects of assisting the staff to improve their competencies. Discipline is also necessary when a staff does not respond to previous attempts to improve or to correct the performance. However, as with everything else in management, documentation and the proper procedures must be followed to ensure fairness and consistency for each staff member and to facilitate the process on behalf of the superior.

It is obvious that supportive counselling should occur before any formal discipline. Each organization and department should have a clearly defined disciplinary process that is applied consistently to all staff. On this basis, the supervisory staff should expect support from their superiors in any disciplinary action—if the action has been done appropriately.

To ensure this, four guidelines should be reviewed with every disciplinary action.

1. The discipline should be based upon provable allegations, which entails having all the facts (not opinions) documented.
2. The discipline should be related to the severity of the misconduct. Organizations and departments should have published guidelines that detail the discipline associated with various types of misconduct. Through this mechanism, the supervisor and the staff know the consequences of misconduct. There is not ambiguity.
3. The misconduct must be job related; disciplinary action cannot be taken for personal reasons, or for behaviors unrelated to job performance.
4. The departmental disciplinary process should be followed.

Again, organizations and departments should publish their disciplinary procedures so that the superior and the staff automatically know what level of discipline can be expected (Stevens, 1976).

It is crucial that supervisory personnel expect and receive support from the nursing administration. Without that support, policies and procedures cannot be consistently enforced. With that support, the nursing supervisor can feel comfortable in applying the process. The nurse-administrator should also expect the supervisor to discipline according to policy and procedure, and to do it in a fair and consistent fashion. Through this reciprocity, each can predict the other's behavior. Furthermore, the trust that develops can reduce the inherent stress of disciplinary action.

Should an employee fail to correct a problem behavior despite repeated counsellings and disciplinary actions, the termination of that employee may become necessary. Documentation throughout the process used to identify the problem behaviors is of utmost importance and serves to protect the interests of the supervisor and the subordinate.

PROGRAM EVALUATION

The evaluation of any program involves a process similar to that previously described for an individual. On a periodic basis (at least annually) the psychiatric–mental health nursing department's performance evaluation program should be reviewed and evaluated. The basis for each evaluation should include the goals and the objectives of the program, demonstrated outcomes, time frames, and the circumstances that may have had an impact on the program's ability to meet predetermined goals. Such circumstances may include changes in client population, budgetary or staffing restraints, regulatory changes, and so forth. Should a program no longer be meeting the needs of the department or the organization, the program's goals and objectives—or the overall program—may need to be revised. Although this may seem to be a tedious task, it is a crucial one needed to ensure that departmental programs are current and reflective of departmental needs and concerns. Without such a review, programs may be outdated, may be misused, or may be dysfunctional.

REFERENCES

Bassford, G.L., & White, H. (1977). Achieving results: Leadership style and small group effectiveness. *Hospital Progress, 60*(4), 83–87, 107.

Benfer, B.A. (1979). Clinical supervision as a support system for the caregiver. *Perspectives in Psychiatric Care, 17*(1), 13–17.

Bernhardt, J., & Schuette, L. (1975). P.E.T.: A method of evaluating professional nurse performance. *Journal of Nursing Administration, 5*(8), 18–21.

Breeden, S.A. (1978). Participative employee evaluation. *Journal of Nursing Administration, 8*(5), 13–19.

Brief, A.P. (1979). Developing a usable performance appraisal system. *Journal of Nursing Administration, 9*(19), 7–10.

Calkin, J.D. (1982). Does an effective clinician make an effective manager? *The Health Care Supervisor, 1*(1), 26–37.

Clark, M.D. (1982). Performance appraisal. *Journal of Nursing Management, 13*(10), 27–29.

Colerick, E.J., Mason, P.B., & Proulx, J.R. (1980). Evaluation of the clinical nurse specialist role: Development and implementation of a dual purpose framework. *Nursing Leadership, 3*(3), 26–34.

Cook, P.A. (1979). Painless performance evaluations—that work. *RN, 42*(10), 75–76, 80, 82, 84–85.

Cooper, J. (1979). Conflict: How to avoid it and what to do when you can't. *Nursing 79, 9*(1), 89–91.

Council, J.D., & Plachy, R.J. (1980). Performance appraisal is not enough. *Journal of Nursing Administration, 10*(10), 20–26.

DeGiovanni, I.S., Gordon, M.E., & Schlesinger, S.E. (1978). Beyond outcomes: Evaluating staff functioning on an inpatient psychiatric ward. *Journal of Psychiatric and Mental Health Services, 16*(4), 28–31.

Deines, E. (1981). Participative management. *Journal of Nursing Management, 12*(11), 51–53.

Diers, D. (1979). Lessons on leadership. *Image, 11*(3), 67.

Edwards, M., & Powers, R. (1982). Turning staff frustration to satisfaction. *Journal of Nursing Management, 13*(1), 51–52.

Fagin, C.M. (1967). The clinical specialist as supervisor. *Nursing Outlook, 15*(1), 34–36.

Feather, R., & Bissell, B. (1979). Clinical supervision versus psychotherapy: The psychiatric/mental health supervisory process. *Perspectives in Psychiatric Care, 17*(6), 266–272.

Foster, C. (1981). You've joined the management team? *Journal of Nursing Management, 12*(10), 16–18.

Fralic, M.F., & O'Connor, A. (1983). A management progression system for nursing administrators, part I. *Journal of Nursing Administration, 13*(4), 9–13.

Hamric, A.B., Gresham, M.L., & Eccard, M. (1978). Staff evaluation of clinical leaders. *Journal of Nursing Administration, 8*(1), 18–26.

Hayes, P.M. (1979). Redefining the role of the clinical supervisor. *Nursing Leadership, 2*(4), 29–30, 33.

Holland, M.G. (1981). Can managerial performance be predicted? *Journal of Nursing Administration, 11*(6), 17–21.

Ignatavicius, D., & Griffith, J. (1982). Job analysis: The basis of effective appraisal. *Journal of Nursing Administration, 12*(7–8), 37–41.

Kepler, T.L. (1980). Mastering people skills. *Journal of Nursing Administration, 10*(11), 15–20.

Lamp, F. (1982). Evening supervision: Too much for too long. *Journal of Nursing Management, 13*(1), 44, 46.

Lerch, E.M. (1982). Criteria-based performance appraisals. *Journal of Nursing Management, 13*(7), 28–31.

Marriner, A. (1982). Managing conflict. *Journal of Nursing Management, 13*(6), 29–31.

McConnell, C.R. (1982). Health care supervision: A special kind of management? *The Health Care Supervisor, 1*(1), 1–13.

McConnell, E.A. (1980). How to choose a leadership style. *Nursing 80, 10*(3), 105–109.

Marshall, J.R., & Schau, E. (1976). An evaluation process for nursing assistants. *Journal of Nursing Administration, 6*(8), 37–40.

Milnar, R. (1981). Performance analysis—a how to. *Supervisor Nurse, 12*(2), 14–15.

Mlynczak, B.A. (1982). Improving management. *Journal of Nursing Management, 13*(7), 45–46, 48–49.

Mullins, A.C., Colavecchio, R.E., & Tescher, B.E. (1979). Peer review: A model for professional accountability. *Journal of Nursing Administration, 9*(12), 25–30.

Munschauer, B.J. (1983). Decentralizing management. *Journal of Nursing Management, 14*(4), 21–22.

Murphy, E.C. (1983). Discipline: Who owns the responsibility? *Journal of Nursing Management, 14*(7), 58–60.

Oermann, M. (1977). Diagnostic supervision. *Supervisor Nurse, 8*(11), 9–11, 14.

O'Loughlin, E.L., & Kaulbach, D. (1981). Peer review: A perspective for performance appraisal. *Journal of Nursing Administration, 11*(9), 22–27.

Schuldt, S. (1978). Supervision and the informal organization. *Journal of Nursing Administration, 8*(7), 21–25.

Sherwood, T. (1982). A case study: Night supervision. *Journal of Nursing Management, 13*(1), 16–19.

South, J.C. (1978). The performance profile: A technique for using appraisals effectively. *Journal of Nursing Administration, 8*(1), 27–31.

Stetler, C.B., Garity, J., Macdonald, M.E., & Smith, S. (1980). A modular approach to management development. *Journal of Nursing Administration, 10*(12), 19–24.

Stevens, B.J. (1979). Improving nurses' managerial skills. *Nursing Outlook, 27*(12), 774–77.

Stevens, B.J. (1976). Performance appraisal: What the nurse executive expects from it. *Journal of Nursing Administration, 6*(8), 26–31.

Trainor, M.A. (1978). A helping model for clinical supervision. *Supervisor Nurse, 9*(1), 30, 32–36.

Walker, J.J. (1976). Counselling sessions that do some good. *Supervisory Management, 21*(11), 10–15.

Wilkinson, W.R. (1981). Effective management. *Supervisor Nurse, 12*(1), 44–45.

Wilsea, M.M. (1980). Nursing leadership crisis: Proposal for solution. *Supervisor Nurse, 11*(4), 47–48.

Worthington, J. (1982). The art of effective communication. *Journal of Nursing Management, 13*(1), 47–49.

Yura, H. Ozimek, D., & Walsh, M.B. (1981). *Nursing leadership: Theory and process.* New York: Appleton-Century-Crofts.

Zaleznik, A. (1981). Managers and leaders: Are they different? *Journal of Nursing Administration, 11*(7), 25–31.

Chapter 9

Clinical Nursing Staff: Roles and Functions

The nursing staff are the direct care providers within the psychiatric–mental health organization. Each staff member has a variety of assumable roles. Any psychiatric–mental health department must include, within its administrative documentation, delineation of the expected clinical roles and the staff who assume these roles. This goal is often accomplished by a department's job descriptions or position statements. However, a job description often contains additional information beyond that of a role definition. In this chapter, the various clinical nursing roles will be examined as they interface with the administrative process.

ASSESSING THE NEED

"A role is a set of . . . expected behavior patterns associated with an individual's function in various . . . groups" (Stuart & Sundeen, 1983, pp. 247–248). Within psychiatric–mental health nursing, a staff member's role would be the behaviors that are associated with that person's functioning as a member of the treatment team. The roles present in an organization would vary, depending upon the needs of the setting.

Whether an annual role review is being conducted or the role requirements are being developed for a new department, the client population being served must be identified. The population often determines the types of roles needed. For example, if the client group being served is primarily geriatric, the staff nurses would be expected to be capable of an in-depth assessment of the client's physical limitations as these may affect the client's ability to assume an active role in the treatment program. In a similar fashion, if the organization provides psychiatric–mental health nursing care to children, the staff nurses would be expected to be competent in the application of therapeutic play activities as part of the milieu.

The organizational environment must also be considered in the initial determination of needed roles. Departmental and staff needs often dictate roles that must be provided in order to ensure quality client care. For example, the nurse-administrator of a general hospital with one inpatient psychiatric unit may find that two clinical specialists in psychiatric–mental health nursing are necessary to provide consultation to the inpatient unit and to the general hospital as a result of the differing consultative needs of the two nursing staffs.

All aspects of care provision must be examined to identify which roles and staff are needed to provide the expected levels of care. This survey encompasses current staff, departmental, and client needs as well as future requirements and plans. By this orientation to the future, the psychiatric–mental health departmental roles can be continually reflective of current organization and client needs.

PLANNING ROLE DEFINITIONS

Registered Nurses

Once the organization and the client population have been assessed, specific roles can be delineated. The staff nurse role is an integral part of the psychiatric–mental health setting. The staff nurse is the person who generally provides, either directly or indirectly, the majority of client care. This role must be closely examined to identify the qualifications needed and the nurses' expected behaviors.

In this examination process, a crucial issue is the relationship among registered nurses from different educational backgrounds—diploma, associate degree, or baccalaureate degree. The ANA's well-known 1985 resolution stated "that . . . by 1985, the baccalaureate degree in nursing [would be] the minimum preparation for entry into professional nursing practice" (McGriff, 1980, p. 365).

Basic to this decision-making process is the fact that "the nursing profession always has recognized the inseparable relationship between the quality of practice and quality of education" (ANA, 1979, p. 3). Hence, the better quality of client care desired, the higher the educational requirements should be for those persons responsible for that care. Differences have been identified in the clinical competence of nurses with different educational degrees. Furthermore, contrary to popular belief, technically-prepared nurses do not gain competencies equivalent to college-prepared nurses after entering the work force (Jacobs, 1980).

In addition, the areas in which baccalaureate-prepared registered nurses are most active are those in which the psychiatric–mental health staff nurse must also be active: "[client] teaching, . . . promotion of psychological well-being, [and] exchanging and recording information about the [client]" (Jacobs, 1980, p. 2). These skills are necessary for a nurse to function as a member of the psychiatric–mental health treatment team. Diploma and associate-degree prepared nurses, in contrast, have not been found to be as involved in these areas, diploma nurses being most active in clinical assessments and responding to emergencies. Of course, role decisions should also couple experience in the relevant psychiatric–mental health settings with educational backgrounds (Jacobs).

Certification

Since 1973, the ANA has recognized nurses' abilities through the certification process. "Certification is a systematic process which recognizes and publicly attests to a person's mastery of knowledge and achievement of skills in a particular specialty. It can be issued by a governmental agency, by an academic institution, or by a professional association" (Tousley, 1982, p. 23). Certification by the ANA implies "documented validation of specific qualifications demonstrated by the individual registered nurse in the provision of professional care in a defined area of practice" (Tousley, p. 24). The objectives of this process are to "(1) assure the public of quality care, (2) provide credentials to expedite employment and third party reimbursement for services rendered, (3) expand opportunities for vertical and horizontal mobility and career advancement, (4) attain greater prestige and peer recognition for achieving clinical expertise, [and] (5) improve clinical practice" (Tousley, p. 25).

Within psychiatric–mental health nursing, there are two levels of certification: the *generalist*, who may be a staff nurse; and the *specialist* in child/adolescent or adult psychiatric nursing, who must have a master's degree in nursing. Staff members should be encouraged to pursue this certification for several reasons. In addition to personal satisfaction, it provides external recognition of their competency in psychiatric–mental health nursing and generates positive reinforcement for professional growth for the involved nurses, their peers, and the organization. Furthermore, it fosters safeguards for the public, ensuring that the nurse has demonstrated competency in psychiatric–mental health nursing practice.

Qualifications of the Staff Nurse and Role Delineation

Consequently, the nursing administrator may wish to hire primarily baccalaureate-prepared nurses. This preference, however, may not always be possible. A baccalaureate-prepared nurse may *not* have had prior psychiatric–mental health nursing experience and an associate-degreed or diploma-prepared nurse may have *had* substantial quality experience within psychiatric–mental health nursing. Therefore, multiple roles may need to exist to accommodate a wide range of qualified persons who work together to provide care of the desired quality.

What means can the psychiatric–mental health nursing administrator use to attain the goal of providing quality care when hiring new staff, while equitably considering this wide range of qualified persons for employment? One method may be to identify the nursing roles of two groups of nurses: nurses and psychiatric–mental health nurses. (This grouping may prove to be similar to that provided by the concepts of primary and associate nurses in other nursing specialties.) The role of a nurse in a psychiatric–mental health setting would include the activities listed in Table 9–1. This role could be filled by nurses with basic nursing education only, regardless of the type of that education. With additional postbasic nursing education or experience, the nurse could assume the role defined as the psychiatric nurse. In some settings, the two roles could be redefined as psychiatric nurse and psychiatric clinical nurse specialist, with the latter having a master's degree in psychiatric–mental health nursing. During this assessment phase, the basic knowledge and skill levels needed within the organization should be identified. This basic knowledge and skill assessment provides direction for orientation or inservice programming, which assists in preparing nurses with a variety of backgrounds for identified roles within the organization.

Three levels of nursing practice within an ambulatory setting are outlined in Table 9–2 and could be transferred into inpatient organizations as well. Within each level are associated educational expectancies, competencies, and responsibilities.

Another method of role definition identified by Benfer (1980) discusses the role of the nurse as a member of the psychiatric–mental health treatment team. In this role, the nurse's responsibilities include

> (1) obtaining a nursing history, making a nursing assessment; (2) implementing planned interventions, assessing effect, and documenting both [client] behavior and the intervention; (3) determining how the needs of the [client] can be met within the milieu; (4) [client] teaching; (5) coordination of the [client's] activities; [and] (6) prediction and prevention. (p. 172)

This concept focuses upon the role of the nurse as a member of an interdisciplinary team that works to provide quality holistic psychiatric–mental health care to each client. Individual functions and responsibilities would be further defined according to organizational and client population needs.

According to Peplau (1978), the roles nurses assume in any psychiatric–mental health setting

> depend upon: (1) the competence brought to work as a consequence of basic or post-basic nursing education, (2) the definition of mental illness and therefore of the work of "mentally ill" [clients] that prevails in a given setting, (3) the extent of consensus around the question of whether each profession should or should not have any discrete, unique, circumscribed roles or whether there can be overlap . . . and if so, to what extent . . . , (4) the cost of certain kinds of care . . . , the difference in status and salary levels, and the numbers of persons needed and available to provide certain kinds of care. (p. 47)

Table 9–1 Role of Nurses and Psychiatric Nurses

Nurses *(Basic Nursing Education Only)*	*Psychiatric Nurses* *(Postbasic Nursing Education)*
Assess patient needs. Develop nursing care plans. Implement nursing care plan: • carry out direct care; • assign and supervise nursing personnel. Evaluate effects of nursing care. Create and maintain an environment in the service unit of benefit to patients. Stimulate patient relationships with family: dyadic patient/visitor conferences with nurse. Carry out medical orders: • pass prescribed medications; • monitor medication effects; • carry out physical procedures. Surveillance of bathing, mouth care, toileting, bed-making, food intake, sleep. General nursing routines, especially for severely retarded and mentally ill psychogeriatric patients. Prepare for or participate in special treatments: • behavior modification, • electroshock, • lobotomy. Referrals to other professions—clergy, social work, etc. Coordination of patient care of other professionals. Schedule patient activities (off the unit): surveillance of adherence to schedule. Arrange and participate in unit "activities of daily living": • ward government; • various modalities of group activity;	Perform all activities listed under "nurse", plus the following: Intake (history taking) Sociological observation of homes Member of mental health team: • Counselling • Individual psychotherapy • Group psychotherapy • Family therapy • Supervisory review of clinical data (own and other) • Discharge planning with team • Follow-up and evaluation of patient outcomes • File case reports "Special" patients in panic Model for constructive intervention in "ward disturbances" Experiential teaching of nurses Writing professional nursing papers *In hospital:* Work with newly admitted patients as indicated above. Work with acutely disturbed patients, especially regarding panic. Work with autistic and otherwise acutely disturbed children. Work with acting-out and otherwise acutely disturbed adolescents. Serve as a resource and consultant to nurses. Present patient data at staff meetings. Arrange supervisory review of clinical data with equally or more experienced professional colleague.

Table 9–1 continued

Nurses (Basic Nursing Education Only)	Psychiatric Nurses (Postbasic Nursing Education)

- remotivation and resocialization groups;
- work groups;
- patient parties.

Make follow-up home visits after discharge.
Talking with patients:

- situational counselling;
- disrupt illness maintenance.

Attend in-service education sessions and ward staff meetings.
Attend outside continuing education meetings.

Source: From "Psychiatric nursing: Role of nurses and psychiatric nurses" by H. Peplau, 1978, *The International Nursing Review*, 25(2), p. 46. © 1978 by the International Nursing Review. Reprinted by permission.

Through an assessment of these factors, the roles needed within the nursing department to support the provision of quality psychiatric–mental health nursing care by the staff nurses can be identified or reviewed. Basic knowledge and skill requirements can be identified for each role and programming can be planned to assist nurses of varying levels of education and experience in assuming the appropriate role. (To aid the nurse-administrator in identifying components of the role of the staff nurse, the authors have included in Appendix 14-C a listing of activities defined as integral to the role of the psychiatric staff nurse.)

ROLE OF THE HEAD NURSE

Another nursing role within many nursing departments is that of the head nurse. Although this position can also be considered a management role, the head nurse is often involved in direct client care and, as such, deserves consideration within the context of this chapter. The ANA (1978) best describes the role of the head nurse as follows:

Nurses at the first-line level of administration are accountable to the middle-level administrator for implementation of the philosophy, goals, and standards of the nursing department on the unit level. Their primary responsibility is the direction of staff members in the delivery of nursing

Table 9–2 Levels of Practice for Psychiatric Nurses in Ambulatory Settings

	Level 1	*Level 2*	*Level 3*
Educational requirements	No formal education necessary other than that for current state licensure	Baccalaureate degree in nursing	Master's degree in psychiatric nursing
Experience requirements	Minimum of 1 year experience in acute psychiatric nursing care	Minimum of 2 years experience in acute psychiatric care settings	Advanced knowledge and expertise in psychiatric care and principles of supervision and consultation
Nature of practice	Supportive treatment	Supportive treatment	Insight treatment
Therapeutic functions	1. Communicating with other professionals and agencies relative to patient care 2. Assisting in assessment and data collection 3. Assisting patients to use environmental resources 4. Assisting in community primary prevention programs	1. Primary responsibility for supportive therapy 2. Assessment of patient functioning 3. Initiation and attendance at conferences regarding her patients 4. Assignment to interdisciplinary teams responsible for delivery of primary mental health care in ambulatory units	1. Primary responsibility for insight-oriented psychotherapy 2. Responsibility for patients cared for by nurses in levels 1 and 2 of practice 3. Assessment of patient pathology 4. Supervision of other health team members 5. Participation in primary community prevention programs 6. Responsibility for obtaining supervision consultation 7. Responsible for assumption of nursing leadership

Source: From *Principles and practice of psychiatric nursing*, 2nd ed., by G.W. Stuart & S.J. Sundeen, 1983, p. 12. C.V. Mosby Co.; © 1983 by C.V. Mosby Co.; modified from K. Gardner *J. Psychiatr. Nurs. 1526*, Sept. 1977. Reprinted by permission.

care. . . . Implementation is the emphasis at the first-line level of nursing management. Such administrators direct and supervise nursing staff in provision of nursing care and assure the availability of support services which facilitate this care. The first-line nurse administrator serves as a resource to staff, interpreting philosophy, goals, standards, policies, and procedures. The nurse administrator at the first-level participates in varying degrees in policy formation and decision making with other members of nursing administration. These administrators are the vital link between nursing management and the staff that delivers care to the client. First-line administrators are responsible for delivering care that is therapeutically effective and safe as well as cost-effective. They accomplish this by effective utilization of resources through the administrative process. The scope of responsibility for the first-line administrator is usually the nursing unit.

Responsibilities of first-line administrative roles typically include: (1) Providing for direct nursing care services to clients. (2) Evaluating nursing care given and assuring appropriate documentation, guidance, and supervision of staff members . (3) Selecting nursing personnel for hire. (4) Evaluating staff, including disciplinary actions and separation from service. (5) Providing for teaching and staff development. (6) Coordinating nursing care with other health services. (7) Participating in and involving staff in nursing research. (8) Providing clinical facilities and learning experiences for students. (pp. 6–7)

Within psychiatric–mental health nursing, the head nurse is instrumental in ensuring that the predetermined level of quality care is provided to the client population. Through this position, management direction is provided that aids in the professional development of psychiatric–mental health nursing at the unit or service level.

ROLE OF LICENSED PRACTICAL NURSES

The licensed practical nurse (LPN) is another member of the health care team who may be included within a nursing department's staff. Many of this nurse's activities are dependent upon a state's Nurse Practice Act, which may define limits for the role. Generally, the LPN is responsible to the registered nurse who delegates identified activities. Most often, the LPN administers medications and provides direct client care under the supervision of a registered nurse. Limitations to this position include the inability legally to receive telephone orders, to assume charge positions, and to function in an independent fashion. In addition, schools for LPNs often do not include psychiatric nursing in their curricula and so their graduates frequently have no exposure to this specialty. The nurse administrator should consider the needs of the department and client population as well as the future goals and directions of the organization before incorporating an LPN as a member of the staff.

ROLE OF THE CLINICAL NURSE SPECIALIST

A role that often varies greatly among psychiatric–mental health settings is that of the clinical nurse specialist. A *clinical nurse specialist* is defined as

> a professional nurse who has completed a master's level program for specialization in a particular nursing area. In the process, . . . some theoretical background in sciences pertaining to that area [has been obtained], as well as cognitive and psychomotor skills required to practice nursing as an applied science. [The nurse] is able to identify and rationalize systematically the nursing needs of [clients], to make relatively precise professional judgements, to devise sophisticated nursing care plans and apply scientific knowledge in [client] care. While performing [client] care activities with a high degree of proficiency, the nurse specialist also acts as a behavioral model of expert clinical nursing and as a resource to others in the [client] unit including nurses, doctors, and students. [This nurse] can explain the rationale of the scientific approach to nursing practice to other nurses, [work with] doctors in planning for a [client], offer advice on [client] care problems, and [assist] other nurses with complex procedures and various aspects of practice. In addition, the specialist has some ability to evaluate the results of nursing research and translate research findings into nursing practice and may have the competence to conduct nursing studies designed to improve care in the [client] unit. (Colerick, Mason, & Proulx, 1980, p. 31)

Organizational Positions

The individual role of the psychiatric–mental health clinical nurse specialist varies from organization to organization and depends, to a great extent, upon organizational and departmental needs (White, 1976). Several issues have impact on the definition of this role. The clinical nurse specialist's position in the organization's chart must be identified (Norton, 1981). The "type of organizational position [the clinical nurse specialist] assumes is largely dependent on . . . personal self-image as a [clinical nurse specialist] and the philosophy of the [psychiatric–mental health] care facility" (Niessner, 1979, p. 28).

Staff Positions

Whether the role of the clinical nurse specialist has been identified as a staff or line role, each has its advantages and disadvantages. An advantage to the clinical nurse specialist being in a staff position is that it "frees the clinical specialist from administrative tasks" (Crabtree, 1979, p. 3) such as requiring the clinical nurse specialist to provide coverage during periods of low staffing. Supporters of this position believe that the clinical nurse specialist "derives authority from expert knowledge and clinical competency" (Crabtree, p. 3), and, therefore, does not need a line position to function with authority.

Disadvantages to this position include the clinical nurse specialist's reliance on the head nurse for implementation of clinical recommendations. If the relationship with the head nurse is strained, the clinical nurse specialist may find all such recommendations are thwarted or sabotaged. Should the clinical nurse specialist work with only a small caseload of clients, influence on the improvement of client care may be minimal and may not prove to be cost-effective. Additionally, a clinical nurse specialist in the staff position may be perceived by the staff as a threat. This threat may cause resistance, which requires much time and energy to resolve.

Drucker believes that a staff position requires persons who "(1) genuinely want others to get the credit, (2) start out with the aim of enabling others to do what they want to do, (3) have the patience to let others learn rather than go and do the work themselves, and (4) will not abuse their position to politic, manipulate and play favorites" (Crabtree, 1979, pp. 4–5). Should a clinical nurse specialist role appear to be incompatible with these attitudes, a line position should be considered. In addition, it must be recognized that the "turnover rate for staff personnel [is] two to four times as great as that for line personnel, particularly if the department has identified either a lack of potential candidates for the position or traditionally has difficulty filling positions due to environmental factors " (Crabtree, p. 5).

Line Positions

Line positions have a basic advantage: the "acquisition of formal authority and reward power" (Crabtree, 1979, p. 5). Through the use of this advantage, the clinical nurse specialist is able to implement programs and procedures that improve the quality of client care without relying totally on others. "The blending of clinical specialist–nursing manager roles into strong leadership positions is critical to the protection of professional nursing practice in institutional settings" (Wallace & Corey, 1983, p. 15). Disadvantages to this type of position may include frustrations due to time limitations for clinical involvement or a lack of administrative educational background. Finally, the clinical nurse specialist may find that the staff members are clinically guarded with a specialist who also functions as their supervisor (Crabtree).

Functional Authority Positions

Erickson has suggested the concept of a functional authority position, which would place the clinical nurse specialist "in a situation equivalent to that of a physician in terms of their rights to give, direct, and order nursing care for their [clients]" (Crabtree, 1979, p. 7). Within psychiatric–mental health nursing, this position would place the clinical nurse specialist in the role of the primary therapist, with physician collaboration for any client medications. This practice would increase the independent role of nursing within the organization but may also have the disadvantage of reducing the number of clients in contact with the clinical specialist. However, in outpatient settings, this role would be advantageous because the nurse could carry a specific caseload of clients.

General Responsibilities of the Role

A second issue to be considered in the role definition of the clinical nurse specialist is the list of responsibilities to be included (Norton, 1981). There must be sufficient time provided for the clinical nurse specialist to be able to realistically complete the required activities. A psychiatric–mental health clinical nurse specialist who is expected to be responsible for in-service as an aspect of staff development must be provided time for the planning, the presentation, and the evaluation of each program. Without this time, the activity cannot be accomplished.

A third issue is departmental needs (Norton, 1981). If the clinical setting includes numerous experienced staff nurses who function as primary nurses to select client caseloads, the clinical nurse specialist needs to provide clinical supervision to these nurses. Again, time and support must be incorporated into the position so that the needs of the clinical setting can be adequately addressed.

A support system must be provided for the clinical nurse specialist within a psychiatric–mental health setting. If the clinical nurse specialist is expected to function to improve the quality of client care through the review, revision, and updating of programs and procedures, the specialist must have the administrative support necessary to ensure the implementation of these changes. Without such support, the specialist must rely solely on persuasive powers over the staff, and these may not be sufficient to bring about the changes.

Finally, a decision must be made as to the number of clients who are to receive this specialized care. If the needs of the organization and the client population are for an additional primary therapist who carries a specific client caseload, the specialist's role is defined in one fashion. The possibility of staff resentment then occurring towards a nurse who, in their opinion, has too light a workload must be recognized (Everson, 1981). If the specialist is expected to have an impact on the quality of care provided to all clients within a system, the role must be constructed to provide for that span of impact.

Once the organization or department has been examined to assess the five areas described above, the major functions expected of the specialist within the department should be identified. Most generally, there are four basic functions defined as typical of the clinical nurse specialist: (1) direct client care, (2) education, (3) consultation (including clinical supervision), and (4) research. Additional functions mentioned in conjunction with the specialist include that of a role model and a change agent (Andrianos & Swain, 1979).

Implementation of the Role

Should the need be identified for a clinical nurse specialist within the psychiatric–mental health department, there may be difficulties in establishing this role as a result of questions about its cost-effectiveness. An unusual method for the introduction of this role is to hire a qualified clinical nurse specialist into an existing position that is currently vacant. Through the support of administrative nursing personnel, the specialist in this situation could demonstrate "justification for the [specialist] role through visible and documented achievements" (Morris & Schweiger, 1979, p. 70).

In situations in which the nurse-administrator prefers to document the need for the role before hiring the specialist, there are three basic phases of this role development that should be used: "role identification, role transition, and role confirmation" (Morris & Schweiger, 1979, p. 71). The need for the role and the position description applicable to the specific psychiatric–mental health setting should both be identified. Once a specialist is hired into the role, a period of transition occurs during which the specialist adapts to the organization. The role is thus further refined and delineated. Role confirmation involves the demonstration of the validity of the role through outcomes. For example, the quality of psychiatric–mental health nursing care may improve 25 percent during the initial year, or incidents involving medications may decrease 15 percent, with all other variables remaining the same.

In planning for the inclusion of the clinical nurse specialist within the organization, several critical questions arise, which, when answered, also facilitate the decision-making process.

> Was a need for a clinical specialist identified by staff nurses? How would the position of clinical specialist fit into the overall objectives of nursing service? Would [the specialist] have a staff or line position? Does [the] staff and rotation pattern realistically allow for increased clinical involvement? What behaviors have highest priority in your proficiency evaluation? What is the clinical specialist's interpretation of how she[/he] would function and how does this interpretation meet . . . specific needs? (Woodrow & Bell, 1971, p. 28)

The cost-effectiveness of the clinical nurse specialist can be demonstrated in a variety of ways. Three initial mechanisms of assessing cost-effectiveness include the assessment of the clinical effectiveness of the specialist, professional growth of the involved staff, or activities within the department which serve to facilitate the delivery of psychiatric–mental health nursing care (Blount, Burge, Crigler, Finkelmeier, & Sanborn, 1981). Examples may include documentation of the evaluation of the clinical competence of the specialist, the number of clients seen within a six-month period, and the resulting improvements in care. Assessment of the professionalism of the nursing staff before and after the inclusion of the specialist into the system would also provide data. The variety of activities in which the specialist was involved and the related outcomes would be assessed to determine the ratio of outcomes to cost savings. A major component of the psychiatric–mental health clinical nurse specialist's role is evaluation of the milieu. Through various activities—alone and in conjunction with staff—the specialist evaluates the short- and the long-term status of the milieu and initiates problem-resolution activities.

Liaison Role

Another role the psychiatric–mental health specialist may assume is that of a liaison within the general hospital. A general hospital, with or without psychiatric units, may use the psychiatric clinical nurse specialist as a support staff for both the patients and the nurses on nonpsychiatric units.

> The nurse has naturally evolved as the most appropriate health care professional to assume this liaison role because of the large number of nurses who provide direct [client] care in nonpsychiatric settings and require assistance in meeting the psychological needs of [clients] (Berarducci, Blandford, & Garant, 1979, p. 66). [While the role requirements may vary, the] responsibilities always include minimizing the amount of anxiety the [client] must tolerate during hospitalization and assisting the staff in dealing effectively with both [clients] with a mental disturbance who have been hospitalized with physical illness and those who find the experience of illness and hospitalization threatening to their usual style of coping with stress. (Berarducci et al., p. 67)

The basic areas of functioning include "consultant to the nursing staff, . . . crisis intervention, . . . teaching nursing staff, . . . liaison with [other departments and disciplines]" (Goldstein, 1979, pp. 34–37).

The psychiatric–mental health clinical nurse specialist has several advantages in providing nurse-to-nurse consultation: (1) understanding of the role of the nurse and the different stresses involved; (2) assessment of nursing strengths and deficiencies and support for professional development; (3) intraprofessional consultation which utilizes professional bonds; (4) availability for formal and informal contacts; (5) awareness of the norms of the system and use of this knowledge in considering alternative solutions to client care problems; and (6) costs of the role—lower than those that involve the use of outside sources (Fife & Lemler, 1983).

Once the nurse administrator in the general hospital has determined that it is desirable to hire a psychiatric–mental health clinical nurse specialist, several questions should be asked to assist in the initial planning before role implementation:

> (1) How much impact has the nursing department had in the system in terms of improving and insuring quality of [client] care? What are the current attitudes toward and understanding of emotional care needs not only within nursing but throughout the system? (2) What departments within the system are united by mutual goals and approaches to administrative and clinical problems? (3) Are there any traditions of territoriality within the system? Are there those who might block the implementation of a psychiatric liaison nurse? Is there acceptance of the philosophy of nurse-to-nurse consultation not only within the nursing department but throughout the system? (4) Have there been any previous attempts to implement the role? . . . Are there any remaining myths or expectations from these previous attempts that may hinder the present attempt to implement the role? (Barbiasz et al., 1982, p. 17)

Emergency Room Role

Another role that may be assumed by a psychiatric–mental health clinical nurse specialist is crisis intervention specialist in the emergency room. The "initial purpose of the position is usually to facilitate psychiatric service to the emergency room" (Andrianos & Swain, 1979, p. 24). In this role, the nursing specialist "provides psychiatric assessment and treatment . . . in the emergency room . . . , serves as a nurse consultant to nursing and medical personnel who carry out psychiatric and medical treatment, and provides screening and therapeutic dispositions for psychiatric [clients] in the emergency room" (Andrianos & Swain, pp. 24–25). To complete these functions, the clinical nurse specialist may also handle referral calls and contacts from the community and provide follow-up reports, participate in research projects, and supervise students (Andrianos & Swain). The specialist who functions in the emergency room does much to extend the ability of the nursing department to provide holistic care to all he organization's clients by directing attention to the emotional needs of each client.

ROLE OF ANCILLARY STAFF

Another role issue is "the dominance of the untrained or poorly educated service personnel [providing] care for the mentally ill" (Sills, 1973, p. 126). Many departments have psychiatric assistants who were hired 10, 15, or 20 years ago when custodial care was the norm rather than the exception. Today the prevalence of a modified version of this role, that of the mental health technician, is increasing. This person often has college preparation in the mental health field, frequently with a completed associate degree as a mental health technician.

Several issues must be examined in terms of this group of personnel in view of nursing's belief in the "inseparable relationship between the quality of practice and the quality of education" (ANA, 1979, p. 3). If the care given is primarily custodial, the psychiatric assistant may function satisfactorily. If the care is noncustodial, regardless of the type of therapeutic treatment program in place, a person with additional mental health or nursing education is needed to provide basic support services to nursing. It should be determined whether the care can be provided by nurses with a variety of educational backgrounds rather than by ancillary staff. Many departments, because of organizational factors or union constraints, are unable to establish this staffing pattern and must continue to use some type of ancillary personnel. Hence, there is need to consider the educational background required for this support position.

If the current department uses the psychiatric assistant, the care provided must be assessed to determine if it is of the quality required by the department and the organization. If it is, there may not be a need for change. However, if the care provided is found to be more custodial than therapeutic, consideration should be given as to whether a change would improve the care given and would be cost-effective over a period of time. Such a change would, naturally, initially prove to be costly. As this cost could be recovered in a variety of ways over a period of time, the change process could be justified. As is true in any change process, substantial research and planning must be undertaken to ensure the success of the change and to accomplish it in a fashion that fosters the dignity of staff and clients.

Should the department determine that this group of ancillary staff is necessary for the provision of quality psychiatric–mental health nursing care, the job descriptions should also be behaviorally based and should lend themselves to the evaluation process. Educational offerings should be provided to aid this group in further enhancing their clinical skills. Furthermore, the expectations of the department for the growth of this group should be consistent with those for other groups of staff providing direct care to clients.

ROLE OF VOLUNTEERS

Many psychiatric–mental health settings use volunteers in a variety of roles in order to improve the quality of care provided by the organization. When volunteers are used in any manner, the same provisions must exist as do for paid staff. Volunteers should be screened just as prospective staff are screened. This screening will provide volunteers with appropriate skills to deliver the identified services. Behaviorally-based position descriptions provide guidelines for the volunteer. A regular evaluation process provides both the volunteer and the organization with an updated appraisal of the volunteer's ability to meet the needs of clients. Continuing education offerings should be open to volunteers with the expectation that they must participate in a predetermined amount of education in order to continue their volunteer work with the psychiatric–mental health client population.

Though volunteers are not paid for their efforts, they can experience stress similar to that of the employed staff. The department must examine the need for a reward and support system that would foster the growth of those volunteers who regularly participate in the program. This reward may be as simple as free attendance at all educational offerings presented by the department and organization, or inclusion in the organization's recreational activities (softball team, etc.). Or, some type of acknowledgment may be offered to exceptional volunteers in order to assist them in maintaining their enthusiasm or, possibly, to prepare them to be eligible for hire in established positions. As in any program within the department, responsible staff from within and outside the department should identify the benefits and the difficulties of a volunteer system. The staff should work with the individual responsible for volunteer services to develop an orientation and evaluation program format that meets the needs of both the organization and the volunteers.

IMPLEMENTING IDENTIFIED ROLES

In implementing new roles or reviewing the effectiveness of current roles, the nursing administrator needs to be assisted by selected staff, for it is difficult to be aware of and to assess all implications that may arise from an individual staff's interpretation of a role. Implementation of new roles follows a process similar to the implementation of a new program. Orientation for those involved, proper documentation, continual evaluation, and an effective communication system enable the transition, though requiring time and energy, to proceed as smoothly as possible.

Within psychiatric–mental health nursing, the impact of designated roles on the treatment modalities used within the organization and on future plans of the department should be considered. Treatment modalities such as team or primary nursing, group therapy, behavior modification, and so on, require the existence of certain educationally prepared staff. Should these staff members not be present within the department, the department may be unable to grow towards a more professional environment. For example, if the department plans to institute a primary nursing pattern of assignment, but does not have sufficient appropriately prepared nurses on staff, the desired assignment pattern will need to be modified or postponed until sufficient staff can be hired. The organization may determine that nurses may participate as co-therapists in a variety of groups, but the staff may be unprepared to assume these roles. The department would then be unable to respond to clinical changes within the organization.

The goals and objectives of the department and organization must also be considered when implementation of roles occurs. If there are objectives that require certain levels of expertise for their achievement, but the staff with these levels of expertise are not available, the objectives or goals will not be met. For example, if the department is committed to a plan of patient education, staff must be available with the expertise, the experience, and the education necessary to plan, organize, implement, and evaluate such a system. Should the staff be ill-prepared in this area, the objective cannot be met now, nor in the near future. Such a problem could, ultimately, affect the future growth of the department or organization and could encourage stagnation rather than progression.

EVALUATING ROLES

Evaluation of roles should occur on an annual basis and should include not only the individual role's impact on the system, but also the system's impact on the role. For example, a clinical nurse specialist may be able to improve the quality of client care substantially but may be faced with outdated organizational impediments. This review can easily be made part of the annual review process, or a protocol can be established to evaluate roles on a more frequent or ongoing basis. Naturally, those persons functioning in the roles should be included in the review process in order to assess the current practices realistically. During this process, roles may be identified that will be needed in the future for the continued growth of the department and continued improvement of client care. The decision can then be made either to plan for the evolution of current roles to meet future needs or to determine that completely new roles are needed. Then, the process to establish the needed roles can be started. Results of any evaluative processes naturally become part of the feedback process of the department and are incorporated into future planning efforts so that the department is future-oriented rather than crisis- or survival-oriented. As psychiatric–mental health nursing continues to develop and grow in its knowledge base, job descriptions and related evaluations will need periodic revision for adequate portrayal of current clinical behaviors. Thus, the stage is set for future clinical improvements.

REFERENCES

American Nurses' Association. (1979). *A case for baccalaureate preparation in nursing.* (NE-6). Kansas City, Mo.: Commission on Nursing Education.

American Nurses' Association. (1978). *Roles, responsibilities and qualifications for nurse administrators.* (NS-23). Kansas City, Mo.: Commission on Nursing Services.

Andrianos, A.F., & Swain, C.R. (1979). Interfacing the role of a psychiatric clinical nurse specialist with a hospital emergency room setting. *Journal of Psychiatric Nursing and Mental Health Services, 17*(4), 24–27.

Barbiasz, J., Blandford, K., Byrne, K., Horvath, K., Levy, J., Lewis, A., Matarazzo, S.P., O'Meara, K., Palmateer, L., & Rossier, M. (1982). Establishing the psychiatric liaison nurse role: Collaboration with the nurse administrator. *The Journal of Nursing Administration, 12*(2), 15–18.

Benfer, B.A. (1980). Defining the role and function of the psychiatric nurse as a member of the team. *Perspectives in Psychiatric Care, 18,* 166–177.

Berarducci, M., Blandford, K., & Garant, C.A. (1979). The psychiatric liaison nurse in the general hospital. *General Hospital Psychiatry, 6*(1), 66–72.

Blount, M., Burge, S., Crigler, L., Finkelmeier, B.A., & Sanborn, C. (1981). Extending the influence of the clinical nurse specialist. *Nursing Administration Quarterly, 6,* 53–63.

Colerick, E.J., Mason, P.B., & Proulx, J.R. (1980). Evaluation of the clinical nurse specialist role: Development and implementation of a dual purpose framework. *Nursing Leadership, 3*(3), 26–34.

Crabtree, M.S. (1979). Effective utilization of clinical specialists within the organizational structure of hospital nursing service. *Nursing Administration Quarterly, 4*(1), 1–11.

Everson, S.J. (1981). Integration of the role of clinical nurse specialist. *The Journal of Continuing Education in Nursing, 12*(2), 16–19.

Fife, B., & Lemler, S. (1983). The psychiatric nurse specialist: A valuable asset in the general hospital. *The Journal of Nursing Administration, 13*(4), 14–17.

Goldstein, S. (1979). The psychiatric clinical specialist in the general hospital. *The Journal of Nursing Administration, 9*(3), 34–37.

Jacobs, A.M. (1980). Clinical competencies of baccalaureate, A.D. and diploma nurses—Are they different? *Issues: National Council of State Boards of Nursing, Inc., 1*(4), 1–3, 6.

McGriff, E.P. (1980). If not the 1985 resolution, then what? An alternative proposal. *Nursing Outlook, 28*(6), 365.

Morris, K.H., & Schweiger, J.A. (1979). Clinical nurse specialist role creation: An achievable goal. *Nursing Administration Quarterly, 4*(1), 67–78.

Niessner, P. (1979). The clinical specialist's contribution to quality nursing care. *Nursing Leadership, 2*(1), 21–30.

Norton, L.C. (1981). The clinical nurse specialist as consultant. *Nursing Administration Quarterly, 6*(1), 69–75.

Peplau, H. (1978). Psychiatric nursing: Role of nurses and psychiatric nurses. *International Nursing Review, 25*(2), 41–47.

Sills, G.M. (1973). Historical developments and issues in psychiatric mental health nursing. In M. Lieninger (Ed.), *Contemporary issues in mental health nursing.* Boston: Little, Brown & Co., 125–136.

Stuart, G.W., & Sundeen, S.J. (1983). *Principles and practice of psychiatric nursing* 2nd ed. St. Louis: The C.V. Mosby Co.

Tousley, M.M. (1982). Certification as a credential: What are the issues? *Perspectives in Psychiatric Care, 20*(1), 23–26.

Wallace, M.A., & Corey, L.J. (1983). The clinical specialist as manager: Myth versus realities. *The Journal of Nursing Administration, 13*(6), 13–15.

White, E.A. (1976). The clinical specialist on the mental health team. *Journal of Psychiatric Nursing and Mental Health Services, 14*(11), 7–12.

Woodrow, M. & Bell, J.A. (1971). Clinical specialization: Conflict between reality and theory. *Journal of Nursing Administration, 1*(11), 23–28.

Chapter 10

Orientation in Psychiatric–Mental Health Nursing

An orientation program for psychiatric–mental health nursing differs from orientation programs for other nursing areas. In 1952, the three functions of the psychiatric–mental health nurse were identified as (1) facilitating client communication, (2) facilitating the client's social interactions, and (3) the fulfilling of client needs (Finkelman, 1980). Although the current focus of psychiatric–mental health nursing care may differ slightly from these statements, these premises are still valid and illuminate the major differences of that nursing area from other nursing areas. These three functions, which assist the clients to regain or to reaffirm their mental health, are abstractions; however, no specific concrete tasks, when performed, can better assist the client. Communication and interpersonal skills can certainly be learned. Nevertheless, when the major tool available to the psychiatric–mental health nurse is the nurse's own ability to use communication skills, everyone does not provide care or complete an interaction in the exact same manner—unlike the expectation when hospital equipment is used or physical care procedures are performed. Therefore, concepts, programs, and plans cannot be transferred from other areas or organizations with the assumption that they will work within a psychiatric–mental health setting. The objectives and general goals of the orientation program may be similar to or, in some instances, the same as those of other nursing areas, but the intent and the focus differ greatly.

As a result of the abstract interpersonal nature of many of the therapeutic interventions of the psychiatric–mental health nurse, the issue of supervision becomes more complex and less easily observed. For example, when catheterizing a client, a newly employed nurse could easily be supervised by a more experienced nurse without causing the client undue anxiety. However, when conducting a one-to-one interaction with a psychiatric–mental health client, the presence of a supervisor might cause nontherapeutic stress to the client, and so it would be contraindicated. Hence, other techniques or arrangements must be made to accommodate this aspect of psychiatric–mental health nursing orientation.

The types of clients seen in psychiatric–mental health organizations also differ substantially from those seen in other nursing areas. These clients usually are in treatment for longer consecutive periods, and are able to develop a therapeutic working relationship with the nurse. In other nursing areas, however, because of the shorter length of treatment, the nurse is not always able to use the nurse-client relationship to assist the physical nursing treatments that occur. Psychiatric clients, because of the depressive nature of many of their illnesses, may also present a suicide potential that is usually absent from clients in other areas of nursing. Any rapid decline in the health of clients outside the psychiatric–mental health nursing practice is usually due to physical causes that are beyond their control. By contrast, death by suicide is very much within the control of the client and, therefore, much more difficult to avert.

Associated with this concept is the use of physical intervention techniques. In addition to being used to protect the client from self-harm, these techniques or strategies are often utilized to protect other clients or the physical surroundings from the agitated client. These techniques may also be present, or needed occasionally in other nursing areas, but not to the extent or the frequency required within psychiatric–mental health nursing. Hence, these strategies must be taught and reviewed with the same frequency as other emergency procedures, such as CPR.

Finally, the orientation coordinator must assess the experiential background of the newly employed nurse. Often, this person has had minimal or no psychiatric–mental health experience. In other areas of nursing, a newly employed person often has had some experience in a related nursing area that can be used during the initial employment phase to ease the transition. As a result of this lack of psychiatric–mental health experience, an orientation program for psychiatric–mental health nursing must provide the acquisition of the basic psychiatric–mental health skills needed by the beginning staff nurse.

Related to this lack of experience are the existing, preconceived ideas that each new nurse brings to the psychiatric–mental health organization. These preconceptions are the result of societal and organizational stereotypes of those persons who experience mental or emotional problems as well as those who treat them within the health care system. These stereotypes must be brought into the open, discussed, and examined in terms of their potential impediment to the individual nurse's success in assisting psychiatric–mental health clients to regain a healthy level of coping with their environment.

ASSESSING INDIVIDUAL LEARNING NEEDS

Based upon the above considerations, the person responsible for planning and coordinating the orientation program for newly employed nurses within a psychiatric–mental health organization must ensure that the resulting program meets the individual needs of the nurses in a fashion that fosters the development of the skills and the abilities needed by a beginning staff nurse. To do this is not an easy project. One strategy is the presentation of the required educational material in learning modules based on progressive educational levels. As certain skills or abilities are mastered, the nurse proceeds to the next module or level. When all modules or levels are completed, the nurse is then ready to assume the full duties and responsibilities of a beginning staff nurse.

Whatever format is finally employed to provide an orientation program, the process must begin with an assessment of the learning needs that must be met through the orientation program. The basis for this assessment must be the philosophy and the behavioral objectives of the orientation program. There should also be an overall plan that can be adjusted and individualized for each new nurse's learning needs. Hence, each new nurse's learning needs, competencies, and learning styles must be assessed, and the overall orientation program must be adjusted for the individual participant.

Identification of such individual learning needs is facilitated by a clear definition of desired competencies. These competencies would be delineated within the behaviorally based documents that provide the foundation for the orientation program. A technique for facilitating this process involves a skill and competency check list (see Appendix 10-A) in which the nurse completes a self-assessment of essential clinical skills and indicates areas or techniques in which learning is needed.

The nurse's self-assessment can be further validated by demonstration or testing in which the nurse demonstrates competence in any questionable areas. The person conducting the orientation must recognize that the nurse's level of confidence may interfere with the accurate self-assessment of skills or competencies (Moran, 1980) and so must allow for such inaccuracies. Studies have indicated that such testing is beneficial in corroborating the nurse's assessment (Kaelin & Bliss, 1979).

For the skills that must be learned, a skills laboratory can be made available in which the nurse can learn through review of self-teaching modules (Kaelin & Bliss, 1979). The nurse can then be evaluated through relevant return demonstrations and role playing. Such verification of knowledge and the learning of basic skills can be accomplished during the first week. When oriented on the nursing unit, the nurse can practice more confidently.

An additional tool that often proves useful is a check list for the nurse's orientation to the nursing unit or service. This tool lists all the priority items and the locations of elements necessary for the nurse to practice efficiently. Through use of this tool, both the orientation coordinator and the participant know what has been reviewed and what still needs to be discussed. The check list would also ensure that all nurses receive the same information when they are oriented.

PLANNING THE ORIENTATION PROGRAM

Personnel and Objectives

Once the assessment of the new nurse has been completed, the nurse begins the orientation process. In developing a program, the psychiatric–mental health nursing administration and all levels of nursing personnel need to be included in the planning stage. As in the case of all other areas of nursing, this early involvement provides knowledge and some degree of control for those personnel who are in contact with the persons receiving orientation. This awareness and control of the orientation process enables these persons to assist the participants more efficiently (del Bueno, Barker, & Christmyer, 1981).

The planners must focus their attention on the desired outcomes of the program or the "achievement of performance expectations" (del Bueno et al., 1981, p. 25). These expectations would be delineated by previously defined and desired competencies and by behaviorally based job descriptions (Moran, 1980). A program that is flexible in content and time and that expects the new nurse to be a self-directed learner uses the orientation coordinator as a facilitator or resource person for the new nurse's learning, rather than as a teacher or a supervisor. The nurse-learner also needs to set behavioral objectives and goals for the orientation period, which would be jointly evaluated by the nurse and the resource person (Borovies & Newman, 1981) throughout the orientation program. This system respects and encourages the self-confident professional to work interdependently with others to progress in the ability to provide quality care.

Content, Methodology, and Criteria

Once the initial planning committee has been established and agreement has been achieved on the program's philosophy and objectives, its content must be identified. The basic content of any orientation program should include the following (Rowland & Rowland, 1980):

- a tour of the organization
- the mission, philosophy, goals, objectives, and standards of the organization and the nursing department
- the structure of the overall organization and the psychiatric–mental health nursing department
- the administrative and departmental policies and procedures
- the personnel policies and procedures
- a discussion of the relationship of the organization to the health care community

- a discussion of interdepartmental and interdisciplinary relationships
- a discussion of nursing personnel categories and job descriptions

(See Appendix 10-B for the orientation of paraprofessionals.) During the planning phase, the presentors and the order of the presentation of the content must also be identified.

The committee must then develop a methodology for meeting the individual differences in the learning needs and styles of each new nurse. This is not to say that there must be a limitless number of programs, but the overall program must allow for the flexible completion of the content.

Finally, the committee must identify criteria for the satisfactory completion of the orientation program (Schroeder, Cantor, & Kurth, 1981). The criteria must be sufficiently general to apply to all units or services, but they must also be specific enough to fit the needs of the individual area. These criteria also must be behaviorally described to provide a means by which all involved (the participants and the coordinator) evaluate the orientation process through the same mechanism.

Throughout the orientation program, the environment should be one that provides a safe outlet for the participants to voice their concerns. Such verbalization clears rumors, decreases anxiety, and aids in the creation of a practice environment in which a nurse feels sufficiently safe to provide quality care creatively. During discussions, nurses are reminded to set realistic goals and expectations for their practice. Unrealistic goals and expectations create unnecessary stress and anxiety that can serve only to hinder the adjustment process (Meisenhelder, 1981). By providing realistic feedback to nurses throughout the orientation process, the orientation coordinator can facilitate a nurse's ability to set realistic goals for self and clients that reflect the capability and the constraints of the organization.

Furthermore, the new nurse must not be counted as a fully practicing staff member until the orientation program is completed. To do so would create a stressful environment that could only serve to hinder the transition of the new nurse into the organization. This hindrance could prolong the time needed for orientation as well as spark a feeling of dissatisfaction, which could result in the nurse prematurely terminating employment.

Newly Graduated Nurses

If the newly employed nurse is also a new graduate, additional issues need to be reviewed and incorporated into the orientation plan. "A generalized orientation program is [usually] not intensive enough to adequately develop [the] new graduate's proficiency in clinical skills and individual functions" (Borovies & Newman, 1981, p. 1832). Schroeder et al. (1981) add, "Many new graduates lack the ability to identify significant nursing care problems, determine appropriate [interventions] and modify care in terms of evaluation of patient conditions" (p. 16). The content of an orientation program should, therefore, include a plan for learning basic skills and a review of the theoretical knowledge required to provide safe quality care (Meisenhelder, 1981). A flexible orientation program that could be adjusted to the individual nurse would address both these needs and the learning needs presented by other newly employed nurses.

The newly graduated nurse has the additional task of attempting to make the transition from an educational environment, with its related values and mores, to the work environment, which often has diametrically opposed values and norms. The new graduate must frequently refocus from the whole-task system that was taught in school to the part-task system of the work place (Kramer & Schmalenberg, 1978). When this transition period is not recognized or is not aided by the organization's orientation program, the new graduate faces additional, unnecessary stress and anxiety that may cause the organization to lose that nurse ultimately through voluntary termination of employment.

The new graduate's integration of this new role and related expectations depends upon such internal factors as the level of preparation and personal characteristics—e.g., self-confidence and self-esteem (Meisenhelder, 1981). The new nurse's self-esteem is particularly important inasmuch as there is a correlation between high self-esteem and a positive work outcome. This concept is based on the existence of three types of self-esteem—chronic, task-specific, and socially influenced—all of which have an impact on the nurse's ability to experience a positive work outcome.

The new graduate frequently feels that adjustment to the work environment is a case of "sink or swim." Feelings exist that a lack of clinical experience may leave the nurse unable to organize and to delegate responsibilities as expected. This insecurity is further compounded by a lack of clarity about the roles, the authority, and the responsibilities of other team members (Borovies & Newman, 1981). Furthermore, in psychiatric–mental health nursing, many role boundaries are frequently unclear. When this ambiguity is compounded by the abstract nature of psychiatric–mental health nursing, the practice environment must seem unclear and confusing to the new graduate. Through a thoughtful, individualized orientation program that recognizes the abstract nature of the psychiatric–mental health practice environment, a new nurse's task-specific and socially influenced self-esteem can be maintained and improved (Friesen & Conahan, 1980).

IMPLEMENTING THE PROGRAM

Phases of Orientation

The process through which a new nurse progresses during the psychiatric–mental health orientation program is fairly predictable and must be considered when one is implementing orientation programs. On the first day, the new nurse anticipates the upcoming experiences but also fears the unknown. This ambivalence should be considered when one is planning the first day activities. The new nurse enters an orientation and "honeymoon" phase which usually lasts from two to four weeks. During this time, the nurse requires frequent free periods to review and to process materials and role expectations. If the nurse is filling a position that has been recently vacated, the previous nurse's behavior and practice expectations are still remembered by the staff and can be compared with those of the new nurse—often, to the detriment of the new nurse.

The third phase of adjustment to a new position can be entitled "proving oneself" (Hanson, 1976, p. 24). During this period of from one to three months, the new nurse begins to identify with certain persons within the organization. The new nurse is learning role expectations and is beginning to act appropriately. Resources and sources of power have also been identified by this time.

A period of creativity and contribution then occurs, which lasts up to six months. During this time, the new nurse is relatively free from anxiety and is feeling comfortable with the new position. The nurse is now able to make constructive suggestions about current nursing practice and should be considered for appointment to nursing committees.

The final stage lasts as long as the nurse remains in the position. The nurse is now functioning within the expected role and has completed the role integration process (Hanson, 1976).

Selected Orientation Program Formats

In order to further a nurse's adjustment to a new psychiatric–mental health organization, an internship or preceptor program may be implemented as a part of the orientation process. Through these programs, the new nurse can more easily adapt to a new position by using the specific support personnel designated to aid in the transition.

Role Transition Program

In order to meet the individualized needs of the newly graduated nurse, a series of meetings that deal with reality shock or role transition and new role integration can be incorporated into orientation programs. Such a program might be composed of three parts: (1) a series of six seminars that enable these nurses to share feelings and concerns about their ongoing experiences, (2) five program modules based on the *Path to Biculturalism,* and (3) conflict resolution workshops. During the completion of the content, the program should also provide for the integration of the new nurse into the organization's social group—a crucial step toward the nurse's successful integration into the new role (Hollefreund, Mlack, Moore, & Jersan, 1981).

The six seminars might focus on the following topics:

1. getting acquainted with each other, and the purpose and outline of this portion of the orientation program,
2. a discussion of reality shock,
3. a comparison of current nursing actions with professional nursing goals,
4. recognizing the various types of feedback that exist and can be used, and
5. identifying value systems of other persons in order to be able to identify potential conflict areas. (Hollefrcund ct al., 1981)

The five program modules would assist the nurses in dealing with the feelings and experiences encountered in their attempts to translate school values into the work situation. The conflict resolution workshops further aid the nurses in the active resolution of conflicts that exist as a result of the nurses' inability to resolve transition issues (Hollefreund et al., 1981).

In this program, new graduates are expected to keep diaries of their feelings and concerns in order to increase their awareness during this transition period. This type of activity is particularly useful in psychiatric–mental health nursing because increasing the nurse's self-awareness is important for the provision of therapeutic care. The information in these diaries not only assists nurses in their participation in the discussion groups; it also facilitates their realization that they are not experiencing these concerns alone—that these concerns are normal during this transition phase. It is the combination of diary sharing and reality shock rap sessions that contributes to the positive psychosocial adaptation of the new graduate (Borovies & Newman, 1981).

By assisting these newly graduated nurses to make the transition from a school environment to a work environment, the organization recognizes that this adjustment phase, if properly handled, can facilitate personal growth. These techniques should also enable the organization to provide the type of professional environment that aids in the retention of nurses.

After the completion of this type of orientation format, the psychiatric–mental health nurse manager of the unit or service should continue to monitor the new nurse closely in order to identify difficulties quickly. By responding to potential difficulties early, the nurse manager can do much to facilitate the nurse's adjustment to the new position (Charron, 1982).

Internship Program

An *internship program* may be defined as a "semi-structured supervised orientation aimed at facilitating the transition from student to staff" (Roell, 1981, p. 29), or from a nurse with no experience in psychiatric–mental health nursing to a practicing staff nurse. This format differs from a general orientation in its "increased presentations of frequently encountered clinical situations" by which new nurses are enabled to identify themselves as working with staff mentors rather than as quasi-students (Chagares, 1980, p. 22).

As in any well-developed orientation program, the nurse's learning needs are identified by self-assessment and verbal clarification. The formally structured classroom component of this program, tailored to the specific orientation, often includes such topics as technical skills, leadership, application of problem-solving or nursing process concepts, philosophy of the organization and department, and special treatment issues (such as milieu management). These nurses are also placed in specific clinical areas for an extended period of time. The nurses are also encouraged to keep a diary of their feelings and concerns (Coco, 1976) and, in a weekly conference with those supervising them, to discuss their progress and the program in general. They also receive periodic evaluations during this process in order to focus their learning experiences. The program may last from 6 weeks to 1 year, the average length being 13 weeks. During this orientation program, the new nurse usually receives less than a full salary. (See Exhibits 10–1 and 10–2.)

The benefits of this type of orientation program have been thoroughly documented. Three recipients benefit from the program: the new nurse, the supervising nurse and related staff, and the organization. The new nurse demonstrates and reports increased confidence and overall job satisfaction, a professional role conception, a sense of security and knowledge about work realities, and a demonstrated improvement in leadership ability (Roell, 1981).

Exhibit 10–1 Internship Program Objectives in Psychiatric–Mental Health Nursing

Each nurse intern will meet the following objectives by the end of the internship program:

1. Identify . . . [the] role in the therapeutic milieu by demonstrating the ability to plan care, initiate care, and evaluate care in the milieu.
2. Identify . . . [the] role in the nurse-patient relationship by establishing a relationship with two patients for six months. Process recordings will be written and discussed with a supervisor.
3. Demonstrate the ability to incorporate general patient care needs, such as nutrition, hygiene, exercise, elimination, and sleep into care planning.
4. Demonstrate the ability to perform the administrative aspects of patient care.
5. Develop skills as a group leader, which will be determined by the ability to conduct a patient group for one month.
6. Demonstrate the ability to be a primary nurse for a variety of patients.
7. Demonstrate the ability to utilize the nursing process in meeting patients' discharge needs by developing three discharge plans.

Source: From *Staff development for the psychiatric nurse* (pp. 60–61) by A.W. Finkelman, 1980, Thorofare, N.J.: Charles B. Slack, Inc. © 1980 by Clarles B. Slack, Inc. Reprinted by permission.

Exhibit 10–2 Internship Program Content in Psychiatric–Mental Health Nursing

At the beginning of the program, each nurse intern would also identify . . . objectives which she[he] plans to complete by the end of the program. As each new graduate comes to the program with different skills and needs, this will allow for more individuality.

Essential content for a psychiatric nurse internship program is as follows:

1. Standards for psychiatric–mental health nursing;
2. The nurse-patient relationship;
3. Nurse's role with families;
4. Nurse's role as a group leader;
5. General patient care;
6. Nurse's role in the therapeutic milieu;
7. Utilization of the nursing process;
8. Discharge planning;
9. Psychopharmacology and administration of medications;
10. Problem oriented medical record;
11. Essential aspects of report and rounds;
12. Communication;
13. Somatic therapies;
14. Care of the assaultive patient;
15. Care of the suicidal patient;
16. Diagnostic categories and relevant nursing care;
17. Administrative aspects of patient care; and
18. Primary nursing care.

Source: From *Staff development for the psychiatric nurse* (pp. 61–62) by A.W. Finkelman, 1980, Thorofare, N.J.: Charles B. Slack, Inc. © 1980 by Clarles B. Slack, Inc. Reprinted by permission.

The supervising nurses benefit from the recognition resulting from being a part of the program and from developing expertise by writing a formal evaluation of a peer (Chagares, 1980). As a result of their peripheral involvement in the program, the other staff members also begin to display an increased interest in the concept of continuing education.

The organization benefits from the increased sense of openness that occurs between the staff and the new nurses and from the associated decrease in related destructive criticisms. The organization further benefits from an increasingly stable staff, improved recruitment and retention, and a decrease in turnover (Roell, 1981).

Preceptorships

In contrast, a preceptor or mentor type of orientation program is a "planned one to one pairing of a [new] nurse with a carefully chosen staff nurse in a clinical setting'' (Friesen & Conahan, 1980, p. 20). This program format assigns clients to this team of two nurses. With this technique, the program becomes cost-effective because the clients are given better quality care when the "experience of the more capable nurse [is] extended" (Atwood, 1979, p. 716). Inasmuch as newly employed nurses are initially action-oriented (Friesen & Conahan), this format allows them to be actively involved in client care within an environment that facilitates their adjustment and learning. Through this team, the mentor and the new nurse develop a unique professional relationship that assists the new nurse to learn routines, to sense the political climate, and to become a partner in decision making (Atwood). Scheduling of both nurses is done for the new nurse's growth and includes weekend, afternoon, and midnight shifts as applicable.

The staff nurses who are chosen to be preceptors are carefully screened. Usually, they are appointed on a voluntary basis by the appropriate head nurse. They are usually "senior staff who [have] demonstrated both attitudes and behaviors consistent with professional nursing practice and clinical competence" in psychiatric–mental health nursing (May, 1980, p. 1824). Their competence should be based upon their use of theoretical knowledge and should be shown through active participation in health team activities. The prospective preceptor should also demonstrate leadership abilities, communication skills, interest in professional growth, constructive resolution of professional or bureaucratic conflicts, and a willingness to work with (and to provide feedback for) new graduates. The preceptor must be one who can ''perceive and interpret accurately the values of work and school'' (Friesen & Conahan, 1980, p. 20).

In return for volunteering as preceptors, nurses are provided with an opportunity for professional growth and development, and experience in peer review (Friesen & Conahan, 1980). They are formally recognized and promoted as being clinically competent at the staff nurse level. Responsible for their individual practice, they are seen as improving the profession as a whole through collegial sharing of knowledge and ideas (May, 1980). If possible, these nurses should also receive tangible rewards for their efforts. These rewards may include such items as improved salary scales or additional conference days (Lee & Raleigh, 1983). It is imperative that suitable recognition be given to preceptors inasmuch as this recognition ''directly reflects the value [the organization's] place[s] on nursing and on excellence in clinical practice and clinical teaching'' (Turnbull, 1983, p. 12). If the department is viewed as not valuing the preceptor's efforts through such recognition, fewer qualified staff members will volunteer for such positions.

Preceptor responsibilities include planning, teaching, role modeling, and the evaluation of their assigned nurse (Friesen & Conahan, 1980). They coach, inspire, and support the new nurse during the difficult transition phase (Atwood, 1979), and facilitate the new nurse's acquisition and practice of teaching and behavioral skills (Friesen & Conahan). The preceptor is encouraged, of course, to call on others as resources because no one is expected to have all the answers.

Through this mechanism, the preceptor demonstrates the support a staff nurse can expect from nursing resource personnel (May, 1980).

In order to educate and to support these nurse-preceptors, each nurse selected to be a preceptor completes a preceptor development program. This program includes a review of principles of teaching and adult-learning theory (May, 1980). During the program, these nurses recall their own orientations and the incidents that facilitated or interfered with their learning. Levels of anxiety are reviewed, including assessment and intervention techniques. Other topics covered include values clarification, cognitive and affective empathy, empathy versus sympathy, and role-play techniques (May). Through completion of this program, the nurses are better prepared to assist the new nurses during their orientation program.

The new-nurse preceptor program usually lasts six months, during which the new nurse gradually assumes more responsibility for client care. Ongoing weekly discussions between the preceptor-mentor and the orientation faculty assist each in adjusting the program to keep pace with the new nurse's progress (Friesen & Conahan, 1980). For example, during the first two weeks, the two nurses work as one staff with an assignment of a group of clients. At this time, the new nurse is introduced to other staff members and begins incorporation into the social group. After these two weeks, the new nurse assumes a more independent practice role, but is still a team with the preceptor-mentor. Both nurses keep logs or diaries to facilitate the assessment and evaluation of the orientation process.

Evaluation conferences are held at predetermined times throughout the orientation, as well as at the end, to provide the new nurse with prompt realistic progress reports. Such evaluations are both verbal and written, and incorporate feedback from the head nurse of the assigned area or service (Friesen & Conahan, 1980).

Promotion Adjustment

When a psychiatric–mental health nurse is promoted, there may or may not be an orientation to the new position; however, there will be an adjustment phase similar to that experienced by the new graduate (Darling & McGrath, April, 1983). Whether this transition process is equally as difficult for the newly promoted psychiatric–mental health nurse (as for the new graduate) depends upon "the extent to which the change . . . is experienced as cutting important social and professional ties; is accompanied with decreased need gratification, and results in feelings of isolation and lack of support" (Darling & McGrath, p. 29). In addition, the newly promoted nurse also experiences an emotional transitional process similar to that of a new graduate upon moving from "uninformed optimism [to] . . . rewarding completion" (Darling & McGrath, p. 29) feelings concerning the new position. An orientation format should be established that facilitates the transition for these nurses (Darling & McGrath, Sept., 1983). The provision of a program that supports and guides newly promoted psychiatric–mental health nurses facilitates their adjustment to their new position and increases the department's retention rate for these nurses.

EVALUATING THE PROGRAM

The evaluation process for a psychiatric–mental health nursing orientation program is similar to the evaluation of other departmental programs. On an annual basis, the content should be reviewed to determine its consistency with the department's orientation philosophy and objectives. Should discrepancies be found, modifications must be made to improve the internal consistency of the program.

In addition, any evaluative review should include feedback from both the nurses who were oriented and those who did the orienting. Through this analysis, deficits and weaknesses can be strengthened and strengths can be maintained. This type of information is particularly crucial inasmuch as it results from the first-hand experience of those for whom the program was designed. The incorporation of these nurses' opinions demonstrates that all staff members are considered important for the success of the department and that their input is valued.

REFERENCES

Atwood, A.H. (1979). The mentor in clinical practice. *Nursing Outlook 27*, 714–717.

Borovies, D.L. & Newman, N.A. (1981). Graduate nurse transition program. *American Journal of Nursing, 81*(10), 1832–1835.

Chagares, R.I. (1980). The nurse internship question revisited. *Supervisor Nurse, 11*(11), 22–24.

Charron, D.C. (1982). Save the new graduate. *Journal of Nursing Management, 13*(11), 45–46.

Coco, C.D. (1976). A report on nurse internship programs. *Supervisor Nurse, 7*(12), 12–16.

Darling, L.A.W., & McGrath, L.G. (1983). The causes and costs of promotion trauma. *Journal of Nursing Administration, 13*(4), 29–33.

Darling, L.A.W., & McGrath, L.G. (1983). Minimizing promotion trauma. *Journal of Nursing Administration, 13*(9), 14–19.

del Bueno, D.J., Barker, F., & Christmyer, C. (1981). Implementing a competency-based orientation program. *Journal of Nursing Administration, 11*(2), 24–29.

Finkelman, A.W. (1980). *Staff development for the psychiatric nurse.* Thorofare, N.J.: Charles B. Slack.

Friesen, L., & Conahan, B.J. (1980). A clinical preceptor program: Strategy for new graduate orientation. *Journal of Nursing Administration, 10*(4), 18–23.

Hanson, S.M.H. (1976). Role orientation and integration. *Journal of Continuing Education in Nursing, 7*(11), 23–26.

Hollefreund, M., Mlack, V., Moore, S., & Jersan, J. (1981). Implementing a reality shock program. *Journal of Nursing Administration, 11*(1), 16–20.

Kaelin, M.S., & Bliss, J.B. (1979). Evaluating newly employed nurses' skills. *Nursing Outlook, 27*, 334–337.

Kramer, M., & Schmalenberg, C.E. (1978). Bicultural training and new graduate role transformation, Part I. *Nursing Digest, 5*(1), 1–47.

Lee, G., & Raleigh, E.D. (1983). A half-way house for the new graduate. *Journal of Nursing Management, 14*(1), 43–45.

May, L. (1980). Clinical preceptors: For new nurses. *American Journal of Nursing, 80,* 1824–1826.

Meisenhelder, J.B. (1981). The new graduate socialization. *Journal of Continuing Education in Nursing, 12*(3), 16–22.

Moran, V. (1980). Notes on continuing education: Individualizing the orientation of staff nurses. *Journal of Continuing Education in Nursing, 11*(2), 54–59.

Roell, S.M. (1981). Nurse intern programs: How they're working. *Nurse Educator, 6*(6), 29–31.

Rowland, H.S., & Rowland, B.L. (1980). *Nursing administration handbook.* Rockville, Md: Aspen Systems.

Schroeder, D.M., Cantor, M.M., & Kurth, S.W. (1981). Learning needs of the new graduate entering hospital nursing. *Nursing Educator, 6*(6), 10–17.

Turnbull, E. (1983). Rewards in nursing: The case of nurse preceptors. *Journal of Nursing Administration, 13*(1), 10–13.

Appendix 10-A

Staff Development
Registered Nurse Check List

STAFF DEVELOPMENT
REGISTERED NURSE CHECK LIST

Name: _____

Education: AD _____ BS _____ Dip _____ MS _____

RN _____ GN _____ Experience: Psychiatric Nursing _____ years

Other Nursing _____ years

Year Graduated _____ Date begin work _____ Unit _____

	Competent and Experienced	Little Experience	No Experience	Theory Only
Conducting Group Psychotherapy				
Conducting Individual Psychotherapy				
Conducting Family Psychotherapy				
Admission of Psychiatric Patient				
Discharge of Psychiatric Patient				
Nursing Care Plans/Psychiatric				
POMR/Psychiatric				
Participation in Milieu Therapy				
Care of Suicidal Patient				
Care of Assaultive Patient				

Source: From *Staff development for the psychiatric nurse* (pp. 58–60) by A.W. Finkelman, 1980, Thorofare, N.J.: Charles B. Slack, Inc. © 1980 by Charles B. Slack, Inc. Reprinted by permission.

STAFF DEVELOPMENT
REGISTERED NURSE CHECK LIST

	Competent and Experienced	Little Experience	No Experience	Theory Only
Care of Alcoholic Patient				
Care of Drug-dependent Patient				
Care of Manic Patient				
Care of Hallucinating Patient				
Medications: Oral				
Sub q				
Z-technique				
Intramuscular				
Rectal				
Case Method				
Functional Method (Indicate # of patients)				
Metric System				
Apothecary System				
Unit Dosage				
Administration of Heparin				
Intravenous Therapy: Use of plastic IV bag				
Add medications to IV bottle				
Add medications to Volutrol				
Change IV bottle or bag				
Time tape IV				
Direct push IV				
Set up Volutrol				
Remove IV catheter				
Venipuncture performance				
Insertion of Foley catheter				
Foley Care				

STAFF DEVELOPMENT
REGISTERED NURSE CHECK LIST

	Competent and Experienced	Little Experience	No Experience	Theory Only
Enema				
Neurological Signs				
Oxygen Administration				
Electronic Thermometer				
Restraints: Abdomen				
Chest				
Wrist and ankle				
Ambu bag				
Cardiopulmonary Resuscitation				
Specimen Collection: Assist with spinal tap				
Urine—Routine				
Fractional				
Acetest				
Clean voided				
Closed drainage				
24 hr				
Stool—Blood				
Ova, parasites				
Sputum—Suction trap				
Primary Nursing				
Team Nursing				
Discharge Planning—Psychiatric				
Lead a group/staff conference				
Giving report				
Receiving report				
Charge Nurse				

Appendix 10-B

Orientation of Nonprofessional Staff

The orientation of a staff nurse has been the major focus of this text due to the trends towards the increasing utilization of registered nurses within psychiatric–mental health nursing settings. Currently, however, nonprofessionals are utilized in a variety of roles within psychiatric–mental health settings. As with the staff nurse, an orientation program must be individually tailored to the role and the organization. The following material details components of an orientation program for nonprofessionals.

Orientation Program

Objectives:
Each orientee will:

1. Identify . . . [the] role on . . . assigned unit by describing it to . . . [the] head nurse.
2. Identify personnel policies relevant to . . . [orientee's] needs.
3. Identify the grievance procedure by describing it in writing.
4. Demonstrate the following on . . . assigned unit:
    a. Location and use of fire equipment.
    b. Location and use of essential equipment.
    c. Use of the telephone and page systems.
5. Describe the following safety procedures to the instructor:
    a. Fire procedure.
    b. Suicide prevention procedure.
    c. Application of restraints.
6. Demonstrate appropriate patient care on assigned unit.

Source: From *Staff development for the psychiatric nurse* (pp. 105–107) by A.W. Finkelman, 1980, Thorofare, N.J.: Charles B. Slack, Inc. © 1980 by Charles B. Slack, Inc. Reprinted by permission.

Orientation Schedule

Monday

8:00–9:30	AM	Welcome and description of orientation, philosophy of patient care
9:00–9:30	AM	Coffee break
9:30–10:00	AM	Introduction of nursing administration staff
10:15–11:30	AM	Orientation to personnel policies

      1. Salary and paychecks
      2. Taxes
      3. Vacation time, sick time, overtime
      4. Full-time and part-time benefits
      5. Holidays
      6. Hours for each shift
      7. Shift differential
      8. Dress code
      9. Insurance
    10. Parking
    11. Educational benefits

11:30 AM–12:30 PM		Lunch
12:30–1:30	PM	Position description
		Description of units and patients
1:30–1:45	PM	Break
1:45–4:00	PM	Administrative organization
		Grievance procedure
		General discussion of orientee's view of psychiatric care

Tuesday

8:00–10:30	AM	Patient management
		Nutrition, sleep, elimination, exercise, hygiene
		(A break is included in this time)
10:30 AM–12:00 M		Communication and observation
12:00 M–1:00	PM	Lunch
1:00–2:00	PM	Tour
2:00–3:00	PM	Patient group activities
3:00–4:00	PM	Nursing care plans

Wednesday

8:00 AM–12:00 M	On assigned unit with a "buddy"
	a. Meet staff
	b. Find equipment
	c. Learn layout of the unit
12:00 M–1:00 PM	Lunch
1:00–4:00 PM	Safety
	a. Fire procedure
	b. Suicide prevention procedure
	c. Application of restraints
	d. Falls
	e. Incident reports
	f. Keys and locked doors

Thursday   Assigned to unit with a "buddy"

Chapter 11

Role of Staff Education in a Psychiatric–Mental Health Organization

OVERVIEW

The staff education component of any psychiatric–mental health nursing department is a most important and vital one. It can vary in scope from the basic orientation of new nursing personnel to responsibility for elaborate organization-wide educational programming that involves coordination of educational efforts in all departments and services. Staff education efforts include in-service education, staff development, and continuing education programs. Each of these three elements addresses specific staff education areas—from individual job-related activities to professional growth and future career development.

In-Service Education

In-service education aims at cultivating those psychiatric–mental health skills necessary for employees to perform their jobs (Yordanoff, 1981). This in-service program includes new job orientation and educational activities centering on policies, procedures, and technical skills. In the psychiatric–mental health setting, the orientation function of in-service education would include basic information about the organization, its treatment philosophy, types of admissions (voluntary or involuntary), fire and other emergency procedures, and other specific job-related policies and procedures specific to each job classification. Orientation would also cover legal aspects of psychiatric–mental health treatment, including privileged communication and client confidentiality, substance abuse confidentiality, state rules governing seclusion and physical restraint, client rights issues, nursing care planning, documentation in the medical record, medication procedures, incident reporting, and so on. Scheduled in-service programs would also further address these topics as a means of a regular review and updating for all staff members.

Other topics related to the practice of psychiatric–mental health nursing would be addressed. These topics might encompass the therapeutic relationship, the manipulative client, psychotic delusional clients, treatment modalities, and other specific client care interventions. The nursing care of clients on special client precautions warrants additional programs on topics that include acute–active suicidal precautions (one-to-one vigilant intervention with the most acutely suicidal clients), other suicide precautions, aggressive or assaultive precautions, and physical management of the aggressive, acting-out clients.

Additional basic in-service programs might include psychotropic medications or safety precautions (e.g., the handling of "sharps"—dangerous or potentially dangerous objects). All of these topics relate to the basic client care activities encountered in a psychiatric–mental health organization.

Staff Development

Staff development focuses on "job enrichment, career development [and] personal and social growth" (Yordanoff, 1981, p. 57). Psychiatric–mental health development offerings would address topics such as decision-making skills, creative management of job stress, current professional issues, career planning, professional or technical writing, creative problem solving, and leadership skills. These sessions would assist the nursing staff in their professional development.

Continuing Education

Those educational activities that improve employees' current skills and prepare the employees for future job opportunities are classified as *continuing education* (Yordanoff, 1981). These activities are frequently offered outside the employing organization and include collegiate coursework, workshops, and conferences. Nurses completing basic degree requirements, master's level programs in psychiatric–mental health nursing, or continuing education programs on selected psychiatric–mental health nursing issues are pursuing continuing education activities.

ORGANIZATIONAL DEFINITION OF STAFF EDUCATION

Psychiatric–mental health nursing staff education efforts must be defined by each organization and must clearly delineate the philosophy of the organization or department about education, the scope of staff education efforts, personnel required, support services needed, and resources available. In large organizations, staff education functions are often handled by an independent staff education department responsible for all areas of staff education. Smaller organizations may have limited staff available, with only part-time educators or consultants to provide educational offerings.

Whatever the scope of staff education in a psychiatric–mental health organization, the support of the nursing and organizational administration is essential. If the intent is to provide all three elements of education (in-service education, staff development, and continuing education opportunities), the organization must be willing to invest in quality personnel and to support those educators' efforts to develop staff members to achieve their individual potentials.

Psychiatric–mental health *staff education* prepares newly hired employees to assume their job responsibilities, assists newly graduated nurses in their transition from student to professional, trouble-shoots when problems in staff performance occur, grooms employees for upward mobility, and coordinates all the educational offerings of an organization. Truly, these tasks are quite varied and demand a high degree of educational skills and preparation.

The staff educators, in conjunction with the nursing administration, can be instrumental in effecting changes deemed necessary to improve the quality of psychiatric–mental health nursing care. Obviously, it is essential that the nursing administration and staff educators work collaboratively to define educational needs and to plan appropriate educational programs designed to meet those needs. Neither the nurse-educator nor the nurse-administrator can independently determine the educational programs to be presented. Both persons can support and assist each other in meeting mutually agreed upon goals.

Therefore, the most effective staff education departments have a representative voice in nursing administrative decisions. A strong relationship with the psychiatric–mental health nursing administrator is also crucial. In this way, the staff educator has an advisory voice in important decision making, hospital, organizational and departmental planning, and related goal setting. Regular meetings with the staff educator and the nurse-administrator are most helpful in maintaining the necessary open communication and in establishing priorities for program scheduling.

ASSESSING STAFF EDUCATION NEEDS

Determining the content of the various psychiatric–mental health nursing education programs can be accomplished through a variety of methods. Periodic staff educational surveys can be helpful in ascertaining the staff's own identified needs and preferences for future programming. Through observation of actual staff performance, nurse-managers can also identify areas that need to be addressed. For example, observation of the seclusion of a client may indicate the need for education about physical management techniques. Careful review and investigation of incident reports is another rich source of determining educational needs. Quality assurance (QA) activities can also reveal educational areas that need attention. Organizational changes such as the purchase of new equipment, the institution or revision of policies and procedures, and advancements in technology and techniques also produce educational needs.

Role of Quality Assurance

QA studies provide a means of identifying the staff's educational needs. Much emphasis is continually placed on the quality of the psychiatric–mental health nursing services being provided. More pressure is exerted because of rising public awareness, cost concerns of third party payers, and regulation and licensing bodies. The psychiatric–mental health staff educator should be an active member of the nursing QA committee, thus assuring their participation in the process of problem identification, educational plans for resolution of the problem, and follow up monitoring for measurement of the improvement of care. If this arrangement is not possible, a communication system could be developed that would ensure that the committee and the educator are well informed.

For example, the staff of an adolescent inpatient unit expressed concerns about client injuries during physical crisis management situations. This problem was referred to the nursing quality assurance committee, which reviewed incident reports of injuries and all seclusion records over a period of several months. As a result, it became apparent that the problem was not client injuries, but staff injuries. Furthermore, the staff injuries seemed related to improper physical management techniques. The staff educator developed a comprehensive program designed to implement a physical crisis team approach to these situations. A video tape of the theoretical basis of physical crisis intervention and demonstrations of physical management techniques was made. Lecture, video tape, and hands-on practice were presented. Team "captains" were assigned. The captain was designated as the person responsible for giving directions to the team when it engaged in any crisis situation requiring physical management. After the team approach had been used for several months, another study was done. The number of injuries was dramatically reduced. This example demonstrates the value of the staff educator in QA activities. In this case, improvement was easily measured and supported the educator's plan of action.

Analysis of Data

Once all the assessment information regarding the educational needs of the psychiatric–mental health nursing staff has been gathered, the next task is to assign priorities to those needs and to determine whether education provides the answer to problems. In many cases, what may have first appeared to be an educational need may actually turn out to be a management problem. Not all performance difficulties, for example, are a result of a deficiency of skills. Non-educational factors may have an impact on the problems and may require alternative actions (Milnar, 1981). These factors may include unrealistic expectations, time problems, or limited resources (including supplies). The best educational program cannot resolve the situation if the basic problem has not been addressed.

For example, the department may have determined that all psychiatric–mental health nursing assessments must be completed within 24 hours of the client's admission. However, no provision was made for the completion of assessments on confused or psychotic clients. Hence, these assessments were not completed within the designated time frame. Education was not needed to correct the problem; rather, a method of assessment that acknowledged this client population needed to be developed.

PLANNING THE PROGRAM

After the psychiatric–mental health nursing staff's educational needs have been prioritized, an overall program plan should be developed. The plan should define the objectives for the program, the type of educational activity best suited for the objectives, and the identified needs. The use of a variety of teaching methods (such as lectures, films, and guest speakers) will provide a balance in approaches and will minimize boredom while maintaining or increasing the staff's participation.

In addition to the educational methods to be used, time frames for the completion of each educational program should be established. Some programs may require only one session, while others may be a series on related topics occurring over many weeks (such as the psychodynamics of various psychiatric illnesses). Educational activities that are routinely repeated at certain established time intervals (e.g., physical intervention techniques, review of special nursing precautions) must be incorporated into the scheduling process.

Changes within the psychiatric–mental health nursing department which require educational programs must be discussed and carefully planned by the nursing administration and the staff educator in a collaborative manner. Large undertakings, such as a change from a team nursing model to primary nursing, require much thought and preparation before any aspect of the change is initiated. In some cases, several years of systematic planning and incremental implementation may be necessary for the plan to succeed. These types of changes can have a great impact on the time and resources of the educator, requiring a far different schedule of educational offerings than previously established. Long-range planning with some flexibility for unknown or unforeseen urgent needs is, therefore, essential if the educational program is to function in an organized fashion.

IMPLEMENTING THE PROGRAM

Instructional Materials and Resources

After establishing the overall program plan, the staff educator should inventory available educational equipment to ensure that the necessary equipment is ready.

Essential to any educational program is audiovisual equipment such as a slide projector, 16-millimeter film projector, tape recorder, overhead projector, video cassette recorder (VCR), video monitor and video projection unit.

Video equipment is rapidly becoming more accessible, financially feasible, and integral to a quality education program. Simple to use, video cassette tapes are more durable than films and are easily stored and shipped. Video monitors and projection units make video material accessible to larger audiences. Video equipment can also be valuable in filming employee participation in such activities as role playing exercises, group process or supervision, and nursing interventions. Individual coaching, based on the strengths and weaknesses identified on the tape recording, can then be given to the employee. The availability of any audiovisual equipment depends of course on the size of the organization, the role of education within the organization, and the funds available for staff education.

Paper supplies, xerographic capabilities, and clerical support are important for efficient, effective, and comprehensive program planning. Absence of any of these elements can greatly hinder the productivity of the staff educator (Horn, 1981). Funds should be allocated for guest speakers as well as for the staff's participation in workshops outside the organization.

Because much emphasis is now being placed on cost-effectiveness, funds for outside education are being drastically reduced in some organizations. Wise choices must, therefore, be made. Consideration must be given to the type of program offered, location, distance to be travelled, value to the staff and organization, and the appropriate staff to attend. Care taken in this area can justify continued organizational support. Because of the value of such programs, interest in continuing the funding for such professional development activities should be promoted.

Other resources to be explored include the skills of employees within as well as outside the psychiatric–mental health nursing department. Staff members who are gifted in certain areas should be encouraged and groomed for providing educational programs that demonstrate their unique skills and knowledge. A nurse who has had several courses in group dynamics, and is involved in group therapy, might be used to help facilitate staff support groups or to teach group techniques.

Shared educational services have the potential for better programming, reduced costs, and increased visibility for the organization. In many parts of the country, continuing education programs specific to psychiatric–mental health nurses' needs are scarce. If an organization cannot develop continuing education programs, it may be able to cosponsor such programs with other organizations, professional groups, or universities. This process would give the staff an opportunity to participate in programs otherwise unavailable or unattainable. The publicity would also enhance the image of the organization in the community, thus aiding in the recruitment of nurses. Guidelines for the approval of programs for continuing education credits can be obtained from state nursing associations or from state boards of nursing (in states with mandatory continuing education expectations).

Learning Modules

Courses composed of several modules can be developed for educational use by individuals or groups of staff. The content for learning modules is compiled according to the purpose of the course, goals and behavioral objectives, assessment of the student's knowledge, media that facilitates the communication of the content, written pre- and post-tests, a student evaluation tool, and evaluation of the learning package (Caine & Ward, 1981). Staff members receive appropriate credit upon successful completion of course material. The use of self-instructional materials requires fewer staff educators and assists persons in meeting their educational needs. Video equipment can also be helpful. The module format can be cost-effective, especially if it is developed and produced within the organization.

Courses that could be developed for use in a psychiatric–mental health organization might include physical assessment, nursing assessment of an emotionally ill client, treatment modalities, psychiatric medications, therapeutic approaches, group dynamics, and so on. Learning modules are also excellent tools for management and supervision courses and in the presentation of preceptor programs for new graduate nurses.

In the following sections, various aspects of the implementation process of staff education programs are presented. The program examples that will be used are the orientation process (see Chapter 10), clinical career ladders, and the use of role modeling by the nursing staff as part of the staff education program. For other aspects of staff education programs, refer to texts that focus on staff education and development.

Clinical Career Ladders

A clinical career ladder program may be investigated as a useful retention or recruitment tool, to provide for professional staff growth and to increase the quality of care delivered. Often, nurses state that they leave an organization because of the lack of recognition for their professional skills or a lack of opportunity to deliver quality care (Gassert, Holt & Pope, 1982). Many are heard to say that they enjoy direct patient care and do not wish to proceed up the administrative ladder. Hence, when additional monetary needs are felt, these nurses may choose to seek other staff nurse employment that offers them the financial support they seek. Or, in some cases, a staff nurse may accept a managerial position for the monetary rewards and not enjoy or be capable of handling this position.

The use of some type of clinical career ladder recognizes the worth and importance of the nurse giving direct patient care and rewards the nurse through recognition, advancement, and, often, monetary benefits. As the nurse advances upward on this ladder, each promotion is associated with a recognition of increased ability, accountability, and responsibility (Nelson & Arford, 1977).

Such advancement further recognizes and expects the nurse at the higher level to have an increased depth of knowledge—"comprehension of specific factors related to care situations" (Knox, 1980, p. 31). The advancement indicates that the nurse is capable of an increased scope of practice (Huey, 1982). Hence, with each advancement, it is understood that there is an increase in the "number and complexity of the variables which the nurse incorporates into the nursing process in [client] care situations" (Knox, 1980, p. 30).

Assessment of Need

Like other programs or projects in the psychiatric–mental health nursing department, the decision to institute a clinical career ladder must occur only after extensive investigation and planning efforts have been accomplished. A clinical career ladder can hope to "enhance the organization's objectives for quality care, promote an environment for clinical development and create salary levels for staff nurses which approach supervisory and administrative pay levels" (Knox, 1980, p. 10). The benefits expected for the department, the client population served, and the organization should be identified before a task force is instituted for its development. The purpose and realistic objectives for this type of program must also be identified. Once these assessments are made, the department and organization should be evaluated to determine what is preventing the achievement of these objectives at the current time (del Bueno, 1982). Will the outcomes of the program justify the costs in time and efforts? Perhaps other less costly and less involved modifications could be made that would achieve the same goals.

Planning

It is hoped that such a career ladder would provide recognition for excellence in clinical practice and that the involved staff nurse would, through intensive clinical practice and a variety of formal and informal learning experiences, become increasingly competent in psychiatric–mental health nursing (Zimmer, 1972). To ensure that a program accomplishes these aims, a task force should be established. The composition of this group should include a variety of nurses from within the department. Representatives from nursing administration, staff education, various levels of nursing supervision, and staff nurses would provide the overall input and feedback to facilitate the success of the project.

Relevant Concepts. This task force would be responsible initially for assessing the department and organization for the presence of concepts, derived from organizational theory, that have proved relevant to career satisfaction and the development and demonstration of competence. These concepts include mutual attractiveness, integrative groups, and professional growth.

To achieve mutual attractiveness, nurses in supervisory positions should be competent in relevant specialty areas, the range of processes used in the nurse-practitioner role, and supervisory relationships. Of course, their education and demonstrated competence must exceed those of the nurses they supervise (Zimmer, 1972). This concept assists in the reduction of conflicts that may be created when clinically advanced staff nurses are supervised by nurse-managers who have few clinical skills and little competence.

The concept of integrative work groups requires that a work group (nursing staff on a particular unit or service) have an ideology that explains the group's current and future activities. An organizational structure that provides for such work groups enhances productivity and facilitates creative ideas. In a psychiatric–mental health nursing department, such work groups would support the clinical efforts of staff nurses and promote their achievement of higher levels of clinical competence.

The final concept of professional growth requires that creativity in practice is possible and encouraged. Four factors contribute to the promotion of this concept: 1) there are persons present in the department who have professionally developed themselves extensively (to serve as role models for the staff nurses), 2) feedback is given on a regular basis about a nurse's work, 3) consistent examination of current nursing practice occurs with an associated evaluation of the quality of that practice, and 4) a feeling of openness exists—i.e., freedom in the use of time, freedom to move through the organization, and the freedom to fail (Zimmer, 1972). The presence of these four factors assists in the creation of a practice environment that fosters the professional growth of staff nurses.

When the presence and support of the above components are ensured, the development of a practice environment that facilitates the growth of career satisfaction within the nursing staff is ensured. Other departmental components that also facilitate career satisfaction are primary nursing and decentralized decision making.

Developing the Ladder. After the appraisal process, the task force would direct its attention to the actual construction of the clinical ladder. It is crucial to identify, during this initial planning, the focus of the ladder's measurement before an attempt is made to define the actual measurement criteria (Knox, 1980).

This focus must aid in distinguishing between the beginning, intermediate, and advanced levels of practice (Zimmer, 1972) and should take note of increasing competence and improvement in quality care as demonstrated in performance criteria and client outcome audits (del Bueno, 1982). Furthermore, the focus should have a "logical relationship to the program's overall purpose and objectives" (del Bueno, 1982, p. 202).

Depending upon the organization, various components of nursing care have been identified as criteria upon which to focus for the development of a ladder:

clinical practice (often divided into the subcomponents of the nursing process), administration, research, education (MacKinnon & Eriksen, 1977), leadership skills (Nelson & Arford, 1977), consulting (Gassert et al., 1982) and professional development (Anderson & Denyes, 1975).

Whichever components are selected for development of specific criteria, the committee should ensure that they relate to psychiatric–mental health nursing competence as well as to skill issues (del Bueno, 1982). A behavioral basis is important (Knox, 1980) because it aids the evaluative process as the nurse progresses up the ladder. Individual units or services can prove helpful in this case, as they can delineate expected behaviors associated with each level of advancement. This process also serves to increase the credibility and validity of the system with nurses working on each unit or service (Gassert et al., 1982).

Tracks and Levels. Another decision that must be made by the committee is the arrangement and number of tracks and levels composing the clinical ladder. For example, it is considered to be increasingly difficult to develop valid criteria as the number of levels rises above three (del Bueno, 1982). Should the organization believe that a five-level ladder fulfills its needs more appropriately, verifying the ladder's reliability will prove to be more time consuming and difficult. To determine the number of tracks desired by an organization, the task force must also evaluate available options to determine which would best suit demonstrated needs. For example, a clinical career ladder may consist of only one clinical advancement track. This single track may be adjusted to provide the choice of a major or minor focus of interest. For example, the first three clinical levels may focus solely upon clinical competence. At Level 4, a major in clinical practice, education, or management may be declared. Each major would require different evaluative criteria (Nelson & Arford, 1977). Another example: the first two levels focus upon clinical competence, while the third level requires a choice on the nurse's part as to whether a clinical or administrative emphasis is desired (Gassert et al., 1982). This model would combine the traditional managerial advancement track—head nurse, supervisor, and so on—with the advancement on a clinical basis.

The task force must then address the issue of job descriptions for each level of the ladder. The clinical ladder provides a framework from which the job descriptions are derived. There are various approaches for this aspect of the program. For a career ladder using criteria that are totally individualized for a unit or service, there may be multiple position descriptions for one level of achievement. An organization that uses broader criteria, however, may have only as many position descriptions as there are levels in the ladder.

Whichever approach, or modification of approach, is used by an organization, each position description should include basic information. One format may include a definition of the role, a statement of accountability, and an outline of expected behaviors (Gassert et al., 1982). Another format may include the position title, description of position, characteristic activities expected, relationships with other positions, and qualifications—required knowledge base, skills, abilities, and education (Anderson & Denyes, 1975).

Evaluation Process. The next task of the task force would be to address the issue of the evaluative process for an applicant for placement at some point on the career ladder. Initial placement on the ladder of nurses currently employed at the institution may present difficult situations. Should every nurse be expected to apply for positioning? Will there be a designated number of positions available at all levels, or will the system encourage and permit every qualified nurse to be placed appropriately? If there are a limited number of positions, how will this initial allocation be determined? Would senior staff members have priority? In such a situation, once positions have been allocated, will monetary benefits need to be adjusted to provide for a consistent gradation? If so, how can this be done on an equitable basis (del Bueno, 1982)? If there are a limited number of positions at each level, how will waiting applications be handled? Throughout this process, the task force must ensure that job security is maintained (Gassert et al., 1982). Should nurses feel that their positions are threatened as a result of the institution of a clinical career ladder, their resistance to its implementation will increase dramatically.

Once these concerns have been discussed and resolved, the task force should develop the routine evaluation process involving a nurse's advancement from one level to another. This process is often begun by establishing the credentials needed by a nurse after that nurse's initiation of a request for promotion (Huey, 1982). This formal request should be accompanied by materials supporting the nurse's exemplary clinical nursing performance. Such documentation could include, but not be limited to, recent evaluations, a personal interview with the review committee, referrals from colleagues and supervisory personnel, recommendation from the nurse's head nurse, and unit documentation that would substantiate the nurse's claim—charting, written papers, self-evaluation, care plans, reports, projects, and conferences (Anderson & Denyes, 1975).

After this self-initiation aspect of the evaluation process, the credentialling committee would review the submitted documents. This standing committee's composition, again, varies according to the organization's philosophy and needs, but it should include such persons as the following: (1) persons chosen by position, area of clinical expertise, and experience with peer review (Anderson & Denyes, 1975); (2) a nursing peer, a nurse at the highest clinical level, and a designated nurse evaluator (Gassert et al., 1982); or (3) an instructor from the staff education department, clinicians, and the applicant's head nurse (Nelson & Arford, 1977). The initial task force should determine whether credentialling committee members are to be named on a permanent or a temporary basis. A decision must also be made as to whether committee members may serve as consultants to applicants (Anderson & Denyes). The credentialling committee would then review the individual nurse's documents and, within a specified time frame, would make a recommendation about the request for promotion. This recommendation should be forwarded to the psychiatric–mental health nursing administrator, who reviews the documents and recommendation and makes the final decision. Should this decision negate the credentialling committee's recommendation, the nurse-administrator should meet with the committee to discuss the decision.

With the final decision, the feedback portion of the evaluation process begins. Within a predetermined time frame, the committee should notify the nurse-applicant of the results of the review process. Each organization determines whether other persons need to receive notification of these results. These persons may include the personnel office, the psychiatric–mental health nursing administrator, the applicant's head nurse, and other persons as needed.

Financial Reimbursement. One of the major issues concerning advancement along a career ladder is the advancement's association with an increase in financial reimbursement. The salary can be a major reason for a nurse's desire to change positions. With the increase in "job demands and associated increases in personal effort [accompanying clinical advancement], direct monetary rewards" are needed (Bracken & Christman, 1978, p. 9). Rationale for this idea can be obtained by referring to Maslow's hierarchy of needs. An employee cannot attend to self-esteem needs when "amounts of energy [must be directed to] satisfying fundamental needs," (Bracken & Christman, p. 9) such as maintaining adequate income to provide for food and housing. A salary is also a tangible reflection of the value placed, in our society, upon achievements. Without such a concrete sign of worth, the advancement may be perceived as a way to obtain more work from employees without increased rewards.

Implementation

After the initial development of the career ladder, additional procedural questions should be answered before implementation is possible. Will ladder advancements be voluntary or mandatory? Will there be a waiting period before one can advance to the next level? Where will a newly hired nurse be placed on the ladder? Based upon whose evaluation? If a nurse demonstrates a consistent decrease in competence level, would the nurse then move down the ladder? Should there be a limited number of opportunities to advance? If an organization uses a float pool or pulls staff to other units or services, should the nurse being sent to the unit or service be at the same level as the nurse being replaced? These questions, plus others unique to each organization, must be answered if the program is to be successful.

Evaluation

Finally, the program itself must be monitored to determine whether expected outcomes have been achieved or whether modifications must be made in the program. Certain benefits may be expected as a result of the implementation of this program. Motivation should be increased for staff nurses, resulting in improvement in client care. This program, which provides improved job satisfaction, should enhance the attractiveness of the organization to registered nurses in the community. Consequently, there would be an increased number of registered nurses employed, increased average length of stay of employment for a registered nurse, increased number of minority nurse applicants, and a decrease in the financial loss to the organization from an increasingly stable work force (Miller, 1975). A procedure must be incorporated into the program to monitor such outcomes and benefits to determine whether the program is functioning at its most effective and efficient level. If not, changes must be made so that the program can meet the objectives for which it was created. (An example of a psychiatric–mental health nursing clinical career ladder is included in Appendix 11-A.)

Role Modeling for Staff Education

Another aspect of staff education is role modeling for all levels of nursing. *Role modeling* occurs "when the individual observes someone else playing a certain role so that she/he is able to understand and emulate the behaviors in that role" (Stuart & Sundeen, 1983, p. 278). Through this technique, members of the psychiatric–mental health nursing staff can learn new and different ways of behaving. By comparing their behaviors with those of the role models, they can institute an evaluative process, with needed corrective actions being identified. This modeling is not limited to nurses in positions of power, but can and should be utilized by all nurses in their attempts to grow professionally.

The psychiatric–mental health organizational environment should be examined, and those areas that would benefit from the use of role modeling should be determined. Because each organization is different, each nursing department should identify areas in which role models currently exist and areas in which such behavior must be encouraged. For example, all nurses may use the nursing process in providing their care. Hence, there is no need for role models to reintroduce this process. Rather, the need may be for role models to support and maintain this behavior. However, if nurses are not viewed as professionally active, this problem must be examined. Role models within the department who are involved in professional activities would need to be supported.

Components of Role Modeling

All psychiatric–mental health nursing staff, particularly those in leadership positions, have the obligation to serve as professional role models to their peers and colleagues. To do this, each nurse should be aware of the aspects that constitute a professional psychiatric–mental health nurse role model: namely, clinical, professional, and personal development. In order to demonstrate clinical development, the psychiatric–mental health nurse should be aware of the current literature and research related to psychiatric–mental health nursing practice and should incorporate this knowledge into the practice area as appropriate. The nurse should demonstrate competent skills in communication and self-awareness and use all opportunities to evaluate and to improve individual practice.

For professional development, the nurse should be active in professional activities that serve to facilitate the profession's ongoing self-awareness and progression. Through these and other community-related activities, the nurse also works with consumers to improve the quality of the psychiatric–mental health care available to the public. The results of these activities should be shared with colleagues at work in order to increase their awareness and involvement in current professional and societal issues.

Finally, each psychiatric–mental health nurse should foster personal development. By cultivating leisure interests and activities, as well as personal relationships, the nurse demonstrates the importance of a well-rounded life style. These activities communicate the importance of both mental and physical health. Such personal development also provides the nurse with a source of energy that aids in dealing with the stresses of the profession and of life in general.

With the staff functioning as the main therapeutic tool in the delivery of care in the psychiatric–mental health setting, it is also important that all levels of nurses be encouraged to support self-awareness. This self-awareness is particularly crucial in the initial development phase of building therapeutic relationships with clients, which serves as a basis for all psychiatric–mental health activities. All the staff should confront and work through feelings involved in working with psychiatric–mental health clients, whether they are children, adolescents, or adults (Wilson & Kneisl, 1979). Through this analysis of self, staff members become more aware of the role they play in the client's continued progress.

Nursing Leaders as Role Models

Within psychiatric–mental health nursing, as in all other nursing areas, the nursing staff need leaders with whom they can share and with whom they can learn (Rowland & Rowland, 1980). As in all other aspects of life, persons use leaders and role models as sources of emulation and motivation to become better. Hence, it "behooves every nurse [leader] to demonstrate, by example, the activities and roles of nursing so that others can emulate them" (Yura, Ozimek & Walsh, 1981, p. 121). Psychiatric–mental health nursing leaders provide challenges, support, and encouragement for those they lead. To function appropriately in the organization, the nurse leaders should be informed as to the needs and concerns of the client population served, as well as those of the staff involved. Such functioning requires that the leaders be clinically knowledgeable and confident regarding the clinical situation and have up-to-date information about aspects of psychiatric–mental health nursing care (Yura, Ozimek & Walsh, 1981).

Although all psychiatric–mental health nursing staff are encouraged and expected to become professional role models for their peers, the leadership positions of head nurse, supervisor, and clinical specialist have additional responsibilities for role modeling in regard to staff development. Because each of these positions is considered a leadership position, each nurse occupying such a position should function on a peer level with leaders in other disciplines (e.g., psychiatrists, certified psychiatric social workers, and clinical psychologists.) Without this equality, nursing becomes a secondary profession in the organization and is handicapped in its attempts to provide quality psychiatric–mental health care. Hence, nursing leaders must treat themselves, their peers, and the leaders in other professions on the same basis. A simple, but often troublesome, example of this inequality would be a head nurse who greets a psychiatrist as Dr. Smith, but who is addressed by the psychiatrist as Jane.

Inasmuch as each organization is different and employs different levels of staff, issues regarding the nurse-leader's role in staff development through role modeling should be individualized. If the nursing department is decentralized (without supervisors) and also does not have clinical specialists, the head nurses must attempt to fulfill additional role model behaviors (as possible), based upon their experience and education. If, however, multiple clinical specialists are available and also function as supervisors, the role of the head nurse should be specifically tailored to that individual unit's or service's needs.

An initial assessment and ongoing reevaluation should be done by nurse-leaders to identify each staff member's strengths and weaknesses. Through this mechanism, limitations can be decreased while, at the same time, each staff member can be supported and encouraged on an individual basis. This information is not only useful during annual evaluations, but it also serves to identify to each staff member that nursing administration is interested in, and concerned with, them as professionals, not just as people who fill positions on an organizational chart. It is hoped that this attitude will also encourage each staff member to assume responsibility for self-growth and, hence, the improvement of client care.

Two important behaviors will result from this ongoing assessment of a staff member's development: consultation and supervision. Both of these components of psychiatric–mental health nursing administration serve to improve a staff's level of functioning and, hence, the quality of care delivered. *Consultation* may be defined as "a process of interaction between two professional persons—the consultant who is a specialist, and the consultee [sic]" (Stuart & Sundeen, 1983, p. 688). The consulter retains control of this process by reserving the right to accept or to reject the ideas offered by the consultant. This process occurs when issues of care require a differing perspective; it, however, does not necessarily occur on an ongoing basis. The procedure usually includes a description of the consulter's perception of the situation, the approaches taken, and "the identification and evaluation of desired outcomes in terms of what is realistic" (Fife, 1983, p. 9). The consultant aids the consulter in evaluating the problem and in establishing goals and plans for attaining goals. Such consultation is generally followed by an evaluation to determine the effectiveness of the consultation (Fife).

Supervision, in contrast, can be defined as "a process whereby a therapist, frequently, but not always a relative beginner, is helped to become a more effective clinician. The goals of supervision are not only to guide the therapist in the successful handling of the supervised case, but to catalyze the therapist's creative and therapeutic use of self" (Stuart & Sundeen, 1983, p. 103). In clinical supervision, all nurses review their individual clinical cases with a selected clinical supervisor (head nurse, supervisor, or clinical specialist—depending on the persons present within the organization and their educational background) in order to improve the level of practice. This activity occurs on a regular basis and serves as a professional growth mechanism for the supervised employee. All psychiatric–mental health personnel should receive this clinical supervision in order to ensure that the care provided is of the best possible quality.

Other role modeling responsibilities for the nurse-leaders include their support of education and research (Fife, 1983). Educational efforts are usually done on an informal and spontaneous basis as a result of clinical situations. The nurse-leader should recognize these kinds of situations when they occur and use them with the involved staff to widen that staff's knowledge base about certain aspects of psychiatric–mental health nursing care.

The nurse-leader, as a role model for staff education, should be certain that the staff perceives research as important. This recognition occurs through various mechanisms. Research should be incorporated into the nurse-leader's practice on a regular basis and incorporated into teaching efforts with the staff. The nurse-leader should also assist staff members in looking at clinical problems as issues that can benefit from the research process. Educative efforts on a more formal basis, such as in-service education and seminars, can strengthen the staff's knowledge base about the research process. The staff can then be encouraged to incorporate research into the clinical setting by examining and attempting to explain why events do, or do not, occur.

Once role modeling has been incorporated into a staff education program, this component must also be evaluated on an ongoing basis. Through observing and evaluating their own behavior, nurse-leaders can ascertain whether all situations were promptly used for staff education. They should also validate with others, both within and outside nursing, that they are perceived as presenting the professional models they believe others should emulate. Through this ongoing self-evaluation, they again demonstrate role modeling behavior and encourage the staff to examine and evaluate their own behavior.

Staff Educator as Liaison

The overall goal of staff education in psychiatric–mental health nursing is to improve the quality of care through the development of staff knowledge and skills. The staff educator is in a unique position to assist both management and the staff, while relying on management for support and feedback. Nursing staff provide information to the educator that may be valuable in defining causes of problems or creative solutions to problems. Often, innovative ideas surface during discussions at educational programs. As a consultant, the educator can also be helpful to the staff who are seeking information about or direction in client care and direction in professional or, in some cases, personal matters.

Nursing administrators are vital to staff education. Their input about unit needs is most important to the educator, and their intervention is often necessary in order to provide a supportive arena in which the staff educator may work. By these means, supplies, supportive (clerical, etc.) services, adequate directions, and explicit standards become available (Sovie, 1981). Adequate staff coverage is also ensured, so that the staff can be scheduled for educational programs without resultant understaffing of the unit or service.

A combined education and management approach is often necessary to resolve staff learning needs. The organization has a responsibility, then, for assisting staff members in maintaining or reaching competency. In situations in which education is not the sole answer, nursing administration may need to intervene. A staff member's failure to perform satisfactorily warrants discussion with nursing management, education, and that employee. If an employee is unable to perform satisfactorily after education has been provided and other contributing factors have been resolved, nursing administration must determine the appropriateness of that employee's remaining in that position. In some cases, a job downgrade or termination may be warranted. This procedure holds true for senior as well as for probationary employees.

There are several means whereby nursing administration and education can further work together to promote staff competence. Priority educational programs, such as cardiopulmonary resuscitation training, physical crisis intervention, and certain client safety programs can be made mandatory for psychiatric–mental health nursing staff. Failure to comply with participation requirements should result in disciplinary action. In-service activities of employees should be recorded in their individual files and should be reviewed during annual performance evaluations (Horn, 1981).

In some states, mandatory continuing education is required for relicensure. This practice can motivate nurses to pursue at least a minimum number of hours of ongoing professional education. The nursing department can use a similar approach by requiring attendance and participation at a minimum number of in-house educational programs within the year. This practice is especially effective when nursing credentialling committees review an individual nurse's overall performance and make appointments for continued employment in the organization.

Organizational Liaison

The staff educator who has responsibility for organization-wide education has the task of coordinating, consulting, and providing programs for other hospital departments. Coordination of all these activities, in addition to the psychiatric–mental health nursing department educational responsibilities, can become unwieldy unless a well-defined plan is developed for managing this effort. Therefore, a clearly defined job description delineating the staff educator's role in relation to the educational needs of other departments is crucial. Program requests from other departments must be assigned priorities; then they must be included in the overall educational calendar. In many instances, psychiatric–mental health program offerings are pertinent for all departments, and participation in these programs should be encouraged for nonnursing employees.

EVALUATING STAFF EDUCATION

Individual Program Components

One mechanism for evaluating the effectiveness of staff education is through the use of pre- and post-tests. These tests assess the learner's knowledge before the educational program and compare it to the learner's knowledge after the program. Although this method is not totally reliable, it does give some clear indication of the learner's knowledge level. If the staff consistently do poorly on post-tests, the source of the problem should be determined. The educator may not provide the necessary information in an understandable and acceptable manner, or the staff may have general difficulty in completing tests. Other problem areas may also be identified. These issues should be resolved in order to facilitate the educational efforts.

Learner knowledge and educator effectiveness can also be demonstrated by use of behavioral objectives established for successful completion of a program (a performance test, such as a return demonstration or other objective testing). Evaluative questionnaires completed by the learners, while not completely evaluating the effectiveness of the program, do provide feedback to the staff educator, indicating acceptance of the program. Other indicators of the effectiveness of the program are the reduction or the elimination of recurrent problems that are addressed by the staff educator or the improved staff performance reflected in performance appraisals.

Overall Program

The staff education program should be reviewed annually and evaluated as to the effectiveness, appropriateness, and timeliness of the programming. Again, goal setting, program planning, and program scheduling must be organized and carefully thought out. Through this review of the overall program, the psychiatric–mental health nursing educator and administrator can modify the program to keep pace with the changing needs of both the staff and the client population.

REFERENCES

Anderson, M.I., & Denyes, M.J. (1975). A ladder for clinical advancement in nursing practice: Implementation. *Journal of Nursing Administration, 5*(2), 16–22.

Bracken, R.L., & Christman, L. (1978). An incentive program designed to develop and reward clinical competence. *Journal of Nursing Administration, 8*(9), 8–18.

Caine, R.M., & Ward, S.F. (1981). Multisensory modularized learning packages. *Journal of Nursing Management, 12*(3), 32–36.

del Bueno, D.J. (1982). A clinical ladder? Maybe! *Journal of Nursing Administration, 12*(9), 19–22.

Fife, B. (1983). The challenge of the medical setting for the clinical specialist in psychiatric nursing. *Journal of Psychosocial Nursing and Mental Health Services, 21*(1), 8–13.

Gassert, C., Holt, C., & Pope, K. (1982). Building a ladder. *American Journal of Nursing, 82*(10), 1527–1530.

Horn, R.S. (1981). Planning inservice education in small hospital. *Supervisor Nurse, 12*(1), 38–41.

Huey, F.L. (1982). Looking at ladders. *American Journal of Nursing, 82*(10), 1520–1526.

Knox, S.L. (1980). A clinical advancement program. *Journal of Nursing Administration, 10*(6), 29–33.

MacKinnon, H.A., & Eriksen, L. (1977). C.A.R.E.—a four track professional nurse classification and performance evaluation system—Jackson Memorial Hospital, Miami, Florida. *Journal of Nursing Administration, 7*(4), 42–44.

Miller, R. (1975). Career ladder program: A problem solving device. *Journal of Nursing Administration, 5*(5), 27–29.

Milnar, R. (1981). Performance analysis—a how to. *Supervisor Nurse, 12*(2), 14–15.

Nelson, C.A., & Arford, P.H. (1977). Strategy for clinical advancement—Department of Clinical Nursing of the Medical University of South Carolina. *Journal of Nursing Administration, 7*(4), 46–51.

Rowland, H.S., & Rowland, B.L. (1980). *Nursing administration handbook*. Rockville, Md: Aspen Systems.

Sovie, M.D. (1981). Investigate before you educate. *Journal of Nursing Administration, 11*(40), 15–21.

Stuart, G.W., & Sundeen, S.J. (1983). *Principles and practice of psychiatric nursing*. St. Louis: C.V. Mosby Co.

Wilson, H.S., & Kneisl, C.R. (1979). *Psychiatric Nursing*. Menlo Park, Calif.: Addison-Wesley.

Yordanoff, D. (1981). When is inservice appropriate. *Journal of Nursing Management, 12*(10), 56–59.

Yura, H., Ozimek, D., & Walsh, M.B. (1981). *Nursing leadership: Theory and process*. New York: Appleton-Century-Crofts.

Zimmer, M.J. (1972). Rationale for a ladder for clinical advancement in nursing practice. *Journal of Nursing Administration, 2*(11), 18–24.

Psychiatric Nursing Clinical Career Ladder

Entry Level. All newly employed nurses for six months unless review of education and experience indicate placement at a Psychiatric–Mental Health Nurse I

Psychiatric–Mental Health Nurse I

Credentials: Education + experience
  Diploma + 3 years
  AD degree + 2 years
  BSN degree + 1 year
Responsible to head nurse
Critical areas
  Clinical practice: Demonstrates competence to be an associate nurse for a specific caseload of patients.
  Administrative: Administers and evaluates delivery of care for a patient caseload, which includes delegation to and clinical supervision of ancillary personnel.
  Research and consultation: Reviews research in psychiatric–mental health nursing. Consults with clinical specialist and with peers.
  Education: Conducts patient education.
  Professional development: Active in professional organization and participates in continuing education activities on a regular basis.

Psychiatric–Mental Health Nurse II

Credentials: Education + experience
  Diploma + 4 years
  AD degree + 3 years
  BSN degree + 2 years
Responsible to head nurse
Critical areas
  Clinical practice: Demonstrates competence to be a primary nurse for a specific caseload of patients.
  Administrative: Administers and evaluates delivery of care for a patient caseload, which includes delegation to and clinical supervision of ancillary personnel; participates in the development and evaluation of unit/service objectives.

Research and consultation: Incorporates research into practice.
  Consults with clinical specialist and with P–MH Nurse I.
Education: Conducts patient and family education.
Professional development: Active in professional organization and participates in continuing education programs frequently and activities on a regular basis.

Psychiatric–Mental Health Nurse III

Credentials: Education + experience
  Diploma + 5 years
  AD degree + 4 years
  BSN + 3 years
Responsible to head nurse
Critical areas
  Clinical practice: Demonstrates competence to be a primary nurse for a specific caseload of patients requiring an advanced level of care.
  Administrative: P–MH Nurse II; and participates in peer review.
  Research and consultation: Participates in research projects.
    Consults with clinical specialist and with P–MH Nurse I and II.
  Education: Conducts staff education with supervision.
    Conducts patient and family education.
  Professional development: Active in professional organizations and participates in continuing education programs and activities on a regular basis.
    Certified in psychiatric–mental health nursing.

Chapter 12

Staff Burnout in Psychiatric–Mental Health Settings

OVERVIEW

In recent years, the literature has been filled with information about a phenomenon known as job burnout. *Burnout* is characterized by a gradual disillusionment with a job, increased feelings of powerlessness to change things, fatigue, cynicism, and frustration—all leading the employee to the point at which job performance is seriously affected. Burnout results from stress that, if over a period of time is not abated, causes a depletion of personal resources.

Work occupies a large portion of a staff member's life. It is important to the staff for personal and economic reasons. Discord between the person and the work setting results in job stress. Because staff members are engaged in their work for such a large part of each day, it is only logical to expect job stress to become a grave concern to the staff and supervisors alike (Pelletier, 1977). Stress is a common part of the staff's life experiences.

Staff members are all under stress every day because they need to adapt constantly to the changes in their personal lives, work, and social situations or environment. Regardless of an employee's position within the psychiatric–mental health organization, that person—with all staff members—is subject to stress. Being subject to stress, they are also candidates for burnout. It is important, then, that the psychiatric–mental health nursing administrator recognize the causes of job stress and the symptoms of burnout so that measures can be taken to prevent this phenomenon from occurring.

McLean (1979) stated, "Our culture places a great deal of emphasis on success. It also teaches us that physical illness is acceptable; mental illness is not" (p. 6). Consequently, when employees cannot succeed in their jobs, prolonged stress results in physical illness. Society and the individual employee can accept this physical illness as rationale for not achieving job expectations. In the past, employers were not responsible for work-related mental illness. Current workers'

167

compensation laws, however, may rule that mental illness that can be attributed to stress on the job is a compensable occupational illness. In areas of the country in which industrialization is high, there is a greater incidence of workers' compensation cases related to job stress. If employment aggravates or precipitates any illness to the point of disability, the employer may be held responsible. In addition to the administration's need to assist employees to deal effectively with stress because of concern for them and a desire to effect quality psychiatric–mental health nursing care, there is the added onus of possible financial responsibility for their mental health.

The staff in the psychiatric–mental health arena are faced with many stressors. Many clients who are acutely ill may not respond to treatment. In addition, clients who do not accept treatment, or even acknowledge the need for help, create a sense of futility and defeat for some staff members. The possibility of explosive, combative, and suicidal situations arising in the milieu increases the acuity of the work setting, compounding stress. As members of an interdisciplinary team, staff members are under stress as a result of conflicts related to roles and role blurring.

In addition to clinical and interpersonal stressors, staff members are faced with the reality of the changing health care environment. Job security has previously been a benefit of employment in health care organizations. Under the team and functional nursing models, paraprofessional staff have been used consistently throughout the years in psychiatric–mental health organizations. With a greater emphasis on improved quality care, the primary nursing model is being implemented. For the first time, health care employees are faced with an added fear— the fear of unemployment, a stressor previously not a part of the psychiatric–mental health arena.

ASSESSING EMPLOYEE STRESS

Employee stress can be demonstrated in a variety of ways, but one of the best indicators is work attendance. Although a few employees may have attendance problems unrelated to stress, escape from stress at work through absenteeism is a common sign of impending burnout. A large turnover of staff, rumors of dissatisfaction, lowered productivity, or high absenteeism may be clues that the environment is contributing to group burnout. Individual burnout and group burnout can be assessed and effectively managed if the psychiatric–mental health nursing manager and nursing administrator are attuned to the symptoms and are willing to take action to rectify the situations contributing to employee stress.

Burnout progresses through several stages. Initially, a new employee may enjoy the challenge of the new job, and accept the related stress as a stimulus for growth. Over time, however, if stress continues, the challenge becomes a problem that results in the burnout process. Veninga (1981) cited the following five warning signals of the depletion of a person's resources and impending burnout: "1) job dissatisfaction, 2) inefficiency at work, 3) fatigue, 4) sleep disturbance, and 5) escape activity" (p. 44).

As employees become less productive, negative attitudes emerge that affect the progress of all staff members. Creative problem solving comes to a standstill, and even minimal changes become overwhelming problems. If unrecognized or avoided, these initial symptoms can become chronic and result in exhaustion, physical illness, anger, or depression. It is not unusual for anger to be overt. Veninga (1981) stated, "when work stress continues unabated, a person's anger often becomes focused. . . . Often [the person] takes on a single conflict. Hatred can center on one or two individuals" (p. 62). An employee may turn a seemingly unimportant situation into a crusade. Another employee, a peer, a subordinate, or a supervisor may become the recipient of the stressed employee's wrath with no apparent grounds for such anger. In both instances, stressed behavior, approaching burnout, is being evidenced.

Once it has been established that the level of stress is having a detrimental effect on an individual person or on a group of employees, the cause of the stress needs to be identified. Plans cannot be made to resolve stressful situations when the cause is not known. Some of the most common causes of stress in psychiatric–mental health nursing are listed in Exhibit 12–1. While other personal factors may also contribute to burnout, these job stressors are the major factors in psychiatric–mental health nursing burnout.

PLANNING AND IMPLEMENTING STRESS MANAGEMENT

Preventive Measures

The best cure for burnout is prevention. Measures can be instituted to provide an environment supportive of psychiatric–mental health nursing practice. A review of current staffing should be made with attention given to the number and mix of staff. Staffing patterns that provide an adequate number of well-prepared staff members to provide the level of care expected need to be determined. Because the physical acting-out behavior of clients is always a potential stressor in the psychiatric–mental health setting, staff members' fears of injury can be reduced with proper staffing and by education in the handling of such clients.

Paperwork has become a monumental part of the nurse's job expectations, and so it, too, is a potential stressor. The entire paperwork system should be analyzed, then, for opportunities to streamline it. Delegation of some of the paperwork to the clerical staff may be possible. Elimination of duplication of efforts and the use of checklists can all help to reduce the amount of time spent on paper tasks. Although streamlining the paperwork may improve the situation, it cannot eliminate it

Exhibit 12–1 Causes of Job Stress

- Conflict with supervisors
- Conflict with coworkers
- Job dissatisfaction
- High, prolonged patient acuity
- Inappropriate nurse:patient ratios
- Too much responsibility
- Too little responsibility
- Inadequate support systems
- Poorly defined job expectations
- Dead-end jobs (especially paraprofessional staff)
- Unrealistic time constraints
- Inadequate or inappropriate staff

entirely. To ensure adequate time for this function is important, then, in the staff's overall work time. Nonnursing tasks performed by nurses should be identified and the delegation of these responsibilities should be made to the appropriate personnel.

Open communication is essential. Staff members at all levels need to have regular opportunities to express their concerns, to be included in plans for the changes under consideration, and to receive support from those in authority. These needs can be accomplished through routine staff meetings as well as interdisciplinary or nursing milieu meetings in which unit concerns are addressed. Furthermore, staff members need recognition for their contributions to client care. Such recognition can be made at meetings as well as individually. Respect for the opinions of others must be fostered, even if there is disagreement with those opinions.

Work schedules should also provide staff members with sufficient time to relax and to regenerate. Both extremes—the long period of successive days scheduled as time off and the "day off–day on–day off" pattern—should be avoided. Besides influencing client care and continuity, extremes in scheduling can increase stress. When possible, the staff should be given an opportunity to have some voice in making their schedules. This opportunity does not mean, of course, that all requests for scheduled days should automatically be approved; rather a mechanism for handling the individual needs of the staff should be in place to allow more flexibility in assisting them to meet their personal needs.

Support groups conducted by qualified persons who are not part of the psychiatric–mental health nursing management team have proven successful. These voluntary groups should be held regularly. The group leader must be nonjudgmental and supportive, helping staff members to ventilate feelings and to look at alternative means of handling their stress. Acting as a liaison between nursing management and staff, the group leader can bring concerns anonymously to the attention of the nurse-administrator for consideration and resolution.

Workshops on stress management can be provided through the staff development or personnel departments. Exercise and nutrition classes offered within the organization or in conjunction with community programs can be a means of providing for the physical well-being of employees. Likewise, consideration should be given to the possibility of providing employee assistance programs geared to referring employees with substance abuse, emotional, personal, or financial problems to appropriate therapists or agencies for help. The absence of staff lounges or lounges that are not comfortable convey a feeling that staff are not important. Attention must be given to this matter so that the staff can feel they are appreciated and valued. The nursing manager has a responsibility to ensure that staff members take time for breaks and meals so that they can remove themselves from a stressful environment to relax and regroup.

Allowing nurses to participate in seminars and workshops away from the organization not only provides some relief from the usual workload, but it acquaints the nurse with valuable information about changes in practice. It also gives the nurse an opportunity to become involved in networking with other nurses engaged in psychiatric–mental health or other areas of nursing. Encouragement by the nurse-administrator for the participation of nurses in the activities of their professional organization can improve professional identification and can provide yet another support system.

In times of increased stress (such as the suicide of a client, program and personnel changes, and union contract negotiations), persons in management positions must be visible and supportive. McLean (1979) underlines this point of view:

> in times of stress, management *must* be there. The presence of authority figures who are available both to answer questions and to lead is essential. Great assurance and reassurance can be drawn from the simple presence of those in command. Dependency needs in times of stress are heightened and a demonstration that one's superior cares and recognizes the impact of stress on the employee under his or her supervision will reap incalculable rewards. (p. 2)

Other methods can be used to prevent or to avert burnout. Allowing an employee to change work responsibilities by rotating to another unit or assuming a different role in the same setting can alleviate the stress of the current job. Oftentimes, becoming involved in a new and challenging program or project can spark enthusiasm and rekindle interest in the job as well.

Most of all, the psychiatric–mental health nursing manager, as well as administrator, needs to be available to listen to the staff. If staff members do not express themselves, for whatever reason, and an assessment of the situation determines it to be stress-related, the nurse-administrator must be direct and express concern to the staff. In this way, the staff may feel more freedom to speak out, thus providing an atmosphere in which dialogue can take place. Staff members often become so immobilized by stress that they cannot recognize resources that are available and close at hand. These resources can be explored and utilized with the help of the nurse-administrator.

Working with the Burned-Out Employee

Stress clearly is a part of everyone's normal living. Even though the psychiatric–mental health nursing administrator may be sensitive to the stressors affecting employees and the steps that can be taken to alleviate stress, it cannot be totally eliminated. Within the department, insignificant, routine changes, as well as planned long-range changes, occur. Nothing stays the same, and employees are always faced with stressful situations, no matter how much is done to minimize the stress involved.

The stress associated with change is known as adaptive stress (Selye, 1976). Everly and Girdano (1980) noted that "change is stressful because it disrupts the psychological and physiological rhythms that accompany all human behavior" (p. 20). Every day we are confronted with stress associated with change. The ultimate outcome of the change, whether for the better or not, is unimportant. The very fact that each person must adjust to a change that causes disruption in personal homeostasis causes stress. Usually, adapting to such change is accomplished with relative ease, but additional or prolonged stages of change and other stressors can all contribute to burnout. Some of the changes within the psychiatric–mental health nursing area that promote adaptive stress include policy and procedural changes, promotions (or demotions), restructuring of the department or organization with a new administration, rotating shifts that alter circadian rhythms, and retirement (Everly & Girdano). Even planning for such changes cannot eliminate the occurrence of adaptive stress.

Another factor in burnout is the employee's personality. For some people, stress is a way of life that cannot be altered. The employee who is burnt out may not be able to recover sufficiently to remain a positive, contributing member of the staff. Persons who are under a great amount of stress have difficulty accepting responsibility for their part in the situation. As a result, blame is often placed on the organization, the supervisor, the physicians, and (in some cases) the clients. The employee has lost all control and relinquishes responsibility for personal unhappiness.

The perfectionist, who is always rushing about and never seems to complete tasks, soon falls into a burnout pattern. Time is wasted, frustration heightened, and failure looms in the background. This employee may have a history of frequent job-hopping. When interviewing job applicants, the nurse-administrator may discover that the reasons for leaving previous positions relate to the lack of support from supervisors and the organization's unconcern for the staff's and the clients' welfare. Although this may well be the case, a pattern may emerge that depicts a person who has difficulty taking responsibility for circumstances that could be controlled in an assertive, realistic manner. Unless employees can alter personal expectations to a realistic level and accept human weaknesses in self and others, they may soon become disenchanted with the job and leave the organization within a short period of time. The nurse-administrator should be alerted to this type of work pattern, because past history will surely repeat itself.

The employee suffering from burnout may need time away from the job to regain equilibrium. Using approaches discussed earlier may assist this employee, but additional time off may be needed. Vacations should be encouraged to allow the employee a break from the job and an opportunity to relax and to put the job into perspective. Career planning may be helpful in providing a more systematic and goal-directed approach to the employee for continued and future employment. The psychiatric–mental health nurse administrator may become directly involved in the development of a career-planning program or may work with the personnel department on such a program. A career-planning program could include such activities as assisting staff members with decisions to return to school for degree completion, graduate or postgraduate education, preparing for ANA certification examinations, and looking at career options for the future.

EVALUATION

Even in the most supportive of work environments, stress can become intolerable. The establishing of plans to prevent and to minimize burnout will not guarantee that staff members will always function optimally and be happy with their work. The psychiatric–mental health nursing administrator must constantly assess the climate, being alert to clues that stress is increasing beyond the staff's ability to cope with it effectively. Modifications in the nursing system must be made as soon as the cause of stress is identified. Support, understanding, receptivity, and flexibility are all keys to providing an environment in which professional practice and personal growth can flourish.

REFERENCES

Everly, G.S., & Girdano, D.A. (1980). *The stress mess solution: The causes and cures of stress on the job.* Bowie, Md: R.J. Brady, Co.

McLean, A.A. (1979). *Work stress.* Reading, Mass.: Addison-Wesley.

Pelletier, K.R. (1977). *Mind as healer, mind as slayer.* New York: Dell Publishing Co.

Selye, H. (1976). *The stress of life*. New York: McGraw-Hill.

Veninga, R.L., & Spradly, J.P. (1981). *The work/stress connection: How to cope with job burnout*. Boston: Little, Brown & Co.

SUGGESTED READINGS

Benson, H. (1975). *The relaxation response*. New York: Morrow.

Forsyth, D.M., & Connady, N.J. (1981). Preventing and alleviating staff burnout through a group. *Journal of Psychosocial Nursing and Mental Health Services, 19*(9), 35–38.

Freudenberger, H.J., & Richelson, G. (1980). *Burnout: The high cost of achievement*. Garden City, N.Y.: Doubleday & Co.

Lavandero, R. (1981). Nurse burnout: What can we learn? *Journal of Nursing Administration, 11*(11/12), 17–22.

Nuernberger, P. (1981). *Freedom from stress: A holistic approach*. Honesdale, Pa.: Himalayan International Institute.

Pines, A., & Maslach, C. (1978). Characteristics of staff burnout in mental health settings. *Hospital & Community Psychiatry, 29*(4), 233–237.

Smith, H.L., & Mitry, N.W. (1983). Nurses' quality of working life. *Journal of Nursing Management, 14*(1), 14–18.

Yee, B.H. (1981). The dynamics and management of burnout. *Journal of Nursing Management, 12*(11), 14–16.

Chapter 13

Staffing

In any health care agency providing psychiatric–mental health care, nursing staff are generally the largest group of employees. Hence, the nursing department is the largest cost center producing the highest workload. The nurse-administrator's role is to facilitate the professional practice of nursing within the organization (Smith & Smith, 1977). As a result, a staffing program must exist that identifies the type and the quantity of nursing personnel necessary to provide nursing care at a predetermined level to a specified client population (Nield, 1975).

The psychiatric–mental health nursing administrator's role in staffing the organization is to ensure the provision of qualified staff in sufficient numbers to provide quality psychiatric–mental health nursing care. Achievement of the organization's and the nursing department's goals depends upon how successfully such staff are provided (Lillesand & Mathews, 1977). To staff effectively, the nurse-administrator applies the nursing process to this aspect of administration. Because psychiatric–mental health nursing differs substantially from other nursing specialty areas, information about the staffing of other areas cannot easily be applied to psychiatric–mental health settings. Hence, such information should be carefully adapted to the specific organization.

In developing a staffing program, the administrator should identify the quality of the desired nursing practice. A prediction must then be made of the number and the levels of nursing personnel needed to ensure that the desired quality and volume of nursing practice can be provided. These staff members must then be selected and organized in specific patterns that create a professional environment in which every nurse can practice. Finally, the efficiency and the effectiveness of the staffing program must be evaluated; subsequent revisions can then be made as needed (Nield, 1975).

ASSESSING STAFFING REQUIREMENTS

Impact of the Psychiatric–Mental Health Environment

The psychiatric–mental health environment presents multiple impediments to the determination of staffing requirements. Care must be provided 24 hours a day, 7 days a week. The client census and acuity change constantly—often within a work shift. This nonroutine, nonpredictable, but highly structured environment does not lend itself easily to staffing programs. The longer period of treatment of a psychiatric–mental health client mandates the need for increased coordination, continuity, and consistency of care. Because of these requirements and the use of the therapeutic relationship, many staffing options that prove useful in other nursing practices are unacceptable for general use in the psychiatric–mental health area. Furthermore, many staffing tools developed and applied in medical–surgical or other nursing specialties cannot be applied to the psychiatric–mental health area because of the abstract nature of this nursing practice.

Furthermore, tools and methodologies appropriate to a specific organization often cannot be applied intact to another organization. Modification is particularly necessary in the case of psychiatric–mental health organizations because of the variety of client populations served by organizations that provide acute care, long-term care, day care, outpatient services, and so on.

Relationship of Standards of Care to Staffing Issues

Professional and regulatory standards provide guidelines for the staffing of an organization. The JCAH advises that staffing should be consistent with client care requirements and with the method of client care delivery (Barham & Schneider, 1980). The American Nurses' Association cautions that comparisons of staffing in various organizations are difficult because of the variances in client needs and requirements, availability of support systems, and qualified staff (ANA, 1977). The psychiatric–mental health nursing department should comply with these and other standards from relevant regulatory agencies.

The organization's and the department's staffing philosophies and goals, as well as internally developed standards, are also components of a comprehensive staffing program. The program selected should be based upon standards of nursing practice that have been agreed upon by the nursing staff. Such standards include job descriptions, related evaluations, and standards of expected practice. Performance times, the classification of nursing hours per client, and other similar statistics can also often serve as standards.

Relationship of Practice Patterns to Staffing Issues

The psychiatric–mental health nursing practice pattern and the associated mix of personnel are components of a documented staffing program. The nurse-administrator should determine through assessment which practice pattern is most applicable to the organization or should evaluate the current pattern to assess its delivery of quality care. One of the most challenging nursing management concerns is the delivery of quality nursing care throughout a 24-hour period and the related accountability for such care (Clark, 1977). Psychiatric–mental health nursing shares this concern. It becomes even more important because of the clients' longer length of treatment and the use of the therapeutic relationship as the primary nursing treatment tool.

The *functional* practice pattern is based upon a nurse's completion of specific duties for a group of clients (e.g., assessments, medications, specific group activities). The head nurse is usually the only nurse who is able to achieve a holistic view of each client. This pattern works well in crisis situations, where much must be accomplished by few, because it is high in efficiency; however, it is low in client and staff satisfaction (Arndt & Huckabay, 1975). In psychiatric–mental health nursing, this system would sabotage the concept of the one-to-one therapeutic relationship. The client would come into contact with multiple staff for short periods of time and would be unable to develop trust, which is such a necessary component of the therapeutic relationship.

Team nursing, another practice pattern, is defined as ''a group of people, led by a qualified nurse, who provide for the health needs of an individual or group of people through collaborative and cooperative efforts'' (Douglas, 1973). The central focus of this practice pattern is total client care, and client assignments are often delegated to those team members who are most capable of meeting specific client needs. The team leader, rather than the head nurse, is often the nurse with the most complete picture of the client. This pattern has demonstrated a higher degree of staff productivity than the functional pattern (Harris, 1970), but this result varies with the skill mix of personnel. Some studies indicate that aides or assistants are used only 65 percent of their total time on the unit, LPNs 95 percent, and RNs 100 percent (Clark, 1977). In psychiatric–mental health nursing, this pattern is more conducive to the development of the therapeutic relationship than is the functional pattern. Still, it often splinters the practice of total client care because of the personnel mix.

The *modular* practice pattern is similar to the team pattern but the team is smaller and has responsibility for a smaller group of clients. An experienced registered nurse acts as the module leader with another registered nurse, an LPN, or a nursing assistant, as the other (one-to-two) module member. Usually, a module (2 to 3 staff) is responsible for 10 to 12 clients who are located adjacent to each other on the unit. As in the case of team nursing, there is an overall loss in unit efficiency; increased time is spent in the coordination of delegated work. There is, however, an increased effectiveness in the delivery of care, which is due to the closer client-nurse relationship that develops (Arndt & Huckabay, 1975).

The *team* or *module* practice patterns are more appropriate for psychiatric–mental health nursing than is the functional pattern; there is greater opportunity for the development of a nurse-client relationship. However, if team or module members are not registered nurses, the registered nurse module leader must spend additional time in the supervision of client care, rather than in the application of that time to the development of the therapeutic client relationships. A therapeutic client relationship may develop with a paraprofessional, but this person is not qualified to develop and to implement an individualized care plan.

The *primary nursing* practice pattern focuses upon the planning of client care rather than upon the actual completion of the needed care (Arndt & Huckabay, 1975). This focus theoretically provides the highest level of professional practice and quality of care that is achievable (Norby & Freund, 1977). The functional and team practice patterns deny clients "sustained contact with nurses, [and, therefore], . . . actually interfere with the nurses' opportunities to employ the intellectual process nursing entails" (Halloran, 1983, p. 17). This opportunity to function more independently allows the nurse more freedom to use nursing judgment, creativity, and the necessary teaching skills (Smith & Smith, 1977). Although efficiency is decreased, care effectiveness is increased substantially, and errors are decreased with the elimination of positions in the chain of command (Arndt & Huckabay). The head nurse is no longer the overseer of client care but a collaborator in the delivery of care.

This practice pattern has been studied in various organizations, thus validating its numerous advantages. There is fixed accountability, increased comprehensiveness, and continuity of care, all of which lead to improved quality of care (Parasuraman, Drake, & Zammuto, 1982). This continuity of care is particularly crucial in psychiatric–mental health nursing. Faster recuperation for selected client populations leads to a decreased length of stay and a resulting decrease in cost per client day (Munson & Clinton, 1979)—an important result in terms of cost containment of health care costs. Clients are more satisfied with nursing practice when the hours of professional nursing care available per client are higher (Abdellah & Levine, 1958). Along with the increased client satisfaction, there is an associated increased client ability to articulate health learning and increased client participation in care. Through such learning, one might also expect an improved compliance-to-treatment rate among patients, which would, again, decrease health care costs by decreasing the need for repeat hospitalizations.

The advantages of the primary nursing pattern are similar for personnel. There is a decrease in errors of commission and omission. The nursing process becomes more visible and is viewed as more important. An increase in the self-esteem of the registered nurse leads to an increase in job satisfaction, which in turn leads to decreased turnover and absenteeism. Interpersonal relationships with other disciplines are improved, and the work environment becomes more consistent with the goals of educational programs and professional nursing ideals (Munson & Clinton, 1979).

Obviously, an assignment system that offers these cost-effective advantages and increased nurse-client contact time would prove beneficial to psychiatric–mental health nursing. Such a practice pattern would foster the therapeutic relationship between nurse and client and would facilitate delivery of the quality of care mandated by many standards and the professions. The primary nursing practice pattern works most effectively to promote a premorbid level of health when the nursing support systems are efficient and the clients have a high degree of "dependence on professional nursing care" (Shukla, 1982, p. 14)—such as the psychiatric–mental health client. Because psychiatric–mental health clients do have an intense need for such professional (RN) nursing care, the efficiency of the organization's nursing support systems should be assessed to determine whether primary nursing should be the practice pattern of choice.

PLANNING A STAFFING PROGRAM

Documentation of the Program

Before the development of an initial psychiatric–mental health staffing program or the revision of an existing format, related organizational and departmental documents should be reviewed. The following concerns should be included in such a review:

- the organization's philosophy, goals, and objectives
- nursing practice philosophy, goals, and objectives
- recruitment policies and procedures
- scheduling policies and procedures
- applicable standards
- assignment patterns—individualized to each unit as necessary
- nursing department budget

If any of these are not documented or not reflective of current organizational and nursing practice, they should be revised.

Documentation of the selected staffing program should begin with a statement of the psychiatric–mental health nursing department's staffing purposes, goals, objectives, and the services to be provided. These should, of course, reflect the organization's mission and goals. The data base for the determination of staffing needs should include the identified client population, with the relevant demographic statistics of age, sex, diagnosis, and length of stay. Staff data about numbers, skill levels, and salary costs should also be included. A specific methodology should be identified and used to determine the number and levels of the staff required and the rationale for the selection of this methodology. Budgetary resources for the supply of staff members should be detailed. Delineated assignment patterns should reflect policy and procedure statements and personnel guidelines. They should also include relevant policies and procedures for each section or unit of the organization. The number and level of required staff should be defined for each unit.

Finally, an evaluation plan should be provided to facilitate the continual review and revision of the overall program (Aydelotte, 1973). Performance standards that provide a method to evaluate the effectiveness and the quality of nursing practice on each unit should be included (ANA, 1977). A system should be identified that monitors the effectiveness of the overall program, examines unit assignment patterns and manpower requirements at specified intervals in view of changing conditions and productivity, and initiates realistic modifications (ANA, 1977).

Once documented, the staffing program will reinforce a conceptual model of nursing practice: a theoretically sound one that reflects the latest trends and research information in the area of psychiatric–mental health nursing (ANA, 1977). Also, assignment patterns will exist that recognize differences in clinical nursing practice needs, variations in style and sophistication of management, organizational environment, and available nursing resources.

Documentation Data

Positive reinforcement should be provided for the creative, effective, and efficient use of nursing staff resources. Staffing personnel should be encouraged to assess and to evaluate staffing issues and concerns in a creative manner. This approach is aided by the staffing program; it provides the information needed for staffing decisions in a concise, clear, and timely fashion (ANA, 1977). Basic information is required about the client population: the level, complexity and duration of care needs; general health status; age; socioeconomic conditions; client expectations; and general factors that influence the perceptions of health needs (Arndt & Huckabay, 1975). Personnel factors that should be included in the documentation are the number and skill mix of required and available personnel, the policies about work hours and shift rotations, job descriptions and role function explanations, education and experience requirement levels, existing competitive markets, and the work ethic prevalent throughout the community (Arndt & Huckabay). Other factors that should be included are average sick time used per skill level of personnel, leaves of absence, vacations, staff development needs, and turnover rates (ANA, 1977).

Because organizational environments vary radically, program documentation must be adapted and applied to information about the specific environment. Such information should include the physical layout of the organization, the number of beds, the services offered, the availability of equipment and supplies, the supportive services from other departments and their response times to requests, the services available to personnel, the existence of automation, the methods of dispensing medications, the size of the clerical support staff, the size and mix of the medical staff (Donovan, 1980), and the budgetary staffing allowances per unit. Organization-specific statistics are also needed about the adjusted client days, the occupancy rates, the total annual admissions, and the average length of stay (Levine, 1973). Department-specific data that is needed includes the average nursing hours per client day, per client classification, per shift, and per personnel mix (Sahney).

Assignment Systems

Once the nursing practice pattern has been selected and sufficient staffing provided, the assignment system must be implemented. This system often depends upon the mix and number of available personnel, the available budget, the training and in-service programs available within the organization, and the policy in regard to professional nursing practice and supervision (Aydelotte, 1973). In considering the assignment pattern to select, the nurse-administrator divides the nursing activities into those that are care-giving and those that involve care-planning.

Organizational decisions should be made as to whether these two groups of activities should be performed by one or many persons and whether this assignment should be continuous or should vary (Munson & Clinton, 1979). The difficulty of the assignments involved should also be considered, and the assessment should be made on the following requirements of assignment: the staff's knowledge and the skill required, the manual dexterity needed, the organizational ability necessary, the problem-solving abilities required, the accessibility to supplies and equipment, the administrative support, the comfort of the client, the usual method of assignment (Norby & Freund, 1977), the position descriptions, the education and experience of staff members, the staff's expectations, the staff's work ethic, the organization's financial resources, the personnel policies, the support systems, and the number of beds per client population (McConnell & Wiley, 1977). Remember that the difficulty of activities increases with the increased activity of the group, the increased intensity of illness of the involved clients, and the increased number of clients (Norby & Freund). Final documentation of the chosen assignment pattern includes the definition of goals, determination of the range of activities included, and the resources needed (Straker & Cummings, 1978).

Cost-Effectiveness

Before the decisions about the staffing program, the assignment system, and the practice pattern are made final, the package must be proved to be cost-effective and to have sufficient support within the organization for acceptance. A cost-effectiveness analysis is often used when benefits are difficult to measure, as in psychiatric–mental health nursing. Certain results or objectives are selected; the goal is to demonstrate the minimum cost of attaining the desired goal or objective. Components of such an analysis include background information about the situation, the desired goal or objective, and the cost of the goal or objective. For example, the following background information is needed to demonstrate the cost-effectiveness of a staffing program: budgeted census, average daily census, budgeted full-time equivalents (FTEs), current FTEs, beds not in use because of inadequate staffing, current FTE per sick-time replacement, current FTE per recruitment and orientation costs and the same costs projected as a result of the suggested staffing program (LJD Associates, 1981). Additional personnel costs that may be needed include FTE changes, salary benefit changes, nursing-hour changes, money-spent-in-recruitment changes, agency-usage change, sick-time and overtime changes, and stress analysis in comparison to a standard level of expected stress.

With this information, the following steps in a cost-effectiveness analysis begin. The desired goal or objective is identified. The program that would enable the achievement of this goal or objective is developed and implemented, often on a trial or pilot basis. The cost of the program per unit is identified—for example, per client day, client visit, client classification. The outcome of the program intervention is then assessed, particularly in terms of projected cost versus actual and previous costs (LJD Associates, 1981).

An outcome of the cost-effectiveness analysis is the itemization of nursing care on a client's bill. For example, separate charges could be listed for one-to-one therapy, group therapy, client education, precautions, and so on. This practice is also facilitated by documentation of the direct care provided by the nursing staff to the client during the course of treatment (Williams, 1977). Costs may be determined that are based upon client care categories, client care delivered, or client days. This technique does facilitate cost-effectiveness analysis and does enable the nursing department to become an income-producing department of an organization, rather than a cost drain. When charging for nursing care, by whichever mechanism, the nurse-administrator should remember that the costs should include administrative time, education, orientation, and research. If these components of nursing practice are not included, the value of nursing practice is underestimated. This devaluation will eventually lead to cost-effectiveness difficulties.

Development of Program Support

As the cost-effectiveness of the staffing program is being documented, the program should be explained to and explored by the nursing staff and supportive services. The nursing department does not function in isolation. As a component of an organization, a single department achieves success or failure depending upon the support it receives—particularly the psychiatric–mental health area. Other departments that come in contact with nursing staff can do much to increase or to decrease the prevalent stress levels. The administration of an organization must be supportive of a staffing program's components, for, without the support of this major group, the psychiatric–mental health nursing department may not have sufficient personnel or the financial resources to supply needed staff.

Another major group whose support is needed is the nursing staff. In order for a staffing program to be successful, nurses must agree that such a program addresses realistic problems by meaningful strategies (Norby & Freund, 1977). Proposed solutions must be presented in an open and direct manner to provide answers to the staff's questions. Approaches must be flexible and must convey a caring attitude (Van Meter, 1982). Such an attitude produces an environment conducive to the delivery of quality psychiatric–mental health nursing care.

IMPLEMENTING A STAFFING PROGRAM

Once the foundation has been established for the psychiatric–mental health staffing program, it should be implemented by those persons accountable for the actual staffing process. These staff members should be encouraged to use the preestablished guidelines as a basis for the provision of the required staff members. A creative atmosphere should exist to facilitate staffing activities appropriate to changing departmental or client needs.

Creative Applications of the Staffing Process

Creative applications involved in the staffing process should include client placement according to staff availability; staff allocation according to client census; planning, budgetary, and quality assurance innovations; and charging for nursing practice (Meyer, 1979). Client placement according to staff availability is also called gate-keeping. This approach requires that all services or units within the organization are similar. If there is only one area that provides for direct nursing care, this alternative is not possible. Admission information must be available and sufficiently complete to enable a designated employee to assign a client to a service or unit that can meet the admission needs of the client. This employee must be kept continually informed about the activities, acuity level, and the staff availability of each service or unit in order to assign the admission properly (Arndt & Huckabay, 1975).

Forecasting Staffing Needs

Forecasting staffing needs is an innovative planning approach that addresses the problem of staffing resources. Generally, an organization's personnel are budgeted at a level adequate to satisfy peak client demands (Meglino, 1979). Most organizations do not have a formal method for accommodating fluctuations in client census on either a daily or a seasonal basis. Prediction of staffing needs may be done on a monthly, quarterly, biannual, or annual basis or on a time frame that is suited for a specific organization. Predictions can also be made on an organization-wide basis or by service or unit.

In large organizations, a forecasting committee may prove to be useful. Members of this group could include a nurse-administrator, a hospital administrator, an admitting department head, a management engineering representative, a staffing coordinator, and several first-line nurse-managers (Althaus, Hardyck, Pierce, & Rodgers, 1982). The wide variety of representation on this committee would enable the group to secure the needed information easily for the prediction of staffing needs. Such information would include

- the staffing history of the organization,
- the budget,
- the number of client beds and services available,
- the nursing hours per client classification,
- the client population,
- the method of nursing practice,
- the available support services,
- the architectural features,
- the skill levels of personnel,
- the client classification system, and
- the staffing policies (Nield, 1975).

A variety of methods are needed for the initial daily calculation of unit workloads. Staffing needs and available resources should be identified. Data about workload requirements and necessary staffing adjustments should be collected daily (Norby & Freund, 1977).

One system for determining baseline data can be outlined as follows:

1. Collect weekly client load data for each unit for a year, along with the number of nursing hours needed to meet the client load.

2. Determine seasonal changes by reviewing admission and discharge figures and client census and classification statistics.
3. Identify a staffing planning period based upon seasonal changes.
4. Predict the daily client load for each unit or service for each shift during the planning period:

   - Identify two-week periods.
   - Calculate the average nursing workloads.
   - Adjust the workloads by the projected change in census.
   - Determine the number of nursing hours needed per shift.
   - Add nonproductive time before determining FTEs.
   - Calculate the average staff needed per shift (Meglino, 1979).
   - For weekends, calculate the number of hours of client care needed per weekend per unit or service; convert this information into the number of employees needed; and multiply this number by two if staff members receive every other weekend off (Lehman & Friesen, 1977).

5. Repeat this process for each planning period.

Once predictions are completed, forecasts must be compared with the current staffing to determine the margin of error in order to make adjustments in future forecasts. Other statistics must be monitored and compared with forecast documentation in order to ensure the accuracy of future forecasts. Such statistics include the client classification totals, the census, and the nursing hours per client classification. Activity changes that include the addition or the deletion of activities to nursing workloads also affect previously determined forecasts (McConnell & Wiley, 1977).

Should the forecast predict a need for higher staffing, alternatives such as part-time or contingency personnel, float pools, overtime, and so on can be used. (These alternatives will be discussed in relation to psychiatric–mental health nursing at a later point.) However, if the forecast predicts overstaffing, existing policies and procedures should be assessed in an attempt to decrease this costly problem. There are, of course, traditional methods of encouraging the staff to use vacation time or to work a shift or a unit or a service in which the need may be greater. However, an alternative that may prove as cost-effective is encouraging staff members to take a day off without pay. This plan would require that the staff involved did not lose any benefits which accrued based upon hours worked. For many nurses, this option would provide the benefit of additional free time without loss of benefits. Like similar benefits, a system would be required (e.g., seniority, shift preference, etc.) that would enable the nurse in charge to administer the benefit fairly.

Supplemental Staffing Methods

Once staffing standards and practice patterns based upon nursing care standards have been established, there will still be a need to supplement the staff because of staff vacancies or client needs. Without such additional staff members, basic nursing care would still be delivered, but the overall quality of such care would suffer. Studies have shown that nurses establish priorities in activities under conditions of marginal or unsatisfactory staffing. The activities completed most consistently are those related to the medical plan of treatment (Williams, 1977). Hence, psychiatric–mental health nursing activities would not necessarily be completed in such situations. For example, the activities most adversely affected by inadequate staffing are observation of the client and communication with the client or the family—two of the most important psychiatric–mental health nursing actions. Furthermore, charge nurse judgments of less than satisfactory staffing are strongly related to perceived decline in their abilities to provide direct care services (Williams, 1977). Obviously, the nurse-administrator should strive to provide adequate staffing for all units or services at all times.

Pulling Staff

There are several staffing alternatives available, but few of them prove totally successful within the psychiatric–mental health setting. One of the most common alternatives used is the concept of *moving* or *pulling* staff from one unit or service to another. This practice is often used in an in-house attempt to redistribute maldistributed staff. However, this action disrupts the working groups that have been established by the nursing staff on the involved units. Moving staff from one unit to another threatens the unity of the involved work group and often leaves the transferred staff angry and insecure (Arndt & Huckabay, 1975).

A work group provides the organization with the advantages of increased security for the group's members, which further provides social satisfaction, improved interpersonal relationships, and increased self-actualization with increased responsibility and incentives. These benefits result in an emotional commitment of the staff to the work group and the unit or service (Price, 1970). It is obvious that these benefits of the work group are also beneficial to psychiatric–mental health nursing practice.

The moving of staff from a work group is not a popular alternative, because it can create conflict. It negatively affects the cohesiveness and morale of the sending group, and the receiving group may be reluctant to accept the staff member (Vestal & Dean, 1981). In addition, the transferred person is in unfamiliar surroundings and has a fear of being unable to give quality care. Should this person have had primary clients, these clients would also experience disruption of care by not receiving care from the staff member most qualified to give it. However, a person's refusal to move may result in disciplinary action—a result that would leave the transferred person with no choice. This feeling of powerlessness causes personnel to function at less than optimum capacity. Furthermore, the nurse-manager is placed in the no-win situation of having to make and to enforce an unpopular, often destructive, decision.

The sending and receiving units or services also experience negative consequences from this staffing alternative. The sending unit is not allowed to enjoy the period of overstaffing that can be a respite from times of understaffing. Or this unit may become understaffed as a result of the pulling action. The receiving unit often has questions about the capability of the transferred staff, and these questions may be interpreted as a lack of confidence in the transferred staff member's ability, creating further insecurity.

Thus, moving staff results in little job satisfaction or continuity of care in psychiatric–mental health nursing (Holle, 1982)—unless the transferred staff member can function in a support capacity, such as medication dispensing or other nonprimary care. With other assignments, this person does little to sustain the quality of care unless the documentation system of the receiving unit or service is extensive, and the staff member is provided time to review the cases of the assigned clients.

In many agencies, however, this alternative is in existence until a more effective method for the provision of staff can be determined. In this situation, there are actions that can be taken to facilitate the process. The nurse-manager involved should make the decision to float a staff member as early as possible and should communicate directly with the involved parties as soon as possible. The situation and the rationale involved should be thoroughly explained in a direct fashion that allows for questions and expressions of concern. This clarification should decrease the anxiety involved and create an environment in which staff or units are perceived as helping each other, rather than as causing disruption (Vestal & Dean, 1981). As far as possible, the sending unit should determine which staff member is to be sent. In most cases, the transferred person should be a registered nurse, because this person provides an overall versatility that cannot be provided by other personnel.

Rotation of Staff

Another internal solution that is often used to provide additional coverage of units or services without resorting to an outside agency is the practice of *rotation*. This is a system whereby staff alternatively work an off-shift (either afternoons or midnights or both) with the day shift. The change of shifts can occur within a week or for longer periods on a regular basis throughout the year. Although such rotations should be distributed on an equal basis to all staff members, it has been found that rotations are often given to those who do not wish to involve themselves and to the less skilled personnel (Georgette, 1970).

When staff members are rotating, the body rhythms of the involved persons need time to adjust. To cope with the psychological and physiological changes involved in the changes in shifts, the staff need an additional day to recycle (Holle, 1982), but it is seldom provided. Changes occur in multiple body systems—temperature, urinary excretion of electrolytes, and the ability of the body to maintain urinary osmolality (Felton, 1975). Sleep is shorter and of poorer quality. It has also been found that a rapid shift in temporal referents—as happens when one is rotating to off-shifts—is a cause of stress (Felton). When a person is working the off-shift, patterns of social routine are also changed. Such dysynchronization of circadian rhythms could lead to psychomotor inefficiency and would exaggerate any feelings of malaise and irritability that arise from the loss of sleep (Felton).

Obviously, rotation works counterproductively to the goals of psychiatric–mental health nursing. For example, the rotating staff would not be able to operate at the optimum level needed for psychiatric–mental health nursing. In addition, rotations work against the therapeutic relationship. When a staff member is rotated to an off-shift, particularly in the unit practicing some form of primary nursing, the staff member is not always able to be assigned to the same group of clients. Hence, the previously developed therapeutic relationship is disrupted. If the clients are assigned to the rotating staff member, the off-shift staff who normally works with those clients must then be reassigned and those therapeutic relationships are disrupted. Furthermore, the client also experiences disorientation when a daytime staff member begins working afternoons or midnights and then is changed back to days. Confusion and disorientation for some clients as well as the retardation of the therapeutic relationship occurs.

If the rotation is to the midnight shift, the therapeutic relationship is totally disrupted unless the client is awake on this shift. Of course, such staff rotation may disrupt the client's sleep cycle, because the client may attempt to remain awake in order to continue working on defined problems with the rotating staff member.

When the unit or service and the organization are committed to this form of staffing coverage and do forecast rotation schedules for the purpose of manipulating client assignments, the expenditure of time and effort and the increased stress and frustration will also have repercussions on the delivery of client care. If such a system were to be used within psychiatric–mental health nursing, the practice pattern of primary nursing would ease some of the inherent difficulties. The primary nurse would be responsible for planning the overall care and would have to work closely with the associate nurse. When a rotation shift was approaching, the primary nurse would have to discuss this with the clients and work through any repercussions. The clients would then be instructed to continue working on the defined problems with the associate nurse who had also been closely involved in this transition phase. Should the client still be hospitalized when the primary nurse returned to the day shift, the entire process would have to be repeated. This routine would add undue and unnecessary stress to a psychiatric client's already stressful treatment course.

Use of Resources External to the Organization

A facility may choose to arrange for additional staffing by an outside staffing resource. Such a resource may be a registry, a supplemental nursing service, or an agency. Each resource provides different services, and each should be assessed in terms of organizational and personnel needs. A supplemental nursing service screens its nurses and verifies their licenses. A registry may be operated by a state nurses' association or a private proprietary company. They screen their nurses but do not provide bonding services, nor do they withhold taxes from paychecks. The nurse contracts with the organization and then pays a percentage of the salary to the registry (Donovan, 1980). An agency, in contrast, places nurses in organizations for a fee or a commission and has no responsibility for bonding the nurses.

The principal reasons for the use of outside staffing resources are cost control and the difficulty in filling vacancies. Permanent employees can be replaced during absences so that staffing levels can be maintained. Emergencies can be met, and hard-to-fill shifts can be covered with a minimum of additional work. In a new organization, outside nurses can be used until permanent staff can be hired and oriented (Jett, 1977). Organizations can also use these nurses for staffing needs due to increased patient census, vacancies, or special or private duty nurse requests (Langford & Prescott, 1979).

Budgetary constraints should be examined in order to determine whether this staffing alternative is truly cost-effective. The total wage package of a nurse should be compared to the wage of the outside nurse to determine if a cost savings is occurring (Anzalone, 1981). In addition to these actual costs, other costs of ensuring competence, orientation, possible staff resentment, ensuring quality client care, and diminished accountability should also be assessed (Nielsen, 1981).

In psychiatric–mental health nursing, the use of outside nurses may be viewed in the same manner as the staffing alternative of moving staff. The outside nurse may be helpful if used in a supportive role, such as medication dispensing. However, unless this person is regularly scheduled on a particular unit or service, the outside nurse cannot function in a full capacity because of the lack of knowledge of the unit or service and a lack of time to develop a therapeutic relationship. Clients cannot establish any level of trust with this person because the nurse may be assigned to that unit or service only once. The outside nurse can provide custodial care, but little else.

However, if a psychiatric–mental health nursing department is forced to rely upon outside resources for staffing, there is much that can be done to attempt to control the quality of practice. The departmental and organizational philosophy should be reevaluated to determine whether the use of outside nurses is consistent with these philosophies. Outside resources should be assessed and periodically reviewed for their compliance with predetermined criteria, such as license verification, CPR training, competency testing, professional liability insurance, and evidence of an annual physical examination that includes TB test or chest x-ray. Documentation about each nurse should include clinical experience, education, skills inventory, references, and evidence of continuing education (Lewin & Brown, 1981). In addition to internally developed standards, compliance with external standards should be ensured. For example, JCAH states that an orientation and evaluation process must occur before the use of these nurses (Lewin & Brown). ANA also has developed guidelines that assist in assuring quality of practice.

Scheduling mechanisms and associated policies should be developed to reflect standards and criteria (Shanks & Potempa, 1981). Such guidelines should indicate that outside nurses must not be relied upon as the core staff or be used to cover for core staff on days off. Attempts should be made, however, to assign the same nurses to the same unit or service in order to increase consistency and decrease orientations needs (Shanks & Potempa). Each nurse should receive an update on client status and be assigned in a fashion that is least disruptive to continuity of care.

One standard of performance should be expected for all nurses. Outside nurses should receive a standard orientation that prepares them to function appropriately. Their evaluation should be based upon defined job expectations. However, if this staffing alternative must be used, consideration should be given to the establishment of an internal nursing resource group. Through this mechanism, the organization might be able to retain nurses who would otherwise leave. Thus, it could provide high quality personnel during times of need. This alternative would satisfy many of the reasons expressed by nurses for seeking employment with an outside staffing resource. They would experience convenience, flexibility, and the opportunity to work on a unit or service that is fully staffed. They would receive the additional benefits of better pay, additional income, and the ability to abstain from the internal politics of a unit or service.

The organization's internal nursing resource group could also eliminate many of the negative aspects of nurses from an outside staffing resource. There would not be a consistent need for orientation, nor would there be a lack of continuity of care or team cohesiveness. Nurses would not need to experience the isolation or the apathetic attitudes that often occur with an associated loss of motivation and professionalism (Donovan, 1980).

Nurses often leave hospital employment because of lack of professional status, poor salaries, few educational opportunities, and inflexible schedules. A psychiatric–mental health organization with an internal nursing resource group could provide the nurse with flexibility of scheduling and could guarantee a certain number of days per week. Salaries would be commensurate with outside staffing resources, but with a small associated package of benefits. Orientation would occur only once, and, with assignment to the same unit or service, nurses would develop cohesiveness and team spirit.

Companion Floor System

Another mechanism to provide additional staffing on a flexible basis is the concept of a *companion floor system* (Arndt & Huckabay, 1975). In this system, two or more similar units or services form a network in order to provide staffing in times of shortage (Bahr, Badour, & Hill, 1977). The benefits arise from the staff's familiarity with the units or services involved and the resulting decrease in anxiety and the increase in ability to provide quality care. This alternative does require the additional time of orienting the staff to more than one unit or service; however, even with such orientation, all stress cannot be reduced because of the usual procedural differences between units or services (Thorpe, 1980).

Again, in psychiatric–mental health nursing, these staff members could function as support staff to free regular personnel to assume additional direct care responsibilities. These staff members can also be expected to provide monitoring and general supervision of the clients after they have been introduced to the involved clients as "someone who is working with them for the day." The companion floor alternative would prove beneficial as a result of the increased familiarity with policies and procedures, as well as an increased comfort level with the clients.

Part-Time Staff

The use of part-time staff is another popular alternative for the provision of additional nursing staff. Part-time staff may work on an on-call or contingency basis, working when they are requested by the organization. Benefits in this case are usually minimal, if any, beyond a basic salary. The number of days to be worked is usually contracted by the organization and the nurse at the inception of the work agreement. Such staff may be asked to work any shift, and may or may not receive on-call pay. This arrangement, again, is defined within the initial work agreement. Generally, some weekend work is expected as part of the original agreement.

A part-time staff member may also work on a per diem basis. If so, there are no additional benefits, but the salary may be adjusted to reflect the lack of benefits and to be competitive with outside staffing resources. Again, weekend work in some form is expected.

For psychiatric–mental health nursing, the part-time staffing alternative is a viable option for the provision of additional staff. When scheduled on a regular basis and when properly included in the assignment of client care, the part-time staff member can do much to sustain the quality and continuity of client care.

Job Sharing

A new form of part-time employment is job sharing—a "voluntary agreement in which two persons share one full-time position" (Bardi, 1981). Each person is paid a salary for the hours worked and receives the fringe benefits of a full-time position, prorated to the actual number of hours employed. This program should be attractive to nurses; it provides the flexibility of a part-time position with more benefits than are usually available. The part-time nature of the work results in increased scheduling flexibility. Because the nurses are able to exert more control over their work environment, absenteeism and turnover are decreased. Productivity is increased as a result of the decreased use of temporary or on-call nurses. Burnout should also be decreased, because of the decrease in stress experienced from the support each job-sharer receives from the partner. The organization would benefit from the decreased recruitment and overtime costs (Bardi).

The question remains whether such a program could prove cost-effective within the organization. This program does require a rather complicated system of record keeping. Hours worked must be correlated with salary and fringe benefits. Costs may increase as a result of adjustments made to the unemployment insurances, worker's compensation, taxes, and the orientation required for two persons rather than one (Bardi, 1981).

Within the psychiatric–mental health area, such an alternative would be useful in providing additional staff if there were clear communication between job-sharers and other personnel by an extensive documentation system. Such activities would be needed to maintain the continuity of care. If done well, such an arrangement might even be used within a primary nursing practice pattern if the job-sharers had primary responsibility for one group of clients. Research may find that such an arrangement may be even more therapeutic than the service of the traditional five-days-per-week primary nurse, because the client would receive seven-days-per-week care that would be consistent in its approach.

Whichever approach is chosen to provide additional staff, the quality and continuity of care must be maintained. Through a careful evaluation of the options available, each option can be reviewed for cost-effectiveness, feasibility, and quality of resulting care. Client care should not be sacrificed in order to provide adequate physical coverage of units or services by the nursing staff.

EVALUATING THE PROGRAM

Regardless of the staffing methodology, the practice pattern, or the staffing alternative selected, the nurse-administrator should be able to demonstrate the system's contribution to the quality of care (see Exhibit 13–1). To determine the effectiveness of a staffing plan, the effects of client conditions must be measured and related to the number of personnel and their cost (Aydelotte, 1973). Although the amount of nursing care that an organization gives is a significant index of the quality of that care (Price, 1970), there is difficulty in defining that quality because of the problem of translating theoretical concepts into measurable behavior (Somers, 1977).

Some attributes of quality care that have been defined include comprehensiveness, continuity and coordination of care, and accountability. The *comprehensiveness* of nursing care is defined as the provision of all aspects of the nursing process—assessing, planning, implementing, and evaluating—in the delivery of nursing care (Munson & Clinton, 1979). Nursing care that demonstrates *continuity* is that care which is client-centered and is uninterrupted in time. When the responsibility for the total nursing care of a particular client resides with an identifiable nurse, as in primary nursing, that nurse is accountable for that client's care. Finally, the collaboration of the health professionals providing client care in order to synthesize a plan ensures the *coordination* aspect of quality care (Munson & Clinton). All these attributes suffer when over- or under-staffing occurs (Norby & Freund, 1977). Hence, the provision of the proper mix of competent nursing personnel facilitates these definable aspects of quality client care.

Concrete evaluation of the nursing care provided can be done by incident reports, study of omitted activities, nursing audits, correlation of client and personnel questionnaires, and daily staffing reports that compare staff available

---

Exhibit 13–1 Criteria for Evaluating a Staffing Program

1. Nursing audits indicate that the objectives of nursing practice are being met. Or, if they are not being met, analysis of the audit findings indicates that nonstaffing factors were the cause of the noncompliance.
2. The nursing staff practices in compliance with preestablished performance standards. If they do not, the reasons for the noncompliance are other than staffing related factors.
3. Staffing patterns for units/services comply with predetermined patterns.
4. Schedules provide documentation of such compliance and any daily variability in staffing numbers falls within acceptable ranges.
5. The nursing staff, via an objectively established evaluation mechanism, express satisfaction with the scheduling and assignment system.
6. The staffing program's costs fall within the established limits.
7. The staffing patterns are reexamined on a regular basis for adequacy in relation to current staffing standards, and changing practices, needs and trends.*

---

*Adapted from *Nursing staff requirements for in-patient health care services* (p. 8) by the American Nurses' Association, 1977, Kansas City, Mo.: Author. © 1977 by the American Nurses' Association. Adapted by permission.

against staff required (Naber, Seizyk, & Wilde, 1977). In order to determine whether a specialized staffing or scheduling alternative plan works, the nursing office can audit charts, incident reports, infection control statistics, sick time and overtime costs, and pre- and post-pilot project results to document the cost-effectiveness of the proposal (Feichtel-Pascuzzo, 1981).

Evaluation of the adequacy of a staffing and scheduling program should be done on a regular basis. When coupled with an evaluation of the quality of the nursing practice within a facility, it provides sound documentation for the maintenance of the current system or, if necessary, the rationale for needed modification. Such documentation will be helpful whether the material is being presented to the administration or to the nursing staff.

REFERENCES

Abdellah, F., & Levine, E. (1958). Effect of nurse staffing on satisfactions with nursing care. *Hospital Monograph Series, 4* (Serial No. G 11258).

Althaus, J.N., Hardyck, N.M., Pierce, P.B., & Rodgers, M.S. (1982). Nurse staffing in a decentralized organization: Part II. *Journal of Nursing Administration, 12*(4), 18–22.

American Nurses' Association. (1977). *Nursing staff requirements for in-patient health care services.* Kansas City, Mo.: Author.

Anzalone, C. (1981). Planned supplemental staffing is a practical alternative. *Hospitals, 55*(6), 70–73.

Arndt, C., & Huckabay, L.M.D. (1975). *Nursing administration theory for practice with a systems approach.* St. Louis, Mo.: C.V. Mosby Co.

Aydelotte, M.K. (1973). Staffing for high quality care. *Hospitals, 47*(2), 58–60, 65.

Bahr, J., Badour, G., & Hill, H.L. (1977). Innovative methodology enhances nursing deployment, cuts costs. *Hospitals, 51*(8), 104–109.

Bardi, C.A. (1981). Job-sharing alternative draws nurses back to the hospital. *Hospitals, 55*(12), 71–72.

Barham, V.Z., & Schneider, W.R. (1980). MATRIX: A unique patient classification system. *Journal of Nursing Administration, 10*(10), 25–31.

Clark, E.L. (1977). A model of nurse staffing for effective patient care. *Journal of Nursing Administration, 7*(2), 22–27.

Donovan, L. (1980). Is temporary staffing worth it? *RN, 43*(9), 37–39.

Douglas, L.M. (1973). *Mosby's comprehensive review series.* St. Louis, Mo.: C.V. Mosby Co.

Feichtel-Pascuzzo, S.A. (1981). The 12 hour day. *Nursing Life, 1*(3), 56–59.

Felton, G. (1975). Body rhythm effects on rotating work shifts. *Journal of Nursing Administration, 5*(3), 16–19.

Georgette, J.K. (1970). Staffing by patient classification. *Nursing Clinics of North America, 5*(2), 329–339.

Halloran, E.J. (1983). Staffing assignment: By task or by patient. *Journal of Nursing Management, 14*(8), 16–18.

Harris, D.H. (1970). Staffing requirements. *Hospitals, 44*(8), 64–70.

Holle, M.L. (1982). Staffing: What the books don't tell you! *Journal of Nursing Management, 13*(3), 14–16.

Jett, M. (1977). Use of temporary nursing personnel as cost-control measures. *Hospital Topics, 55*(7), 48–50.

Langford, T.L., & Prescott, P.A. (1979). Hospitals and supplemental nursing agencies: An uneasy balance. *Journal of Nursing Administration, 9*(10), 16–20.

Lehman, M.W., & Friesen, Q.J. (1977). Centralized control system cuts costs, boosts morale. *Hospitals, 51*(10), 75–76, 78, 80.

Levine, E. (Ed.). (1973). *Research on nurse staffing in hospitals, report of the conference on May, 1972.* (NIH, DHEW Publication No. 73–434.) Washington, D.C.: U.S. Government Printing Office.

Lewin, B.A., & Brown, L.E. (1981). Monitoring supplemental staffing agencies. *Journal of Nursing Management, 12*(9), 56–60, 62–63.

Lillesand, K., & Mathews, L.L. (1977). The staffing function and management techniques. *Nursing Administration Quarterly, 1*(4), 27–30.

LJD Associates. (1981). *Cost effectiveness analysis of nurse staffing systems.* Program #2. Colorado Springs, Colo.: Author.

McConnell, E., & Wiley, L. (1977). Staffing should be spelled $taffing or how many staff nurses are enough? *Nursing 77, 7*(11), 97–101.

Meglino, B. (1979). A methodology for nurse staffing. *California Management Review, 21*(3), 82–93.

Meyer, D. (1979, March). *A comprehensive approach to staffing.* Paper presented at the Journal of Nursing Administration Conference, Los Angeles, California.

Munson, F., & Clinton, J. (1979). Defining nursing assignment patterns. *Nursing Research, 28*(4), 243–248.

Naber, M., Seizyk, J., & Wilde, N. (1977). Standards + nursing care needs = staffing methodology. *Nursing Administration Quarterly, 1*(5), 1–11.

Nield, M. (1975). Developing a projected nurse staffing program. *Supervisor Nurse, 6*(7), 17–24.

Nielsen, B. (1981). Agencies fill a need but are not the answer. *Hospitals, 55*(6), 66–69.

Norby, R., & Freund, L.E. (1977). A model for nurse staffing and organizational analysis. *Nursing Administration Quarterly, 1*(4), 1–13.

Parasuraman, S., Drake, B.H., & Zammuto, R.F. (1982). The effect of nursing care modalities and shift assignments on nurses' work experiences and job attitudes. *Nursing Research, 31*(6), 364–367.

Price, E.M. (1970). *Staffing for patient care: A guide for nursing service based on a research report.* New York: Springer-Verlag.

Sahney, V. *Nurse staffing: A brief description of issues.* Unpublished report, Wayne State University, Detroit, Mich.

Shanks, K., & Potempa, K. (1981). A system for using supplemental staff. *Journal of Nursing Administration, 11*(8), 41–46.

Shukla, R.K. (1982). Primary or team nursing? Two conditions determine the choice. *Journal of Nursing Administration, 12*(11), 12–15.

Smith, E., & Smith, V.F. (1977). Mobilizing human resources. *Nursing Administration Quarterly, 1*(4), 43–46.

Somers, J.B. (1977). Purpose and performance: A system analysis of nursing staffing. *Journal of Nursing Administration, 7*(2), 4–9.

Straker, M., & Cummings, J. (1978). Staffing patterns and team composition. *Hospital and Community Psychiatry, 29*(4), 243–245.

Thorpe, R. (1980). Cross-training program for nurses: A solution to a staffing program. *Supervisor Nurse, 11*(10), 65, 67.

Van Meter, M. (1982). A "magic" solution for all our staffing ills. *RN, 45*(1), 48–53.

Vestal, K.W., & Dean, D. (1981). Pulling staff: Problem or solution? *Journal of Nursing Management, 12*(9), 44–46.

Williams, M.A. (1977). Quantification of direct nursing care activities. *Journal of Nursing Administration, 7*(8), 15–18, 49–51.

Chapter 14

Client Classification Systems

The degree of illness of the clients should be considered when attempting to determine the desired staffing level. It is obvious that additional staff must be scheduled in order to care for clients who are more acutely ill. The question becomes, then, What acuity of illness warrants additional staff? This task has been a challenge to the nursing profession for many years and continues to present problems. How do you decide a client's degree of illness? This decision is particularly difficult in psychiatric–mental health nursing settings inasmuch as there are few concrete indicators of a client's acuity of illness. Nevertheless, in spite of the difficulty, a client classification system (CCS) based on acuities can be used to determine the number of necessary staff members.

A *client classification system* is a ''categorization of [clients] according to some assessment of their nursing care requirements over a specified period of time, . . . the identification and classification of [clients] into care groups or categories, and . . . the quantification of these categories as a measure of the nursing effort required'' (Giovannetti, 1979, p. 4). Its purpose is to classify clients according to their need for nursing care (Reinert & Grant, 1981). Inasmuch as the number of clients on a unit is less of a determinant of the staffing needed than is the variance in the amount of nursing care required by these clients (Pardee, 1968), it is essential to use a system that determines the classification of nursing care required by clients.

The areas of medical and surgical nursing have done much to develop, to pilot, and to use CCSs of various styles and types. However, little has been published about the application of this method to the area of psychiatric–mental health nursing. Hence, each organization and nurse-administrator must originate a system or develop it by modifying preexisting systems from other nursing areas.

The JCAH standards state that the number of registered nurses and ancillary staff for each unit should be determined by evaluating client care requirements and matching them with staff expertise (Cleland, 1982). Within a psychiatric–mental health organization, the only effective system of assessing the number of staff members needed is by the realistic determination of the clients' needs (Christie, 1974). The CCS should enable individualized client needs to be qualified and quantified to determine accurately staffing needs for the organization.

For a CCS to be consistent and effective, however, it must be based upon an interpretation of clients' needs and must be considered as a tool for the planning and evaluation of client care. It cannot be used solely as an administrative tool for determining fiscal responsibility (MacDonell, 1976); the staff will not see the validity of such an instrument, and will soon lose interest in its accurate completion.

The information presented in this chapter can serve as a foundation for the use of a CCS within psychiatric–mental health nursing. Two systems currently used within psychiatric–mental health nursing are included in Appendix 14-A and Appendix 14-B. The nurse-administrator is cautioned, however, about assuming there is no need for modification of these systems. Information, formulas, and plans must be reviewed in terms of each organization's individual client population, philosophy, purposes, goals, budgetary constraints, personnel, and organizational environment. These systems may be used as pilot projects, barring any major conflicts, and then evaluated to identify modifications needed for the individual organization.

ASSESSING NEEDS

Types of Systems

Several types of CCSs have been used in medical-surgical settings and may prove adaptable to the area of psychiatric–mental health nursing. The *prototype evaluation system* identifies categories, establishes parameters for each category, and assigns clients to a category as care needs indicate. This method can be subjective, and there have been problems with reliability. It is easy to explain to the staff; but planning for emotional, teaching, and discharge needs is often overlooked. These areas are often crucial in the delivery of psychiatric–mental health nursing care, which makes this system difficult to transfer to psychiatric–mental health settings. It has the additional drawback of being difficult to monitor.

In the case of the *factor-evaluation system*, predetermined descriptors of care are identified, and each client is rated separately for each descriptor. The ratings are then combined to determine the category of care needed for the client. Although this system is more objective than the prototype evaluation method, it involves substantial paperwork and is, therefore, often not attractive to the staff (Reinert & Grant, 1981).

The *GRASP system* of client classification (Meyer, 1978) can also be used to factor out nursing care costs. This system involves an "accurate assessment of total [client] care needs'' (Meyer, p. 83). Nursing activities required by clients are assigned points based upon the amount of time required to complete each activity. In this system, one point equals 6.5 minutes. The points for each activity are increased by 12 percent over the required time to cover unpredictable delays. The formula for determining the total care time for a client is

$$\text{Total care} = \frac{6.5 \text{ min./point} \times \text{number of points}}{.85}$$
$$+ 38.0 \text{ min. (indirect client care)}$$
$$+ 14.5 \text{ min. (teaching and emotional support) *}$$

This method usually requires two minutes per day for the completion of all components of the system once the staff members have been properly oriented and have adapted to the paperwork. By assuming the delivery of high quality client care, this system enhances staff satisfaction by enabling them to deliver such care in a stable and balanced workload (Meyer, 1978).

The following *Aberdeen formula* for a different CCS is based upon the degree of client dependency:

$$W = N\left[F\,(B + T) + A + D + M\right]$$

W = average weekly nursing workload in hours
N = average number of clients on unit
F = client dependency factor for unit specialty
B = time in hours/week required to maintain the standard of basic nursing care for a totally helpless, bedfast client
T = time required for technical nursing of the unit specialty expressed in a percentage of the time spent on basic nursing
A = time/client/week for administrative duties
D = time/client/week for housekeeping duties
M = time/client/week for miscellaneous duties**

This formula has been used extensively throughout England for a variety of nursing specialties.

A *matrix client classification system* can be borrowed from industrial engineering. This method uses validated time allowances and a coordinated development of a computerized data reporting system. All client care needs are identified and assigned to appropriate skill levels of the staff, and the necessary amount of time to perform related activities is allocated. Thus, a client is not limited to one level of

---

*From "Workload measurement system ensures stable nurse-patient ratio" by D. Meyer, 1978, *Hospitals, 52*(5), p. 84. © 1978 by American Hospital Publishing Co. Reprinted by permission.

**Reprinted from "The Aberdeen formula" by H.M. Cromptom, H. Mitchell, and J. McCameron, 1976, *Nursing Times, 72*(34), p. 122, © 1976. Macmillan Journals Ltd. Reprinted by permission.

care. The data produced are nursing-hour requirements rather than acuity levels of clients. As a result, four levels of nursing-hour requirements are developed. One daily assessment can project client needs and staff requirements for three shifts. This system, which also recognizes psychosocial interactions and the teaching needs of clients (Barham, 1980), could prove adaptable to psychiatric–mental health nursing settings.

System Requirements for a Psychiatric–Mental Health Nursing Organization

Before selecting a CCS model as being appropriate to a particular psychiatric–mental health organization, it should be determined whether the model meets the preestablished objectives for such a system. The CCS should, of course, meet regulatory agency requirements. In addition, the system must be congruent with organizational and departmental objectives.

Ideally, according to Alward (1983), a CCS appropriate to a psychiatric–mental health nursing department would meet the following requirements:

1. Match [client] needs and nursing resources;
2. Project staffing needs for the nursing budget;
3. Measure efficiency of nurse managers;
4. Justify temporary and permanent changes in staffing; and
5. Provide a basis for nursing charges. (p. 15)

Through accomplishing these activities, the CCS can aid the psychiatric–mental health nursing administrator in coping with the financial limitations imposed on the nursing department by current cost control measures (Tomsky, 1983).

In the case of psychiatric–mental health nursing, it has been difficult to develop a client classification tool because of the ambiguity and abstract nature of the nursing interventions and client needs. Often, an organization has not developed a conceptual definition of psychiatric–mental health nursing, which it must do before it can develop a classification system.

The purpose of a psychiatric–mental health CCS is similar to that of other areas—the determining of staffing requirements (Schroder, 1982). The nurse-administrator must be concerned with the maintenance of the quality and the content of the program, equitable workloads, prescribed individualized care plans, and the appropriate skill-mix levels (Grazman, 1981). The system should be based on standard terminology that can be easily understood by all staff involved, and should be easy to update and to audit (Vaughn & MacLeod, 1980). The nurse-administrator must also consider the time required for the completion of each component of the system, and should consider how often it should be done and by whom (Schroder).

PLANNING A PSYCHIATRIC–MENTAL HEALTH NURSING CCS

Developing the System

In order to devise a CCS that can measure client needs and the resultant staffing required, the client population should be assessed (Cohen, 1981) and the characteristics of the clients most often seen at the organization should be identified. Such characteristics include the total number of clients, their degree of dependency, the content and sequencing of physician orders (often used as an estimate of total workload), length of treatment, legal requirements, and the hospital mission and philosophy (Levine & Phillip, 1975). The nature of the client's needs and the duration of those needs must also be determined (Bahr, Badour, & Hill, 1977).

Client Classification Indicators

A select number of client classification indicators must be determined. Aspects of client care that occur most frequently throughout the treatment of the client, these indicators must also reflect the nonroutine occurrences that require substantial nursing time. Although there should be a critical number of indicators, they need not restrict the possibilities for the categorization of clients (Giovannetti, 1979). These indicators should also be verified for accuracy and inclusiveness, simplicity of format, and division of work (Schroder, 1982). Appendix 14-C presents a list of the nursing activities most often found within psychiatric–mental health nursing and that can often be used as indicators for a proposed CCS. A list of nursing activities must be exhaustive, specific, and mutually exclusive. Moreover, they should be weighed in terms of the average time required for their completion, or the performance times for each activity should be developed.

Performance Time Requirements

Standard times for the performance of nursing activities may be defined as the "average time that a nursing task or procedure requires plus a twenty percent allowance for fatigue, preparation, travel time, waiting time and individual variance" (Williams, 1977, p. 49). The nursing practice time requirements for a client category or each specific nursing activity should be identified within a CCS (Giovannetti, 1979).

Performance time requirements for specific psychiatric–mental health nursing activities may be developed in a variety of ways. (This text reviews only a select number of techniques, referring the reader to other texts for more in-depth methodologies.) Standard times that have previously been developed and documented should be examined and, if found relevant, adopted for organizational use. The nurse-administrator must remember that a specific client classification tool may be adaptable to various organizations, but the quantification data may not be transferable (Giovannetti, 1979).

Time-motion studies may be conducted within the organization by experts inside the organization's nursing department or by experts from consulting firms in the community. Two basic approaches characterize this system: observation and self-recording. Both techniques for conducting the studies may be done on a continuous basis or at intervals. However, time-motion studies have multiple limitations that must be considered before the technique's implementation (Williams, 1977).

- How can simultaneous activities be timed?
- Is it possible to secure the large sampling needed in the time frame required by the organization?
- Time-motion studies emphasize the time factor aspect of nursing care, which is not necessarily relevant to psychiatric–mental health nursing.
- There is a question of reliability in the data produced.
- When the self-recording version is used, nurses may forget to record data.

A more subjective method is to have the nurse estimate the time required for each activity and to allow the pilot project to determine the validity of these estimated times.

An example of one determination of standard hours per client-day per classification in the medical-surgical area is 4.5 hours of nursing care per client in the case of Category-2 clients (Georgette, 1970). Furthermore, the same group determined a ratio between the client categories:

- Category 1 (clients needing the least amount of care) require × 0.65.
- Category 2 require × 1.0.
- Category 3 require × 1.35.
- Category 4 (clients needing the most amount of care) require × 2.0.

These numbers indicate that a Category-4 client would require 2.0 times 4.5 hours of nursing care per day or nine hours of nursing care per day. The hours required for other categories can be determined in a similar fashion. However, another study determined that a Category-3 client (similar to the Category-4 client of the above example) required 2.5 times the care of a Category-2 client and five times the care of a Category-1 client (Aydelotte, 1973); therefore, it is always necessary to validate study results within one's own organization.

Whichever technique is used to determine time requirements for nursing activities, time should be allowed for activities that are less well defined. Administrative time must be included as well as education, training, research, and consultation times. Performance times must also include a fatigue factor, which does not include meals (Schroder, 1982). Without these allowances, the performance times would greatly underestimate the amount of time required by a particular client during a specified period of time.

Computing Client Care Hours

"Until tasks are done, nursing cannot function on a professional basis" (Poland, English, Thornton, & Owens, 1970, p. 1482). These tasks most often determine the amount of nursing care a client receives. Tasks, too, are difficult to define within the area of psychiatric–mental health nursing because of its abstract nature; however, they are often essential for the computation of client care hours. *Client care hours* represent "the time required by each shift for actual hands-on nursing care by a group of" clients, whereas *nursing hours* are the "budgeted nursing staff assigned to a nursing unit based upon the average daily census" (LJD, 1981, p. 56).

The initial determination of client care hours per category depends upon multiple variables within an organization (Harris, 1970):

- organizational structure
- units of service
- assignment methods
- scope of nursing responsibility
- care and treatment policies
- client mixture
- other factors

All these factors have an impact upon the amount of nursing care time required by a client identified as belonging within a particular category of the CCS. Time should also be included for the assessment, the planning, the documentation, and the evaluation of client care. Unless these factors are considered, the resulting times will not accurately reflect the time spent in the nursing process.

Another problem associated with this task is the determination of levels of responsibility for each personnel skill level along with the resulting determination of assignments for each staff member. One of the first tasks of a nurse-administrator is the definition of the upper and lower limits of the abilities of a category of personnel. "How many [client] care hours should be provided by professional nurses? will never be adequately answered if [client] classification continues to be made only according to the type and number of procedures and treatments a [client] requires" (Rahr, 1973, p. 66). Because clients with high emotional-cognitive needs (psychiatric–mental health clients) require more professional nursing contact (Grant, Bellinger, & Sweda, 1982, p. 81), it is particularly important to identify the distinction between professional and nonprofessional levels of psychiatric–mental health care. Furthermore, poor use of staff members and associated job dissatisfaction often result in high turnover rates and absenteeism (Smith, 1977).

Client care requirements identified on a particular shift must be divided among the various types of personnel available. This division is based upon organizational goals, the complexity of care activities (see Appendix 14-D), client acuity, the knowledge and skill of available staff (Norby, Freund, & Wagner, 1977), efficiency in the use of personnel, plus the defined expected standard of quality care (Arndt & Huckabay, 1975). For example, one author determined that, for nonpsychiatric clients, 4.7 hours were required per client per day. The ideal staffing pattern suggested by that author was 2.5 hours of care given by a registered nurse and 2.2 hours of care given by other nursing personnel (Abdellah & Levine, 1958).

Another method for determining the limits of ability for categories of personnel is to decide whether an activity requires care giving or care planning and management (Munson & Clinton, 1979). An activity that is solely care giving and has no associated planning component may be delegated. Any activity that requires care planning or care management as any aspect of its delivery must be completed by a registered nurse.

Client care hours must not be determined in isolation. All levels of personnel must be consulted to ascertain the range of abilities of each level of the nursing staff. All staff members must be well informed of these ranges and any modifications that may occur in them.

Standard hours of client care per category equal the time required for direct care per category, plus the time required for indirect care per category, plus telephone time per category, plus errand time per category (Reinert & Grant, 1981). Quantification of standard times for specific nursing procedures provides the information about direct care requirements. Indirect care time must include those administrative activities that a nurse must perform or that are more economical for a nurse to perform (Clark, 1977). Depending upon the organization, this indirect care time may also include telephone and errand time. "Indirect care varies directly with the census while direct care varies with the intensity of care required" (Clark, p. 26). Hence, indirect care time should be more standardized than direct care time.

The average client care hours per client per category can now be determined by using the following formula:

$$\text{Average client care hours per category} = A_1 + B_1$$
$$A_1 = \text{Average direct-care hours for a Category-1 client}$$
$$B_1 = \text{Average indirect-care hours for a Category-1 client}$$

Nonproductive time should also be factored into the figures. Generally, this time is considered to be 25 percent of the staff time (meals, rest, and meetings) (Chagnon, Audette, Librien, & Tilquin, 1978). Cohen (1981), in a nonpsychiatric setting, identified these client care hours per client per category as follows:

- Category 1 require 2.5 care hours/client.
- Category 2 require 3.5 care hours/client.
- Category 3 require 4.5 care hours/client.
- Category 4 require 5 care hours/client.
- Category 5 require 6 care hours/client.

Another author, Meglino (1979), determined that an extension factor existed for specialty units. The factor for psychiatric–mental health clients was 1.5, which can be inserted into the following equation:

Patient care hours for psychiatric–mental health Category-1 client = (Average care hours per Category-1 client for other nursing units) × 1.5

The result is the average client care hours for a specific category of psychiatric–mental health clients. Again, such a figure's validity should be verified for the specific organization.

The total number of client care hours needed per unit per service per shift can be identified from the average client care hours per category per shift. Exhibit 14–1 provides the formula for making the calculation. The number of staff members required is then determined by dividing the total client care hours per shift by the number of hours a staff is available per shift (LJD, 1981):

$$\frac{\text{Total client care hours}}{\text{Nursing hours per shift}} = \text{Number of staff}$$

One author has suggested using 360 minutes per shift per staff as the amount of productive time that can be expected (Chagnon et al., 1978). The above formula would then be as follows:

$$\frac{\text{Total client care hours}}{\text{Six hours}} = \text{Number of staff}$$

Of course, the mix of personnel would, then, need to be determined.

The formula point at which an additional staff member must be obtained must also be determined. For example, if the total client care hours are 54, then nine staff members would be needed. If the formula point had been preset at four, then total client care hours of 58 would require ten staff members.

Exhibit 14–1 Number of Client Care Hours Needed per Unit or Service per Shift

Total Client Care Hours _____   _____
                              unit/service   shift

Census _____

Category	Average Hours	Client/Category	Total
1	_____ ×	_____ =	_____
2	_____ ×	_____ =	_____
3	_____ ×	_____ =	_____
etc.	_____ ×	_____ =	_____

Source: From *Cost-effectiveness analysis of nurse staffing systems*, by LJD Associates, 1981, Program #2. Colorado Springs, Colo. © 1981 LJD Associates. Reprinted by permission.

In projecting the average required staffing, the average client care hour requirement per shift per day over a month's time would be identified. This number would again be divided by the number of nursing hours per staff to identify the average required staffing. (These figures should be calculated on the basis of a minimum of a month's figures and should be used only to project staffing needs during similar times.) For example, if the average client care hour requirement per day for the day shift is 48, the average daily staffing requirement would be 8 ($48 \div 6 = 8$). However, because 1.4 staff members are needed to fill one position for seven days a week (Table 14–1), 11.2 staff members would be needed to provide 8 staff members per day shift for seven days per week ($1.4 \times 8 = 11.2$). This staffing pattern would require 11 full-time staff members and 1 part-time staff member who works one day a week or the equivalent.

Whichever method is used for determining client care hour requirements, the staff must perceive it as actually measuring the true requirements (Jelinek, Zinn, and Byra, 1973). If the staff is included in the development of the methodology, they will recognize that many factors have been included, as well as

Table 14–1 Full- and Part-Time Equivalents to Determine Staffing Needs

Classification	Number of Staff	Number of Days/Week
Full-time	1.4	7
	1.0	5
Part-time	0.8	4
	0.6	3
	0.4	2
	0.2	1

direct-care activities. They must be reminded, however, that these figures do not identify individual client needs, nor do they indicate which staff can be expected to be available (McConnell & Wiley, 1977). Other data are needed to delineate an accurate staffing picture.

Client Care Category Guidelines

In addition to the client indicators, nursing activities and performance times, a profile of the unit and the client care category guidelines is also needed in order to develop a CCS (Naber, Seizyk, & Wilde, 1977). Client care category guidelines depend upon the type of CCS selected and range from three to five categories. Table 14–2 depicts a system based on the number of hours of nursing care needed per day.

Clinical Application of a CCS

The clinical application of a CCS must be incorporated into the original implementation. Then, when needs have been identified, the staff can receive orientation and education that will facilitate their adjustment and the adoption of the system.

In the clinical area, the use of such an instrument can increase the staff's focus upon client care so that time is spent in the actual assessment and validation of the client's daily condition. The tool can be used to teach the staff by pinpointing the differences in their perceptions of clients. It can also be used during supervision conferences for identifying areas of concern and validating assessments. The tool is also useful for program evaluation because it identifies problems, areas of stress, and in-service needs. Program evaluation can also be assisted through the instrument's use in comparing programs and the impact of programmatic changes.

The tool can further provide a basis for the development of a comprehensive care plan and, through the enhancement of the nursing process, can increase the

---

Table 14–2 Client Care Category Guidelines

Category	Hours/Day	Title
1	1.0–2	Self-care
2	2.1–4	Minimum care
3	4.1–6	Intermediate care
4	6.1–8	Moderate care
5	8.1–14	Intensive care

Source: Adapted from "Variables affecting staffing," by A. Marriner, 1979, *Supervisor Nurse, 10*(9), p. 62. © 1979 by S-N Publications, Inc. Adapted by permission.

meaningfulness of the classification system. Finally, the instrument can serve as a quality control tool by aiding in the comparison of prescribed client care with documentation of the actual care given (Reinert & Grant, 1981).

IMPLEMENTING THE SYSTEM

Once the CCS is developed, a procedure or routine for the completion of the tool must also be developed. This procedure should be as clear, concise, and simple as possible in order to facilitate the completion of the instrument without causing undue stress or time loss for the staff. The documentation of the procedure should include the determination of those who complete the tool, the documentation formats, the process for the translation of acuity data into staff requirements, and the process for evaluation of the system.

Usually, the tool is completed by one shift to determine the following shift's staffing needs; through this technique, potential bias and padding is limited (Naber, 1977). The staff completing the instrument should be predetermined and should be persons who are familiar with all the clients. This assignment should be as consistent as possible in order to decrease any potential sources of discrepancy. If a computer is available, calculation of client acuity can be done by using a program tailored to the specific organization. Such usage would certainly facilitate daily calculations of acuity and also encourage the use of those data in research projects.

One technique suggested for the actual documentation is the use of a wall chart, covered with a clear covering so that the changes in acuities can be done with a grease pencil (Meyer, 1978). Categories that remain the same would require no additional documentation. The location of this chart would depend upon the clients' involvement in the process; it may need to be placed out of their line of vision. The classification should be visible to all staff members, because use of the system could then be increased. Should written documentation of the tool be required for other purposes, the unit clerk or secretary could transcribe this chart onto a form that could be sent to the nursing administration as required.

Interpreting the Data

The nursing office should develop tables that translate client acuity into the number of nursing hours required per shift. The number of nursing hours required can then be converted to staffing needs, which would also include the skill levels of personnel ("Variable staffing," 1973). This calculation can assist the persons responsible for providing corrective coverage by enabling them to determine whether additional staff are needed, and at what level (Edgecumbe, 1965). Each unit or service can thereby quickly identify areas of over- or understaffing and make adjustments.

Implementation Problems

Even with the most thorough planning, the psychiatric–mental health nursing administrator can be faced with obstacles in implementing the system. Huckabay and Skonieczny (1981) found the following rank-ordered areas to be problematic:

(1) recruitment; (2) complaints of staff; (3) stress to staff; (4) resistance to change; (5) reliability [of the tool]; (6) [frequency of] classification; (7) [difficulty] select[ing a client] classification system; (8) conduct[ing] research; (9) stress to administrative nursing personnel; (10) budget; (11) cheat[ing]; (12) motivat[ing] staff; (13) lack of control over the situation; [and] (14) difficulty training in-service education instructors. (pp. 89, 93)

Problems that may arise within the department should be anticipated and interventions planned. If there are not sufficient staff members to provide adequate coverage, adjustments should be made to decrease the presence of this stressor.

Even when the CCS has been tailor-made to the organization and has been validated by a pilot project as being accurate, useful, and easily completed, difficulties may still be encountered. When it is a newly introduced system or form, the staff, understandably, may be resistant to the change. They may find that the tool requests too many data, or that it is too time consuming to complete. The staff may also use the tool to demonstrate how stressed they are. In order to receive additional staff, they may pad the information about the acuity of clients when they feel this is the only available way to receive support.

One of the easiest methods of dealing with these concerns and of decreasing resistance is to involve the staff in the implementation of this process from the beginning. By meeting with a variety of staff members from all levels, seeking their opinions and feedback, and involving them in all phases of the project, the nurse-administrator can do much to improve the project's chances of success. Rumors can be clarified, false information can be corrected, and staff members have an opportunity to feel they have had an impact on the project. The nurse-administrator also has the opportunity to demonstrate the ability to be open and to respond to constructive criticism in a fashion that serves to strengthen the legitimacy of the program.

Uses of a CCS

Once developed and in place, a CCS can be used in many ways. It may be used to justify staffing changes and needs based upon objective data about the clients' acuity of illnesses rather than upon subjective predictions. The tool may also be of assistance in the determination of equipment and supply needs (Price, 1981). In addition, the tool may prove to be helpful in analyzing the client census in relation to client acuity, thereby providing additional data for forecasting staffing needs (LJD, 1981).

Furthermore, the classification system may be used as an indicator of increased stress levels by demonstrating discrepancies between required staff and available staff. Based upon the overall acuity levels of the units or services available, the system may also be used to distribute client admissions to those units or services better staffed to handle them. The system may assist in the development of reimbursement strategies and as resource data for budget review and revision.

EVALUATING THE CCS

Determining the Instrument's Reliability and Validity

After the CCS is developed, its reliability must be ensured. The general definition of *reliability* as "consistency or repeatability of a measured instrument" (Giovannetti, 1979) identifies several components that should be present if an instrument is to demonstrate reliability. The concept of *stability* ensures that the tool will demonstrate consistency of measures on repeated applications. *Homogeneity* requires that a person's responses to the various items or components of the instrument are consistent. A tool demonstrates *equivalence* when different investigators using one instrument to measure the same person at the same time or a different instrument applied to the same person at the same time obtain consistent results (Giovannetti, 1979).

Another major aspect of a newly developed tool that must be documented is validity. *Validity* may be defined as the ability of an instrument to actually measure that which it states it measures (Giovannetti, 1979). Three components must be present before the tool demonstrates overall validity: content validity, face validity, and criterion validity. *Content validity* is demonstrated when the tool adequately represents the domain it purports to measure. The instrument demonstrates *face validity* when there is agreement that the instrument seems reasonable and obtains reasonable data—a judgment made by selected experts in the field. *Criterion validity* consists of concurrent and predictive aspects and refers to the extent to which the tool corresponds to some other observation that accurately measures the phenomena of interest (Giovannetti, 1979).

It may seem difficult or superfluous to ensure these aspects of a classification tool. They are important, however, if the system is going to be recognized as a legitimate tool of nursing practice.

In order to include a CCS as a part of an organization's staffing plan, the system is tested by the use of a pilot project that incorporates information about the client population and the staff. Extensive orientation and in-service training for all personnel involved is needed in order to facilitate the adequate testing of such a time-limited project. Upon its completion, the project is reviewed for its reliability and validity and the necessary modifications are made to the system (Schroder, 1982).

Evaluative Audits

The final step in the implementation of a client classification tool is the evaluation process. At first, the system must be examined to determine its validity and reliability. Initially, audits should be done three times per week on different shifts. Once the data indicate consistency of results, the audits may be decreased to three times per month on different shifts. Finally, they may be decreased to quarterly (LJD, 1981).

The results of these audits can be used for teaching in much the same way as the tool itself is used. Differing degrees of structure in the environment can be identified and analyzed. The acting-out behavior of the clients can be related to staffing variances, as well as to degrees of structure, and examined. The rate-of-incident reports can also be examined in relation to staffing variances. Finally, care plans can be examined to determine their reflection of acuity ratings; then these ratings can be used to verify the predicted results of care plan modifications (Schroder, 1982).

The evaluation process, like any tool or program, is never truly completed. Continuing audits serve to monitor the system's ability to continue to meet the needs of the organization, the department, and client populations. Without such ongoing review, a system can be quickly outdated as external and internal changes make their impact upon nursing practice within an organization.

REFERENCES

Abdellah, F.G., & Levine, E. (1958). Effect of nurse staffing on satisfactions with nursing care. *Hospital Monograph Series* (4, Serial No. G11258).

Alward, R.R. (1983). Patient classification systems: The ideal versus reality. *Journal of Nursing Administration, 13*(2), 14–19.

Arndt, C., & Huckabay, L.M.D. (1975). *Nursing administration: theory for practice with a systems approach.* St. Louis: C.V. Mosby Co.

Aydelotte, M.K. (1973). Staffing for high quality care. *Hospitals, 47*(2), pp. 58–60, 65.

Bahr, J., Badour, G., & Hill, H.L. (1977). Innovative methodology enhances nursing deployment, cuts costs. *Hospitals 51*(8), 104–109.

Barham, V.Z., & Schneider, W.R. (1980). MATRIX: A unique patient classification system. *Journal of Nursing Administration, 10*(12), 25–31.

Chagnon, M., Audette, L., Librien, L., & Tilquin, C. (1978). A patient classification system by level of nursing care requirements. *Nursing Research, 27*(2), 107–112.

Christie, L.S. (1974). Researching staffing needs in psychiatric hospitals. *Nursing Times, 70*(48), 1870–1871.

Clark, E.L. (1977). A model of nurse staffing for effective patient care. *Journal of Nursing Administration, 7*(2), 22–27.

Cleland, V. (1982). Relating nursing staff quality to patients' needs. *Journal of Nursing Administration, 12*(4), 32–37.

Cohen, A. (1981). Putting together an applicable patient categorization system for a hospital and nursing home. *Hospital Topics, 59*(1), 16–21.

Crompton, H.M., Mitchell, H., & McCameron, J. (1976). The Aberdeen formula. *Nursing Times, 72*(34), 121–123.

Edgecumbe, R.H. (1965). The CASH approach to hospital management engineering. *Hospitals, 39*(6), 70–74.

Georgette, J.K. (1970). Staffing by patient classification. *Nursing Clinics of North America, 5*(2), 329–339.

Giovannetti, P. (1979). Understanding patient classification systems. *Journal of Nursing Administration, 9*(2), 4–9.

Grant, S.E., Bellinger, A.C., & Sweda, B.L. (1982). Measuring productivity through patient classification. *Nursing Administration Quarterly, 6*(3), 77–83.

Grazman, T.E. (1981). Nurse staffing dilemma: Analyzing objectives, recognizing constraints. *Hospital Progress, 64*(4), 58–61.

Harris, D.H. (1970). Staffing requirements. *Hospitals, 44*(8), 64–70.

Huckabay, L.M.D., & Skonieczny, R. (1981). Patient classification systems: The problems faced. *Nursing & Health Care, 2*(2), 89–102.

Jelinek, R.C., Zinn, T.K., & Byra, J.R. (1973). Tell the computers how sick the patients are and it will tell how many nurses they need. *Modern Hospitals, 121*(12), 81–85.

Levine, J.D., & Phillip, P.J. (1975). *Factors affecting staffing levels and patterns of nursing personnel* (U.S. Public Health Service Publication, HRA No. 75–76). Washington, D.C.: U.S. Government Printing Office.

LJD Associates. (1981). *Cost-effectiveness analysis of nurse staffing systems*. Program #2. Colorado Springs, Colo: Author.

MacDonell, J.A. (1976). Canadian experience with patient care classification. *Medical Care, 14*(5), 134–137.

McConnell, E., & Wiley, L. (1977). Staffing should be spelled $taffing or How many staff nurses are enough? *Nursing 77, 7*(11), 97–101.

Marriner, A. (1979). Variables affecting staffing. *Supervisor Nurse 10*(9), 62–65.

Meglino, B. (1979). A methodology for nurse staffing. *California Management Review, 21*(3), 82–93.

Meyer, D. (1978). Workload measurement system ensures stable nurse-patient ratio. *Hospitals, 52*(5), pp. 81–82, 84–85.

Munson, F., & Clinton, J. (1979). Defining nursing assignment patterns. *Nursing Research, 28*(4), 243–248.

Naber, M., Seizyk, J., & Wilde, N. (1977). Standards + nursing care = staffing methodology. *Nursing Administration Quarterly, 2*(1), 1–11.

Norby, R.B., Freund, L.E., & Wagner, B. (1977). A nurse staffing system based upon assignment difficulty. *Journal of Nursing Administration, 7*(9), 2–24.

Pardee, G. (1968). Classifying patients to predict staff requirements. *American Journal of Nursing, 68*(3), 517–520.

Poland, M., English, N., Thornton, N., & Owens, D. (1970). PETO: A system for assessing and meeting patient care needs. *American Journal of Nursing, 70*(7), 1479–1482.

Price, E.M. (1981). Seven days on and seven days off. *American Journal of Nursing, 81*(6), 1142–1143.

Plutchik, R., Conte, H.R., Wells, W., & Karasu, T.B. (1976). Role of the psychiatric nurse. *Journal of Psychiatric Nursing & Mental Health Services, 14*(9), 38–43.

Rahr, V. (1973). Rationale for determining staffing pattern—What's missing? *Supervisor Nurse, 4*(5), pp. 61–62, 64, 66.

Reinert, P., & Grant, D.R. (1981). A classification system to meet today's needs. *Journal of Nursing Administration, 11*(1), 21–25.

Schroder, P.J. (1982). *Patient classification in a psychiatric setting.* Presentation at Harper-Grace Hospital, Detroit, Mich.

Smith, E.J., & Smith, V.F. (1977). Mobilizing human resources. *Nursing Administration Quarterly, 1*(4), 43–46.

Tomsky, C.N. (1983). Acuity based staffing controls costs. *Journal of Nursing Management, 14*(10), 36–37.

Vaughan, R.G., & MacLeod, V. (1980). Nurse staffing studies: No need to reinvent the wheel. *Journal of Nursing Administration, 10*(3), 9–15.

Williams, M.A. (1977). Quantification of direct nursing care activities. *Journal of Nursing Administration, 7*(8), 15–18, 49–51.

Variable staffing adds up the patient needs to determine how many nurses should provide the care. (1973). *Modern Hospital, 121*(6), 87–88.

Appendix 14-A

Categories of Nursing Care Needs of Patients

1. Intensive Care
1. Gross disorientation
2. Assaultive & destructive behavior
3. Bizarre behavior
4. Poor impulse control
5. Acute suicide prevention
6. 1:1
7. Seclusion
8. Severely impaired judgment
9. Day of admission

2. Modified Intensive Care
1. Moderate disorientation
2. General suicide precaution
3. Elopement precaution
4. Seizure precaution
5. Motivation limited
6. Needs frequent supervision for ADL

3. Intermediate Care
1. Behavior pattern deviates moderately; requires moderate control of activity.
2. Requires only periodic observation & treatment.

4. Minimal Care
1. Awaiting discharge
2. Needing only slight control of activity
3. LOA or pass

Source: Reprinted with permission of Kingswood Hospital, Ferndale, Mich.

SPECIAL CONDITION NOTE: Patients having one or more of the following conditions shall be classified at one higher step of nursing care needs.

1. Isolation for communicable or infectious disease
2. Handicap (blind, deaf, dumb, amputee)
3. Senility, confusion, or general debility of age and patients over 65 years of age
4. Temperature above 102°F times three
5. Unstable blood pressure
6. Haldol titration
7. Signs of drug ingestion
8. Day of ECT treatment
9. Intellectually impaired

C.F. Menninger Memorial Hospital Patient Classification System

Levels of Acuity

I. *Minimal*
1. Independent in functioning
2. Self-directed activities, ADL, leisure
3. Teaching completed
4. Medication regime established

II. *Moderate*
1. Limited or periodic restriction of activity
2. Minimal supervision needed
3. Teaching done within established learning goals
4. Direction limited to support and encouragement
5. Medication regime established

III. *Active*
1. ADL, routine activities, health and dietary needs monitored
2. Teaching needs established, but affect a variety of areas
3. Demands for staff time high, but sporadic
4. Regular monitoring of medication

IV. *Intensive*
1. ADL require frequent monitoring and assistance
2. Teaching goals and methods are being established
3. Demands for staff time are high and constant
4. Team treatment plan requires frequent modification, increased communication
5. Physical treatment needs are present

Source: Reprinted with permission of the Menninger Foundation, © 1981.

V. *Critical*
1. ADL require total monitoring and assistance
2. Teaching is primarily via specific explanation
3. Staff time required on 1:1 basis
4. Team treatment plan requires frequent communication, modification
5. Frequent physical treatment required
6. Special restricted status

C. F. Menninger Memorial Hospital

Nursing patient classification form

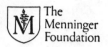

The Menninger Foundation

Unit   Team   Date

Routine

	Patient initials																		
Supervision	1 to 1	4																	
	Watchfulness	3																	
	Awareness	3																	
	Frequent check	2																	
	Routine	1																	
Meals	Trays	3																	
	Group dining	2																	
	Unmonitored dining	1																	
Hygiene	Direct assistance	3																	
	Needs urging/monitoring	2																	
	Cares for self	1																	
Activities	Activities in room only	3																	
	On unit only	3																	
	Scheduled activities	2																	
	Routine and leisure	1																	
LOR	Unit confinement	4																	
	Individual accompaniment	3																	
	Group accompaniment	2																	
	Buddy accompaniment	2																	
	Alone to scheduled appt.	1																	
	Full responsibility	1																	·
Risk	Suicidal or combative, high	4																	
	Suicidal or combative, mod.	3																	
	Suicidal or combative, min.	2																	
	No overt suicidal risk	1																	
Meds	Meds reluctantly	3																	
R	Meds willingly/frequent	3																	
	Meds willingly/few or prn	2																	
	No meds	1																	
Physical problems	Secondary physical symptoms unusual (extra care)	3																	
	Secondary physical symptoms usual (routine care)	2																	
	No physical problems	1																	

Extra

Behavioral	Demanding of time or anxious	2																	
	Angry or weeping	3																	
	Withdrawn	2																	
	Assaultive	3																	
	Other acting out	3																	
	Elopement risk	2																	
	Disorganized	3																	
	Receiving extra teaching	3																	
	Cold wet sheet packs	4																	
	Seclusion or restraints	4																	
	Room restricted	3																	
Extra demands	Off-campus appointments with accompaniment	3																	
	Family conference	2																	
	On grounds appointments	1																	
	New admission	2																	
	Conference (extra paper)	3																	
	Discharge	2																	

Explanation sheet for patient classification

General instructions

1. The first half of the ratings are for routine care—check *one* in *each* category ☑.

2. The second half of the ratings are for *extra* things; check only and as many as apply.

3. Consider the time frame for reference as this week (i.e., if admitted this week, or going to be discharged this week, or the conference is this week). One form is filled out for each week.

Specific instructions

Supervision: The amount of checking on, monitoring, etc., specified on care plan.

Meals: Self-explanatory. (Buddy dining would be listed as unmonitored, since staff is not with them.)

Hygiene: The amount of staff involvement in getting patient to carry out activities of daily living.

Level of responsibility: As identified in the team plan.

Medication: An indication of how much time nursing staff need to give to medication (frequent is defined as 4 or more times per day, few or PRN is anything less than 4 times per day).

Risk: *High* (suicidal and/or combative, not necessarily both). Is the patient on one type of precaution, at watchfulness or precaution level for suicide or one who is an active threat? *Moderate* is one who is on awareness or the team is being alert to potential. *Minimal* is one where suicidal or combative behavior is not seen as a current factor. *No overt risk* is for the patient seen as not a suicide risk at all.

Physical problems: Extra care includes dressings, colostomy care, monitoring during detox, potential hypertensive crisis, diabetic reactions (equate to the type of care a patient would receive in a general hospital).

Secondary physical symptoms considered "routine" would be such things as patients with colds, minor cuts, headaches, sprains, etc.

Extra category
Conceptually, we want you to mark the behaviors or issues that nursing has had to deal with during the week, not isolated instances that may have happened only once. For instance, as a general rule, most patients would not be marked in demanding of time or anxious, angry or weeping, and withdrawn all simultaneously, although there may be a few who fit this. It is important to note that this is not what you think a patient might do, or what they were like on admission, but what they were like actually, this week. In other words, *current* behavior, not historical information.

With the category "*receiving extra teaching*," I think we can all agree most of our patients need this, but was it an active process where we were spending time doing this in a concerted way?

Family conference: An indicator of where nursing had to be actively involved in working with the patient and/or families or where the patient is under increased stress due to visit as well as when family visits once or twice a week.

On grounds appointments: Reflect time spent by nursing in escorting the patient to such appointments, not buddy or self-escorted appointments nor dining room. Do not mark this if on unit confinement; appointments only on the unit do not count as on grounds appointment.

Discharge: If the patient is discharged during the week being rated. (Work toward discharge which is ongoing is picked up in other areas and is a built-in extra.)

Conference: Mark this if a diagnostic conference, etc., is held during the week.

Appendix 14-C

Psychiatric Nursing Activities

Assess patients' emotional needs.
Respond to patients' crises.
Intervene to reduce panic of disturbed patients.
Make sure patients' rights are safeguarded.
Assess the effect of somatic therapies on patients.
Set limits on patients' behavior.
Provide leadership and clinical assistance to other nursing personnel.
Serve as a role model to other staff.
Try to initiate improvements in the programs of the service.
Encourage independent behavior in patients.
Collaborate with members of other disciplines in treatment of patients.
Interview patients to gain information about them.
Implement a nursing care plan.
Serve as a role model to patients.
Assess patients' physical needs.
Develop a nursing care plan.
Work with patients on activities of daily living.
Assess the noise level of the ward and take steps to improve it.
Put the principles of TC into practice.
Encourage patients to try out more constructive patterns of living.
Teach patients appropriate social behavior.
Participate in policy making for the service.
Serve as a clinical teacher to paraprofessionals.
Help improve patients' social competence.

Source: From Role of the psychiatric nurse by R. Plutchik, H.R. Conte, W. Wells, & T.B. Karasu, 1976, in *Journal of Psychiatric Nursing & Mental Health Services, 14*(9), p. 40, 41. © 1976 by Charles B. Slack, Inc. Reprinted by permission.

Participate in research involving patients.
Use community resources such as the Visiting Nurse Association.
Do family psychotherapy with patients.
Do group psychotherapy with patients.
Help improve patients' recreational skills.
Do individual psychotherapy with patients.
Collaborate in planning of research projects involving staff.
Collaborate in research projects involving patients.
Initiate research.

Appendix 14-D

Complexity Listing of Psychiatric Nursing Activities

The following activities are listed in three columns—the first column containing the least complex activities and the last column, the most complex activities.

Assist with ADL
Escort patient
Housekeeping
Laundry tasks
Initial orientation
Shave patient
Specimen collection
Supply monitoring
Talking with patients
Vital signs
Weights

Group activities
   supervision
Medical procedures &
   treatments
Monitoring patient
   safety:
   Elopement
   Homicide
   Suicide
Reality orientation
Supervise recreation
Redirection of patient
Sharps: monitoring

Admission procedures
Care planning
Charting
Discharge procedures
ECT
Family therapy
Group activities:
   Direct
   Plan
Group therapy
Medications
Narcoanalysis
Nursing rounds
One-to-one
Patient classification and
   categorization
Patient education
Psychotherapy
Restraints:
   Application
   Monitor
Shift report
Socialization teaching
Transfer procedures

Chapter 15

Treatment Modalities: Their Impact for Psychiatric Nursing Administrators

The administration of psychiatric–mental health nursing frequently differs from other specialty areas of nursing as a result of the treatment modalities used. Therefore, the psychiatric–mental health nursing administrator should have a psychiatric–mental health clinical background and be aware of issues that are unique to this practice environment. Such treatment modalities as the therapeutic milieu and the interdisciplinary treatment teams exist primarily in this specialty area and, as such, mandate that the nurse-administrator be familiar with their uniqueness. The following chapter discusses these demands and their implications.

ASSESSING AND PLANNING FOR INTERFACING WITH SELECTED TREATMENT MODALITIES

Client Population

To plan for the therapeutic interfacing of nursing with various treatment modalities, the psychiatric–mental health nursing administrator begins with an assessment of the client population. This assessment is necessary in order to ensure that the treatment program is designed to meet the clients' needs. For example, if the client population served consists of chronically mentally ill clients, the treatment program should focus on supportive attempts to aid these clients in remaining within the community as much as is feasible. If the client population is concerned with primary crisis intervention, the program needs to focus upon short-term treatment, perhaps on an inpatient basis, to aid the client in the reestablishment of pre-illness mental health levels.

The client population served should be reviewed on an annual basis for basic demographic data: age, sex, race, presenting problems, and so on. Through this annual review, the level of nursing care provided can be assessed and compared with the level and type needed. Forecasts in this area are particularly beneficial. Through these efforts, the psychiatric–mental health nursing administrator can take steps to ensure that the treatment program changes with the population, not in response to changes.

It is also important to communicate such knowledge to all levels of psychiatric nursing personnel for several reasons. The staff will view the program in a more holistic manner as they recognize that the program is designed for the clients served and that the clients are not forced to adapt to preexisting treatment plans. The staff will also recognize the need for program and treatment changes as population characteristics change. Through an ongoing assessment of client population and programs, quality psychiatric–mental health nursing care is maintained.

Therapeutic Milieu

A primary treatment approach used in psychiatric nursing is the therapeutic milieu. *Milieu therapy* can be defined as "a scientific manipulation of the environment aimed at producing changes in the personality of the client" (Stuart & Sundeen, 1983, p. 580). In this modality, all interactions with the client have the potential for therapeutically aiding the client in the progression towards defined treatment goals. Most psychiatric inpatient programs today subscribe to the therapeutic milieu program format for the delivery of care. This emphasis is in contrast to the historical emphasis on a custodial approach.

In much of the literature, psychiatric–mental health nurses are identified as having the primary responsibility for the maintenance of the therapeutic milieu. Whether they do or do not depends on the ability of the nurse-administrator to provide a practice environment in which nurses can assume this responsibility. Hence, the nurse administrator is responsible to "establish, maintain, and coordinate a patient-centered program" (Lathrop, 1978, p. 677) that uses the nursing process, the appropriate nursing models, and the psychiatric–mental health nursing standards to aid clients in identifying and realizing their potentials (Lathrop).

Treatment Teams

An important treatment component of the therapeutic milieu is the clinical treatment team. A *team* can be defined as "a group of people, each of whom possesses particular expertise; each of whom is responsible for making individual decisions; who together hold a common purpose; who meet together to communicate, collaborate and consolidate knowledge, from which plans are made, actions determined and future decisions influenced" (Benfer, 1980, p. 166). Within this team, the nurse must function as a colleague in order to provide quality nursing care. The treatment team most often experienced in psychiatric–mental health nursing may include the following persons: the psychiatric–mental health nurse, the psychiatrist, the psychologist, the psychiatric social worker, the psychiatric assistant or mental health technician, the occupational therapist, the recreational therapist, the creative arts therapist, the dietician, and auxiliary personnel. An organization may have all or only some of these team members available for collaboration (Stuart & Sundeen, 1983). The disciplines that comprise the treatment in a particular setting should be clearly identified.

Although most teams are classified as multidisciplinary or interdisciplinary synonymously, the two terms are not the same. A multidisciplinary team is composed of persons from a variety of disciplines who provide discipline-specific components of one patient's treatment plan to that patient. The term *interdisciplinary team* refers to "members of different disciplines meaningfully involved in a formal team arrangement that maximizes opportunities for educational interchange and service delivery" (Benfer, 1980, p. 166). It would seem logical, therefore, that one would aim to create inter- rather than multidisciplinary teams if one wished to focus upon the holistic approach to health care so prevalent in nursing.

Three components are crucial for the smooth functioning of the psychiatric treatment team: collaboration, cooperation, and leadership. The extent to which each component exists within the organization should be identified. The purpose of collaboration is "to use the different abilities of a team member to give the client the most effective services available" (Wilson & Kneisl, 1979, p. 79). Without collaboration, the care delivered will be fragmented at best and contradictory at the worst. Constant communication is needed to ensure that the plan developed for the patient is composed of complementary parts. Hence, cooperation is mandatory for the team.

Competition may hinder cooperation should communication become dysfunctional or roles blurred. Such role blurring or confusion may also result in feelings of anxiety or personal threat in individual members of the team (Wilson & Kneisl, 1979). Such role confusion and blurred disciplinary boundaries are common within the psychiatric–mental health setting (Carser, 1981) and are sources of potential conflicts between staff members and between disciplines. Unless these conflicts are verbalized and thereby resolved, much confusion and conflict will be perpetuated and will, ultimately, affect the care received by clients.

By having a clearly defined purpose, philosophy, and goal statements, as well as position descriptions, the nurse-administrator provides a foundation for nursing staff members' delineation of their roles. This process also serves to clarify to other disciplines the roles the nurses will assume. Role blurring can also be decreased by clearly defined position and discipline descriptions for all disciplines, which are made available to all members of the treatment team. Briefly stated, the psychiatrist is responsible for the medical care of the client, while the psychologist handles the administration and interpretation of psychological testing and serves as a consultant for behavior modification programs. In certain organizations, psychologists may also conduct group and individual therapy sessions. The psychiatric social worker focuses upon the family of the patient and may assume responsibility for family and group therapy, discharge planning, and community referrals. The occupational therapist addresses the psychological components of rehabilitation through the use of arts and crafts, while the recreational therapist attends to the improvement of social skills and the use of leisure time through recreational activities (Stuart & Sundeen, 1983). The activity therapist is responsible for activity programming (Benfer, 1980), while the creative arts therapist utilizes art, music, dance, and poetry to improve the client's communication, self-esteem, and social skills (Wilson & Kneisl, 1979). The dietitian has primary responsibility for assisting the client in the planning and achieving of a healthy nutritional status.

The registered nurse is responsible for the maintenance of the clients' milieu and the delivery of psychiatric–mental health nursing care. A clinical specialist prepared in psychiatric nursing is also involved in individual, group, and family psychotherapy. Within nursing, the psychiatric aide, the assistant, and the mental health technician perform duties delegated by the registered nurse according to legal and organizational policy. Auxiliary personnel, such as volunteers, also generally fall under the aegis of nursing and provide supportive care to clients, as established by the volunteer program of the organization.

The final component crucial for the smooth functioning of a treatment team is leadership. In traditional settings, the psychiatrist is often designated as the leader. However, because the leader functions as the coordinator of care, practitioners of other disciplines may emerge as leaders within the team. A more crucial concern is the type of leadership of the designated staff member. Openness, collaboration, and the sharing of ideas must be fostered in order to ensure that all alternatives to client care have been examined in the formulation of an individualized treatment plan. In a team in which discussion or disagreement is discouraged, clients are unlikely to receive individualized care unique to their needs. Instead, the stereotyped plan for the identified diagnosis or the favorite plan of the leader will be instituted. Hence, it is imperative that the identified leader be a person capable of guiding the treatment team as an interdisciplinary team. The psychiatric nurse-administrator should support nurses as members of the treatment team.

Primary Therapists

Because nurses do function as members of an interdisciplinary team and because a client's primary therapist is selected from those team members, nurses can be expected to function as primary therapists to a caseload of clients. However, not all members of the nursing staff will be able to be primary therapists.

The psychiatric–mental health nursing administrator, within the context of professional standards of practice and legal constraints, develops criteria that should be followed in selecting nurses as primary therapists. Usually, education and experience in this area would be the determining factors; for example, clinical nurse specialists with master's degrees are routinely qualified to be primary therapists (Leib, Underwood, & Glick, 1976).

Other factors may also be considered, depending upon the uniqueness of the organizational environment. Three personal characteristics are also thought to be relevant in identifying persons as therapists: being

> nondefensive and authentic or genuine in the therapeutic encounter; . . .
> able to provide a nonthreatening, safe, trusting atmosphere through . . .
> acceptance, positive regard, nonpossessive warmth for the client; and
> . . . able to understand, "be with," "grasp the meaning of," or have a
> high degree of empathic understanding of the client on a moment by
> moment [sic] basis. (Balgopal & Vassil, 1978, p. 133)

Another concern is the question of supervision. Many organizations automatically assume that the psychiatrist will do the clinical supervision of all primary therapists. This expectation may not be realistic, however, because different perspectives are held by the various disciplines. It would seem logical that primary therapists should be supervised by qualified persons within the same discipline. Hence, nurses who are primary therapists would be clinically supervised by a nurse who is qualified to provide such supervision. For example, certification standards of various disciplines usually indicate the qualifications a person needs to provide supervision. A certified clinical nurse specialist in adult psychiatric–mental health nursing could provide supervision to nurses who have been identified as qualified to function as primary therapists in that area of nursing. Should such a person not be available within the institution, plans could be made to contract with someone within the community who can provide such services to the nursing department.

Social Learning

Another concept integrally tied with therapeutic milieu programs is social learning. *Social learning* can be defined as "learning from others what is and is not acceptable behavior" (Carruth, 1976, p. 1804). As managers and facilitators of the therapeutic milieu, nurses should be familiar with this theory. In-service or continuing education can be planned to assist nurses to recognize social learning's applications within the department and organization. By combining the nurses' awareness of their roles as members of groups (i.e., the treatment team) through the use of social learning theory, they improve their abilities to deliver care and to assist clients in the improvement of their level of functioning.

Group Dynamics

Because much of the activity of the therapeutic milieu occurs in groups, the importance of knowledge about group dynamics should be recognized and plans should be made for the attainment of this knowledge by the nursing staff. Such information naturally includes theories and concepts of group process, but it also requires that members of the nursing staff recognize the social or moral values of their clients, client groups, and themselves in attempting to plan care (Wolf, 1978). Without such knowledge and understanding, a staff member will be severely handicapped in responding to the everyday issues and concerns in the delivery of quality psychiatric client care. When attempting to evaluate the functioning of the therapeutic milieu from the perspective of nursing administration, aspects of group evaluation, team functioning, and interpersonal relationship skills of the nurses should be incorporated in order to evaluate the quality of care provided or to identify areas for needed improvement.

Treatment Modalities within the Milieu

Treatment modalities used with clients within the milieu vary with both the client and the primary therapist. The treatment may focus on the individual client or on the client as a member of a group or family. Knowledge of the various treatment modalities should be incorporated into the assessment and planning for the maintenance of the therapeutic milieu.

Each organization should have detailed descriptions of the components of psychotherapy as they are understood within that organization, including treatment modalities that may be used and that have been found to be beneficial to the patient population served. Such treatment modalities may then be used by members of the disciplines functioning as primary therapists within that organization. The psychiatric–mental health nursing administrator should have a working knowledge of each treatment modality in order to assess and plan with the nurses for the evaluation of the client care given. This text does not intend to be a reference for these modalities; it briefly describes only the focus and the central techniques involved in each modality so that the nurse-administrator can refresh previous knowledge or begin an increasing awareness of the modalities used within the organization.

Individual Psychotherapy

Psychological Growth Therapies or Existential Therapeutic Processes. Treatment modalities are usually divided into different groups, depending upon the primary focus of the modality. The psychological growth therapies or existential therapeutic processes include such modalities as gestalt, logotherapy, rational-emotive, reality, encounter groups, and transactional analysis. These modalities focus upon the here and now of the client's situation (Stuart & Sundeen, 1983). Problems in behaviors are thought to result when the individual is "out of touch with . . . self or . . . environment which has resulted from the inhibitions or restrictions which the person has placed upon . . . self" (Stuart & Sundeen, p. 41). The focus is usually on the "encounter, a meeting of two or more people and their appreciation of one another" (Stuart & Sundeen).

Gestalt Therapy focuses on the resolution of important emotional experiences and improvement in the client's ability to select experiences. To do this, the client concentrates on feeling-related bodily sensations. It is believed that the identification of feelings improves self-awareness, which, in turn, improves self-acceptance. The techniques used in this modality include "fantasy, role playing, emotional catharsis, group work, discussing dreams and body language" (Wilson & Kneisl, 1979, p. 678).

Logotherapy focuses upon the future. The goal is to aid the client in becoming a responsible person. Clients are helped to take control of their life and to determine its meaning (Stuart & Sundeen, 1983).

Rational-emotive therapy focuses on the eradication of irrational beliefs and should result in change in specific behavior. The therapist uses confrontation to force clients to claim responsibility for their behavior. In this cognitive-oriented therapy, clients are encouraged to accept themselves as they are and not as the result of behaviors. Central to this modality are the techniques of "explaining irrational beliefs, positive reinforcement of effective behavior, and group marathon encounters" (Wilson & Kneisl, 1979, p. 679). "Action is emphasized for both the client and the therapist" (Stuart & Sundeen, 1983, p. 41).

Reality therapy focuses upon the improvement of the client's sense of identity through the satisfaction of self-esteem and love needs in a responsible fashion. Clients are aided by the therapist in identifying their life's goals and the manner in which these goals have not been attained. Current alternatives are explored, because clients are free to discuss any topic that focuses upon behaviors rather than on feelings (Stuart & Sundeen, 1983). Central techniques for this modality are techniques of "involvement with the therapist, which [lead] to ability to care for others with increased awareness of effectiveness and social acceptability of one's own current behavior" (Wilson & Kneisl, 1979, p. 678).

The goal of *encounter therapy* is to improve the client's abilities for honest communication. Encounter therapy attends to the here and now, utilizing interactions within groups. This type of modality can be conducted with a regular group format or through group marathon sessions. The norm of the group requires that members be responsible for their behavior. The emphasis is placed on members' feelings, and intellectualization is discouraged (Stuart & Sundeen, 1983). Central techniques for this modality include "nonverbal techniques and structured interpersonal experiences to break down personality defenses" (Wilson & Kneisl, 1979, p. 678).

Transactional analysis works to increase the client's self-esteem, improve the ability for social interaction, and develop intimacy. Through the analysis of three frames of reference in communication, the client is aided to identify and to eradicate destructive types of interactions (Wilson & Kneisl, 1979).

Behavioral Therapies. The behavioral therapies focus on clients' actions rather than on their thoughts and feelings. It is believed that a change in a client's behavior results in changes in the client's cognitive and affective spheres. Behavior problems are seen as habits that can be changed through the use of learning theory. Several modalities can be included in this category: desensitization, assertiveness and aversion therapies, and the token economy (Stuart & Sundeen, 1983).

Desensitization therapy relies on the use of relaxation techniques to aid the client in gradually increasing a tolerance to something that was previously anxiety-producing.

Assertiveness training focuses on aiding the client in directly addressing concerns with others without infringing on the rights of others.

Aversion therapy uses a painful stimulus to create an avoidance of another stimulus. For example, many stop-smoking programs incorporate either physically or visually painful stimuli to create an aversion to cigarettes or smoking. These stimuli are intended to cause the client to break this habit.

A *token economy* is used for positive reinforcement of socially acceptable behavior in chronically hospitalized clients. Clients receive tokens when their behavior is socially acceptable. They may then save these tokens to purchase something they find rewarding. Hence, socially acceptable behavior is rewarded and reinforced (Stuart & Sundeen, 1983).

Art and Play Therapies. There are additional treatment modalities that may be used by the nurse-therapist. *Art therapy* is "based upon the belief that conscious and unconscious feelings or thoughts can be expressed graphically and that everyone has the ability to project inner conflicts on paper" (Labarca, 1979, p. 118). Inasmuch as defense mechanisms are not easily transferred to paper, the drawing will more directly express the client's feelings. The art therapist aids the client by offering interpretations of the drawing, which serve to associate nonverbal and verbal communications (Labarca).

In *play therapy,* the therapist provides the child with opportunities to create situations in play that lend themselves to the resolution of conscious and unverbalized conflicts. Through play therapy the nurse can provide the child with opportunities for "object constancy, opportunities that promote predictability and opportunities for the child to use toys that help symbolically in projecting anger and in developing other defense mechanisms" (Stuart & Sundeen, 1979, p. 485). The functions of play therapy include helping children to assimilate "past experiences that they had no control over, communicate with the unconscious, communicate with others, explore . . . while learning how to relate to self, the world and others, and compromise between the demands of drives and the dictates of reality" (Wilson & Kneisl, 1979, p. 508). The role of the therapist is nondirective and accepting. This approach allows the personality of the child to evolve. Ideally, a playroom should be available with an appropriate selection of toys based upon the client population. There is importance not only in how the child plays, but also in the toys selected (Kranz, 1978).

This list is, by no means, an exhaustive list of the treatment modalities a nurse-therapist may use when working with individual clients. Hence, the nurse-administrator must be familiar with those modalities that are sanctioned by the organization and that are most beneficial for the client population. This knowledge is used then to guide program and educational planning to support the efforts and practices of the nurses involved in direct therapy.

Group Psychotherapy

In addition to working with individual clients, the psychiatric–mental health nurse may be functioning as a therapist within a group. *Group psychotherapy* may be defined as "the treatment of emotional stress and disorder through the means of a group method and group process" (Stuart & Sundeen, 1983, p. 709). Within psychiatric–mental health treatment settings, the intent of group therapy is to provide the client with a safe environment that will support the client in attempts to deal with identified problems (Slimmer, 1978). The specific goals of group therapy should be clearly delineated, because they determine many of the practice guidelines of a particular group (White, 1974). Group therapy differs from individual therapy in that the group, in addition to the therapist, serves as a therapeutic tool. Within a group format, the therapist may use other treatment modalities such as transactional analysis and psychoanalytic understandings.

As is the case with those who function in other therapeutic strategies, a group therapist must be qualified to function in that capacity. This therapist should have an educational and experiential background in group theory and dynamics and human behavior and should be provided with clinical supervision (Wilson & Kneisl, 1979). Of course, any group therapist, like any therapist, must be "aware of and examine the effects of his [or her] behavior and beliefs on the group, and must be able to communicate a sense of acceptance, accurate empathy, honesty and genuineness to the group members" (White, 1974, p. 578).

A single therapist may conduct group therapy, or the group may be run by co-therapists. Certain issues should be addressed that are unique to this type of therapy leadership. The selection, pairing, and preparation of the co-therapists is important. Factors such as age, sex, personality characteristics, and interpersonal relationship styles should be considered when a co-therapy team is being established. Generally, the therapists should be of equal status to function well in group therapy. Therapists of unequal status may experience relationship difficulties that would impede their ability to function jointly as therapists.

Certain considerations must be discussed by the co-therapists before they form a therapy team. For co-therapists to be successful, they must be willing and able to communicate clearly with each other. Their relationship is crucial to the success of the group. Each co-therapist should expect to assess and to analyze the group process, the behaviors of the group members, and themselves. They need to be able to function consistently as a team, not in competition with each other. They must seek supervision or consultation for the group process and their relationship (Williams, 1976).

Types of Group Therapies. Group therapies have been historically categorized through a variety of methods. Traditionally, they were categorized according to the therapeutic goals of the group such as "regressive-reconstructive, repressive-constructive, activity level of the therapists, and the level of analysis in terms of insight achieved" (White, 1974, p. 576). Recently, groups have been divided into categories according to six main approaches: (1) reeducative group therapy, (2) psychodrama groups, (3) experiential-existential group therapy, (4) group-dynamic group therapy, (5) psychoanalytic group therapy, and (6) intensive interactional group therapy (White, 1974).

Reeducative and remotivation groups were designed to assist institutionalized persons become more socially skillful (Wilson & Kneisl, 1979). They generally use behavior therapy, lectures, and discussions to provide information and support and to improve the client's defenses (White, 1974).

Psychodrama groups "utilize psychoanalytic principles and theories, combined with structured dramatization of a [client's] interpersonal and intrapersonal emotional difficulties" (White, 1974, p. 577). This type provides more intensive experiences than those usually available in psychotherapy. It is concerned with individual problems and provides therapy in which nonverbal and verbal communication may be jointly used. While designated group members portray situations, other members (alter egos) verbalize what they determine the actors might be thinking or feeling. All members are encouraged to function in various roles.

Sociodrama is similar to psychodrama, but its emphasis is on common societal roles rather than on individual problems. It may be defined as an "action-oriented laboratory for observing verbal and nonverbal communication and for studying and solving problems in interpersonal relationships" (Wilson & Kneisl, 1979, p. 475). Sociodrama provides a safe environment in which group members can experiment with problem solving in interpersonal relationships (Wilson & Kneisl, 1979).

Experiential-existential group therapy "emphasizes the experiencing of immediate feelings, with the therapist participating as a full member of the group" (White, 1974, p. 577).

Group-dynamic group therapy focuses on the group rather than on the individual and examines group processes as they happen (White, 1974).

Psychoanalytic group therapy uses the philosophy and the techniques of psychoanalysis (White, 1974). Personality reconstruction groups are of this type. The focus is on the analysis of individual persons within the group. Interpersonal interactions of the members are of secondary importance and are examined only in terms of how they demonstrate individual members' concerns (Wilson & Kneisl, 1979). The goals of these groups are for persons to understand and to modify their behavioral patterns and coping mechanisms (Stuart & Sundeen, 1983).

Finally, *intensive interactional group therapy* places primary emphasis on the here and now by use of the group's processes (Wilson & Kneisl, 1979). Its aims are "the correction of distortions, the development of more satisfying relationships, the use of consensual validation and the development of interpersonal learning" (White, 1974, p. 577). The group is helped by the therapist to focus on group process rather than group content and is expected to use this process in the course of therapy.

Family Psychotherapy

In addition to group therapies, a nurse may work with families. This treatment has been defined as one that posits that "the emotional symptoms of problems of an individual are an expression of emotional symptoms or problems in a family, with the family system being viewed as the unit of treatment" (Wilson & Kneisl, 1979, p. 565). In order to become involved in this modality, the nurse must have an educational and experiential background in family therapy. Family therapy focuses on the here and now in its use of utilizing family processes to improve the functioning of the family system. The persons involved in family therapy may vary according to the goals of treatment. For example, a family therapy session may include a husband and wife, a parent and child, or the extended family.

IMPLEMENTING TREATMENT MODALITIES WITHIN THE THERAPEUTIC MILIEU

After assessing the treatment modalities used within a psychiatric–mental health treatment setting and planning for their therapeutic incorporation as part of the milieu, the psychiatric–mental health nursing administrator works with the nurses within the department in the maintenance of a therapeutic milieu. Multiple treatment strategies exist that provide for and support the concept of the therapeutic milieu. For the purposes of this text, the authors have selected the following strategies or techniques as those that, most frequently, may have an impact on the nurse's ability to structure the milieu in a therapeutic manner:

- team building
- pharmacology
- electroconvulsive therapy
- physical intervention with clients

Team Building

When a nurse-administrator recognizes the existence of dysfunctional teams within the organization, a team-building approach should be explored as a possible solution. *Team building* "aims at improving the problem-solving ability of team members by working through the specific task and interpersonal issues that prevent a team from effective functioning" (Laszlo, 1978, p. 11). Through this process, several goals, depending upon the organization and the team involved, can be established: improved group process communication; more effective problem solving and decision making; group goal clarification with an associated commitment of the team to these goals; and improved awareness of conflicts within the group and strategies for conflict resolution (Laszlo, 1978). If this mechanism is to be successful, it is important that the leaders be objective and qualified to lead this type of experience. Often, it may be found more helpful to have nonteam members lead the team building efforts to ensure objectivity.

The process may be conducted in a series of eight workshops or in an all-day workshop with follow-up sessions. Often, the team may find it helpful to hold these meetings away from the organization. Two facilitators begin by conducting diagnostic interviews with each team member. In these interviews, the team members are questioned about their perceptions of each team member and the team as a whole. All members are asked the same questions to ensure consistency and validity, and all answers are kept in strict confidence to facilitate the obtaining of honest answers. The information gathered from these interviews is then combined and organized into general issues and concerns, and specific topic areas are identified: roles, cooperative efforts, group process, communication, and so on. Each team member then receives a copy of the topic listing to stimulate discussion.

In addition to the diagnostic interviews, each team member also receives a group climate questionnaire. The results of this questionnaire are tabulated and presented to the group. Analysis of the results is based on the concepts of the understanding, acceptance, valuing, and genuineness shown to each member by the work group or team.

The team members are then ready to attend the all-day workshop. The day is divided by the lunch hour, with the morning devoted to group feedback and the afternoon to individual feedback. The group facilitators begin by presenting to the group the purposes of constructive feedback and nonthreatening methods of communication that tend to facilitate provision of this feedback. During the morning, the team discusses the group climate questionnaire. Team members compare and contrast findings with individual beliefs and identify problems that should be addressed in future problem-solving meetings. During the afternoon session, each team member is instructed to speak with all other team members for five minutes per person, giving them feedback about their individual behavior in the work setting. Such feedback is to be given in the following format: "When you (a description of what the person says or does) in (where the behavior occurs) it (the effects that are observed) and it makes me feel (a description of feelings)" (Laszlo, 1978, p. 12).

This system lends itself to psychiatric–mental health nursing where nurses are constantly working within teams—interdisciplinary and nursing teams. Through clarification of group problems and concerns, team members can become increasingly comfortable in assessing not only their role as a member of the team, but in identifying ways to help other team members perform to their optimal capacity.

Nurse-Physician Relationships

The nurse-physician relationship is an important subgrouping within the treatment team. These two persons are often required to work more closely together than are the other team members. Hence, any dysfunction in this relationship can cause a decrease in the quality of care provided by the overall treatment team. It is important, then, that the status of the nurse-physician relationships within the particular setting be assessed. Should improvements be necessary, the following strategies can be facilitative:

- "Avoid 'charged' words" (Johnston, 1983, p. 19). Use neutral, objective terms when describing efforts to improve client care.
- "Build nurses' clinical competence and clinical credibility" (Johnston, p. 19). Through detailed job descriptions and relevant in-service programming, the psychiatric–mental health nursing department demonstrates clinical competence. When increasing competence is demonstrated, a nurse's credibility is also increased.
- "Create a prospective problem-solving structure" (Johnston, p. 20). Should problems arise in nurse-physician relationships, joint supportive problem-solving efforts by the parties involved should be facilitated.
- Opportunities should exist for nurses and physicians to work together routinely on a formal basis to solve client care problems.
- "Support the nurses" (Johnston, p. 20). Nursing management and administration must support the nurses in their clinical decision-making efforts by providing an environment in which clinical judgement is valued and clinical decision making encouraged.

- "Stop blaming the doctors—and start listening" (Johnston, p. 20). Throughout the department, nurses must view physicians' concerns objectively rather than defensively.

By implementing these and other relevant strategies, the nurse-administrator supports a practice environment in which different disciplines can work collaboratively in the best interest of the client.

Pharmacology

As is true in any nursing setting, clients in the psychiatric–mental health setting are often receiving medications as an aid to facilitate their return to mental health. Thus, nurses should recognize their need to assume appropriate responsibility for this component of the treatment plan. "The professional nurse must maintain responsibility for the medication regimen whether [personally] administer[ing] the medication . . . or delegat[ing] that function" (Boettcher & Anderson, 1982, p. 12). This responsibility must be stressed so that the nurse assumes this duty and does not treat it in a perfunctory fashion. "To use the nursing process effectively in relation to psychotropic medication therapy, the nurse must have solid interpersonal communication skills, knowledge of the psychodynamics of human behavior, and an awareness of current technical information about psychotropic medications" (Boettcher & Anderson, p. 12).

The hospital formulary is particularly useful because it identifies and delineates a substantial amount of technical information. As the organization's pharmacy and therapeutics committee generally develops and monitors the formulary, nurses should be members of this committee. Through nursing's involvement, the formulary can become a useful tool for nurses administering medications throughout the organization.

Within psychiatric–mental health nursing, the nurse has additional responsibilities related to the suspicious, the acting out, or the suicidal client. Each of these categories of clients requires uniquely individualized nursing care. The suspicious client and the acting out client may not take their medications in a fashion that will enable those medications to function as they were intended. The nurse should recognize the client's concerns but must emphasize the medication's role as one part of the treatment regimen that will help the client to return to a premorbid level of functioning. The suicidal client presents a different problem. This client could be placed at serious risk should a nurse be less than diligent in monitoring the administration of medications. Hence, additional precautions are needed with a suicidal client to ensure that the medications ordered are ingested and not saved.

In the above-named categories, as well as with other clients, the nurse must recognize the importance of teaching. Clients should recognize their role in their health care. This understanding includes "knowing when they are ill, how they are ill, and what to do about it" (Lane, 1981, p. 28). As is the case with other health problems, the client must recognize the role that medications play in the treatment of the illness and that the alleviation of symptoms does not automatically signal the end of the need for medication. As the clients recognize the important role medications may play in their return to health, their compliance with the medication regimen will improve. Such compliance is mandatory so the client can maintain a healthy status independent of the organization. Without it, clients are often readmitted to the hospital because of the lack of follow-through on this component of their treatment.

Several ways in which a client's responsibility for self and compliance with medications can be increased include the incorporation of medication groups or self-medication programs as part of the overall treatment program. Medication groups are "designed to help clients understand the role that psychotropic medications play in maintaining mental health. A problem-solving, task-oriented approach helps clients gain insight into their own feelings about taking medications" (Cohen & Amdur, 1981, p. 343). Through their increase in understanding and insight, the clients recognize the importance of medications as part of their treatment and are likely to comply with the regimen.

Self-medication of clients is another practice that may be incorporated into a treatment program. Through this system, the nurse monitors clients' ability to dispense their own medications under supervised conditions. Through this involvement in self-care, clients are more likely to demonstrate similar behavior once they are at home.

A final technique that may prove useful in helping clients to assume responsibility for their medications is the use of PRN medications. Traditionally, it was the nurse who determined whether clients required additional medication. In a team approach that would involve clients in their own care, clients would seek out the assigned nurse, discuss their concerns, and explore alternatives to medication. The nurse and the client would then jointly decide whether medication would be most helpful at that time. This approach alleviates the impression that medications are a cure-all, maintains the client's role in this aspect of nursing care, and helps the client to discuss the events that have led to the request for additional medication.

Electroconvulsive Therapy

Another treatment modality that has impact on the nurse's ability to structure the milieu is electroconvulsive therapy (ECT). *ECT* is a treatment in which a seizure is artificially caused by passing a current through electrodes applied to the client's temples (Stuart & Sundeen, 1983). Usually, there are six to ten treatments occurring three times per week on alternate days. The clients who are most likely to benefit from ECT are those with the following medical diagnoses: "(1) endogenous morphic depression, (2) acute catatonic excitement, (3) severe catatonic withdrawal, (4) unipolar or bipolar affective disorders, (5) acute schizophrenia [that is] unresponsive to appropriate trials of psychotropic medications, and (6) organic mental syndrome with psychosis secondary to atherosclerosis or senility" (Wilson & Kneisl, 1979, p. 607).

The handling of ECT should be considered as similar to a surgical procedure, both in the consent needed and in pre- and posttreatment monitoring by the nurse. Although the actual procedure may be done in any room, certain equipment should be available such as a hospital bed, oxygen, suction equipment, intravenous (IV) apparatus, cardiac resuscitation equipment, and the ECT machine. An anesthesiologist should also be available to assist in the procedure.

Because this procedure is a specialized one, all nurses should be familiar and comfortable with it in order to be able to accompany and to assist their clients, should the need for ECT arise. Hence, ECT training should be included as part of the regular educational programs throughout the organization. Nurses should also be aware of the need for teaching and communicating with their clients. Through such interventions, the nurse can do much to alleviate the clients' and the families' concerns and anxieties and so enable the procedure to be completed as smoothly as possible. Post-ECT, the nurse needs to remain with the client to be of assistance during the transition to an active level on the unit. Additional staffing may be needed for those days on which a client is scheduled for ECT.

Physical Intervention

Physical intervention is another treatment modality of which the psychiatric nursing administrator should have knowledge. Physical intervention may be defined as any procedure by which the staff helps the client to reestablish self-control of behavior by providing some degree of external control. Physical intervention procedures may range from nonverbal limit-setting to the use of seclusion and restraints.

Basic to facilitating the use of this modality is the nursing department's documented philosophy, which addresses physical intervention. This document provides a basic set of beliefs for all staff about physical intervention. In addition to this document, procedures are outlined to provide the staff with specific guidelines for the provision of physical intervention. Such guidelines serve as a basis for the planning of care by all staff members, and should be adapted for the individual client and situation.

Inherent to these procedures are two concepts: communication with the client and participation of all the staff in the designated intervention. The client should be kept informed about what is happening, what is going to happen, and why it will happen. Because physical intervention can often be a frightening event to a client who does not understand what is happening, such communication can do much to decrease this unknown. Through this type of intervention, the staff may be able to avoid more physical interventions inasmuch as the client may be able to reestablish internal self-control and no longer need external controls.

Participation by all staff members in any form of physical intervention is crucial for the effective functioning of the treatment team. Should any team member (aide, social worker, one particular nurse) be exempt without reason from the more active forms of intervention (restraints, seclusion), the degree of trust among the team members is weakened, and the clients will not believe that all staff present will provide the needed controls when necessary. This dichotomy, particularly within a therapeutic milieu setting, can be counterproductive to the original premises of the milieu.

Two other related areas in which the nurse-administrator has a role are the admissions policy and the physical plan of the particular unit or service. The admitting policy should recognize situations in which a unit or service may be unable, for a variety of reasons, to handle an acting-out client therapeutically. Thus, that client would be admitted to a unit or service that could more easily provide the controls the client needs at that time. Admitting a hostile, aggressive client to a unit or service on which there are many hostile, aggressive clients not only adds additional stress to that milieu, but does not provide the newly-admitted client with the best treatment environment possible (Karshmer, 1978).

The physical plan of a unit or service is also particularly crucial to the provision of therapeutic physical interventions. A unit or service must have sufficient areas in which the client can seek privacy in order to reestablish and to support internal controls. There must be quiet areas for conversation in which the nurse can be alone with the client. This also aids intervention in the regaining of such controls. In addition, based upon the philosophy of the organization and department, provision must be made for quiet rooms or seclusion rooms so that those interventions may be most therapeutically used with a minimum of distress to both the involved and uninvolved clients. Planning for the provision of private areas is most easily done when a new facility is being designed; however, assessment of existing facilities should be made to ensure that such areas are as available as the client population warrants.

Patients' Rights

A physical intervention issue that should be considered is that of patients' rights. (See also Chapter 4.) Legal requirements vary from state to state, and the nurse-administrator should check with the organization's legal staff to determine which regulations are applicable in which circumstances. However, the Task Force on Behavior Therapy has addressed the issue of coercive treatment and has delineated three criteria that may be used in its justification:

(1) the patient must be judged to be dangerous to himself or others, (2) it must be believed by those administering treatment that it has a reasonable chance to benefit the patient and those related to him, [and] (3) the patient must be judged to be incompetent to evaluate the necessity of the treatment. . . . The patient should not be deceived. He[/she] should be informed as to what will be done to him/her, the reasons for it, and its probable effects. (Stuart & Sundeen, 1983, p. 526)

These criteria, of course, refer to the latter phases of physical intervention (restraints and seclusion), but these criteria would be helpful when policies and procedures dealing with treatment against the client's verbal wishes are being developed. It must also be made clear that all forms of physical intervention are to be done in accordance with the client's treatment plan and not as a means of punishment. Use of physical intervention by the staff as a form of punishment would be cause for immediate disciplinary action.

Physical Interventions

Monitoring. Physical intervention begins with monitoring. The nursing staff should be educated and reeducated about the importance of early intervention. By being aware of each client as an individual, the nursing staff can recognize a situation in which a client is beginning to have difficulty or needs assistance in maintaining control. Early intervention can also encourage these clients to leave the highly populated areas of the unit for quieter locations to allow them, with the nursing staff, to regain more easily control of their own behavior.

Not only do such clients pose a threat to their own self-control, but they can also be extremely disruptive to the therapeutic milieu. Therapeutic removal of a client can do much to reassure other clients that the staff are also available to aid them should this type of intervention be needed. This action also reassures clients that their safety is secure, even if another client should begin to act out. Their degree of trust and security in the milieu and the associated staff is increased and provides them more freedom to examine their own emotions and behaviors, secure in the knowledge that assistance will be provided when it is needed.

Psychopharmacology. Psychopharmacology is the next level of physical intervention that may be beneficial for the client in regaining internal controls. Such medication, individualized to the client, should be offered when it is recognized that it would be helpful to assist the client in regaining self-control. Offering the medication would also assist the client in recognizing the mechanisms that can be used to aid in the regaining of internal control and would reflect the role medications can play in the client's treatment plan. The medication should be offered in an honest, straightforward manner, presented as a temporary aid for the client.

Restraints and Seclusion. Should all previous means of physical intervention prove unsuccessful, the client may require the use of restraints or quiet (seclusion) rooms. Organizations vary in their opinions as to which of the two formats is sanctioned, and the rationale for the option selected, as well as the client population, should be examined to determine which would prove most beneficial to the clients.

Several principles support the use of restraints or seclusion time as a component of treatment for a client. The *containment* principle refers to the "restriction of a [client's] movement to the extent that the [client] is safe from both self-injury or injury to others" (Whaley & Ramirez, 1980, p. 13). *Isolation* addresses the problem experienced by seriously ill clients in the area of interpersonal relationships. The seclusion room provides the opportunity for maintaining control over an identified small area, as well as a chance to be temporarily freed from the stress of such relationships. "The principle of *decrease in sensory input* is related to the so-called 'hyperesthesia' of the psychotic state for which the seclusion room may provide a relative monotony resulting in relief from the sensory overload" (Whaley & Ramirez, 1980, p. 14).

Five other specific behaviors may serve as indicators for the institution of restraints or seclusion time. This assistance should be initiated when the client demonstrates: (1) inability to control violent behavior when psychotic; (2) "the presence of marked agitation, thought disorder and severe confusion in a [client] whose physical condition prevents or seriously limits the use of antipsychotic medications; (3) presence of hyperactivity, insomnia, decreased food and fluid intake and grossly impaired judgment; (4) decrease in sensory input" (Whaley & Ramirez, 1980, p. 14); and (5) a request on behalf of the client for this intervention.

Another potentially difficult issue is the rationale for the termination of such interventions. The following criteria may serve as guidelines for making the decision to terminate the treatment: "(1) decrease in restlessness and anxiety, (2) stabilization of mood, (3) increased attention to space and orientation, (4) improvement in reality testing and judgment, (5) regulation of food intake, (6) regulation of sleep patterns, and (7) normalization of blood pressure and metabolic processes" (Whaley & Ramirez, 1980, p. 14). The use of a gradual release from this treatment should also include continual discussion with the client to ensure that the self-control previously in jeopardy has been regained. Releasing the client too soon may predispose the client to failure.

A related issue is that of surveillance cameras in the quiet or seclusion rooms or areas in which restraints are used. This use may have an impact upon the rights of the involved clients, and the organization's legal staff should be consulted to determine proper protocol. For some clients, the use of cameras to monitor behavior and to prevent unnecessary extended uses of the intervention may be clinically indicated.

A final issue to be considered is the postintervention meeting by the staff. Provision should be made in the workday to have such a meeting so that the staff can discuss and evaluate the intervention. It is imperative that the staff recognize their role in the situation (Loomis, 1970), and this is difficult to do when the day proceeds as if nothing has happened. It has been determined that the interventions of restraints and seclusion create multiple feelings in staff that must be recognized and discussed. Feelings that occur include anxiety, hopelessness, frustration, vengeance, feeling used, feeling drained, and other feelings that may have an impact upon the involved staff's ability to respond therapeutically in future situations (DiFabio, 1981). By meeting immediately after the conclusion of the intervention, the staff will be able to recognize and to discuss these feelings, to solve problems about the situation, and to discuss whether other interventions might have proved more suitable. This meeting is also the time for the staff to examine their information and beliefs about the client (DiFabio, 1981) and to evaluate the treatment plan, making appropriate modifications if needed. Such a time of sharing and evaluation can serve to facilitate the maintenance of the quality of nursing care provided during these interventions. The nurse-administrator should also encourage the staff to use these times to review the requirements for the initiation, monitoring, and discontinuation of restraints and seclusion that are mandated by the state departments of mental health and by JCAH.

EVALUATING IMPACT OF THE MODALITIES

During the evaluation process, the impact of the various treatment modalities on the therapeutic milieu is determined. The organization and the department should have previously developed criteria that, when present, indicate that the milieu is functioning at an optimal level. If these criteria are evident and in sufficient quantity, the treatment modalities used should be supportive of the therapeutic milieu. If, however, these criteria are absent or have decreased in quality since the last review, the causes of this change should be identified. Treatment modalities which are found to have negative impact on the milieu should be reassessed as to their applicability to the setting. The modalities may then be deleted or may be adapted so that they may better suit the organization's, department's, and clients' needs. These modifications would result from the collaborative efforts of members of all clinical disciplines, who would then continue to monitor the future suitability of the modalities on a regular basis.

REFERENCES

Balgopal, P.R., & Vassil, T.V. (1979). The group psychotherapist: A new breed. *Perspectives in Psychiatric Care, 17*(3), 132–135, 141–142.

Benfer, B. (1980). Defining the role and function of the psychiatric nurse as a member of the team. *Perspectives in Psychiatric Care, 18*(4), 166–177.

Boettcher, E.G., & Alderson, S.F. (1982). Psychotropic medications and the nursing process. *Journal of Psychosocial Nursing and Mental Health Services, 20*(11), 12–16.

Carruth, B.F. (1976). Modifying behavior through social learning. *American Journal of Nursing, 76,* 1804–1806.

Carser, D. (1981). Primary nursing in the milieu. *Journal of Psychosocial Nursing and Mental Health Services, 19*(2), 35–41.

Cohen, M., & Amdur, M. (1981). Medication groups for psychiatric patients. *American Journal of Nursing, 81,* 343–345.

DiFabio, S. (1981). Nurses' reactions to restraining patients. *American Journal of Nursing, 81,* 973–975.

Johnston, P.F. (1983). Improving the nurse-physician relationship. *The Journal of Nursing Administration, 13*(3), 19–20.

Karshmer, J.F. (1978). The application of social learning theory to aggression. *Perspectives in Psychiatric Care, 16*(5–6), 223–227.

Kranz, P.L. (1978). The play therapist: The student, the struggle, the process. *Journal of Psychiatric Nursing and Mental Health Services, 16*(11), 29–31.

Labarca, J.R. (1979). Communication through art therapy. *Perspectives in Psychiatric Care, 17*(3), 118–124.

Lane, D.E. (1981). Self-medication of psychiatric patients. *Journal of Psychosocial Nursing and Mental Health Services, 19*(5), 27–28.

Laszlo, S.S. (1978). Team building in a psychiatric hospital. *Journal of Psychiatric Nursing and Mental Health Services, 16*(2), 11–13.

Lathrop, V.G. (1978). A nurse-directed psychiatric intensive treatment unit. *Nursing Clinics of North America, 13,* 673–683.

Leib, A.C., Underwood, I.G., & Glick, I.D. (1976). The staff nurse as primary therapist: A pilot study. *Journal of Psychiatric Nursing and Mental Health Services, 14*(10), 11–18.

Loomis, M.E. (1970). Nursing management of acting-out behaviors. *Perspectives in Psychiatric Care, 8*(4), 168–173.

Slimmer, L.W. (1978). Use of the nursing process to facilitate group therapy. *Journal of Psychiatric Nursing and Mental Health Services, 16*(2), 42–44.

Stuart, G.W., & Sundeen, S.J. (1983). *Principles and practices of psychiatric nursing.* 2nd Edition. St. Louis, Mo.: C.V. Mosby Co.

Whaley, M.S., & Ramirez, L.F. (1980). The use of seclusion rooms and physical restraints in the treatment of psychiatric patients. *Journal of Psychiatric Nursing and Mental Health Services, 18*(1), 13–16.

White, E.M. (1974). Psychotherapy. In M.E. Kalkman & A.J. Davis (Eds.), *New dimensions in mental health psychiatric nursing.* New York: McGraw-Hill Book Co.

Williams, R.A. (1976). A contract for co-therapists in group psychotherapy. *Journal of Psychiatric Nursing and Mental Health Services, 14*(6), 11–14.

Wilson, H.S., & Kneisl, C.R. (1979). *Psychiatric Nursing.* Menlo Park, Calif.: Addison-Wesley Publishing Co.

Wolf, M.S. (1978). The effect of education on nurses' views of a therapeutic milieu. *Journal of Psychiatric Nursing and Mental Health Services, 16*(8), 29–33.

Chapter 16

Quality Assurance in the Psychiatric–Mental Health Organization

One of the major responsibilities of the psychiatric–mental health nursing administrator is the provision of quality client care based upon preestablished standards of care. Over the course of time, the focus of regulatory agencies has placed emphasis on the provision of safe, comprehensive client care. This approach stresses a holistic view of client care that uses all available resources in the most appropriate and efficient manner as a means of securing individualized therapeutic treatment. The nurse-administrator not only has a legal and moral responsibility, but also is ethically accountable to ensure that the clients are receiving the highest quality of care available for their health care dollar. To carry out this responsibility, the nurse-administrator must adequately assess the organization and must develop a quality assurance (QA) plan that appropriately meets the needs of the organization, the department, and the client population served. The QA for psychiatric–mental health nursing is a component of the organization's overall QA program. It complements the organizational QA program and addresses care issues specific to psychiatric–mental health nursing practice.

ASSESSMENT OF NEEDS

The psychiatric–mental health nursing administrator must begin the planning process with a thorough assessment of the organization and the department and a determination of the meaning of QA within that organization. *Quality assurance* can be defined as "a program executed to make secure or certain the excellence of health care" (ANA, 1977, p. 30). Within psychiatric–mental health nursing, quality assurance may involve a variety of activities, which may include evaluating the effectiveness of nursing interventions with specific client populations, identification of problems with subsequent problem resolution, or monitoring of the outcomes of changes implemented to correct problem or deficient areas in the care-giving system.

The QA plan is the established guideline that determines the scope of the QA program, the methods employed, and the means of evaluating that program. The QA plan must be consistent with the mission statement, the philosophy, and the goals and objectives of both the organization and the psychiatric–mental health nursing department. In addition, the QA plan must address specific departmental needs.

To assure that QA issues are addressed, the JCAH, in January, 1981, established a QA standard that—

- emphasizes the value of a coordinated, facility-wide quality assurance program; allows greater flexibility in approaches to problem identification, assessment, and resolution;
- emphasizes the importance of focusing quality assurance activity on problems whose resolution will have a significant impact on [client] care and outcomes;
- emphasizes the importance of focusing quality assurance activity on areas where demonstrable problem resolution is possible;
- encourages the use of multiple data sources to identify problems; and
- discourages the use of quality assurance studies only for the purpose of documenting high quality care. (p. ix)

Using these guidelines, the psychiatric–mental health nurse administrator is charged with the responsibility of establishing and implementing a departmental QA program that can be a meaningful tool for the constant and consistent striving for higher-quality, more economical client care. As a result of the problem-focused approach to QA, the department may well improve the care being rendered, streamline procedures, and reduce staff time spent in repetitious or useless activities.

In developing a specific problem-focused departmental QA plan, the nurse-administrator must consider many questions. The Commission on Professional and Hospital Activities has identified 17 (see Exhibit 16–1). Reviewing these questions can assist the nurse-administrator in determining some of the existing supports that can contribute to the successful implementation of the QA plan.

In the development of a QA plan, for either a newly established department or an existing one, the psychiatric–mental health nursing administrator must have realistic expectations for the QA plan. For example, the time and cost of QA studies must be economically feasible, and there must be adequate staff available to carry out the studies. Again, the QA plan cannot be formulated in a vacuum if it is expected to meet the department's needs. It must be established with attention to the administrator's knowledge of departmental budget, staffing, and other available resources.

Exhibit 16–1 Questions to Be Asked in Quality Assurance Planning

Does your [department]—

1. Have a person whose word "goes"?
2. Have a meeting which has a cross-section of your professional staff?
3. Have a mechanism by which results of any studies or evaluations are shared with appropriate staff?
4. Have a mechanism whereby one person or committee receives all reports of evaluation activities?
5. Receive periodic appraisals and recommendations from outside monitoring agencies?
6. Have a mechanism for receiving feedback or complaints from clients/patients or the community?
7. Have a meeting where staff concerns are likely to be voiced?
8. Keep minutes of the various committee meetings?
9. Have a policy and procedure manual?
10. Have a mechanism which identifies any potential situations which could lead to a law suit?
11. Fill out incident reports for accidents/incidents involving staff or clients?
12. Have written job description for each position?
13. Do periodic performance appraisals of all . . . staff?
14. Budget for professional staff continuing education?
15. Have a mechanism by which client/patient care is evaluated for comprehensiveness and appropriateness?
16. Have a mechanism for reviewing those cases which pose problems in treatment?
17. Have a staff member/s who is/are sought out for advice and consultation without necessarily having official authority?

Source: From *Quality assurance practicum for mental health and substance abuse facilities* (p. 5) by Commission on Professional and Hospital Activities, 1981, Ann Arbor, Mich.: Author. © 1981 by Commission on Professional and Hospital Activities. Reprinted by permission.

DEVELOPING A QUALITY ASSURANCE PLAN

Fundamental Principles for a Facility-Wide Plan

"A quality assurance plan should present a clear picture of the quality assurance program so that the program can be easily understood by both staff and external reviewers" (JCAH, 1981, p. 28). The QA plan is a tool that is used to achieve the goals of the QA program. The psychiatric–mental health nursing QA plan can be developed only after goals for the QA program have been identified. Once these goals are established, the means for reaching the goals are delineated in a specific individualized plan that is appropriate to the department and the organization.

The means for reaching the QA goals of an organization may be established in one of two ways. The department or service may have individual specific QA plans that articulate with a general organizational QA plan. The responsibility for the development of each QA plan lies within each respective department or service. In a second manner, the overall QA plan of the organization may mandate QA activities for each department or service. Thus, QA activities would be similarly generated from each department or service.

In either case, because QA is concerned with the scope and quality of all services rendered within the organization, it is important that QA activities be coordinated to decrease duplication of efforts and to enhance interdisciplinary cooperation. Joint QA may be appropriate and highly desirable if effectiveness of the interdisciplinary treatment team is being assessed. An activity such as inter-disciplinary client care monitoring may provide the department and the organi-zation with a meaningful exchange of information, enrichment of treatment approaches, and an augmentation of services to clients. Nursing may be involved in joint QA activities (such as a study of medication errors) performed in conjunc-tion with the organization's Pharmacy and Therapeutics Medical Staff Commit-tee. Joint activities such as these could be done separately, but the time, effort, and use of support services would be duplicated.

Coordination of the QA program within the organization may be accomplished by the establishment of a separate QA department, the designation of a QA coordinator, or the use of a coordinating committee. The QA department would use the skills of its employees to coordinate, to assist, and to perform QA functions in a large organization. The department's sole purpose would be responsibility for QA in all departments and services. A member of the department would be assigned as the resource person for psychiatric–mental health nursing and would assist the nurse-administrator with QA plan development, methods for determin-ing problems in psychiatric–mental health nursing care, establishment of priorities of problems, methodologies to be employed, and coordination of efforts with other components of the QA program (such as medical staff committees like utilization review or pharmacy and therapeutics). The QA liaison person could also provide statistical assistance to nursing, retrieve data for studies undertaken in nursing, and generate all QA reports. This process would relieve psychiatric–men-tal health nursing of the additional burden of staff time, especially for nonprofes-sional activities such as data retrieval and typing. The QA department approach would be far too expensive for a small organization but could well be cost-effective in a large, complex organization in which general, overall QA activities are so numerous that a single QA coordinator or a part-time committee simply could not handle the workload.

A QA coordinator has responsibility similar to that of a QA department but works within a smaller context. The QA coordinator would attend QA meetings of all departments, services, and medical staff committees, providing assistance and direction. The amount of direct help, such as data retrieval and the preparation of reports, would vary according to the amount of work within the organization. In some organizations, the QA coordinator may have responsibilities for QA on a part-time basis, with additional responsibilities such as utilization review coordination or medical records tasks. Although in such a case, the QA coordinator may provide coordination and some assistance to the components of the nursing QA program, the burden of QA work in this situation may fall upon the psychiatric–mental health nursing department.

The coordination of the QA program by means of a committee may be employed either facility-wide or on a departmental basis. The composition of the committee would be determined by the organization or department as the best possible way to promote the QA program and to accomplish its goals. Representatives from various disciplines or departments would thus function as a clearing house for the QA activities of the overall organization. Members of a QA committee might include the following persons:

- Chairperson of the Incident Review Committee
- Chairperson of the Professional Staff
- Chairperson of the Accreditation Committee
- Chairperson of the Utilization Review Committee
- Chairperson of the Infection Control Committee
- Representatives of discipline chiefs
- Director of Inpatient Treatment
- Director of Community Rehabilitative Services
- Director of Human Resources Management
- Coordinator of Discharge Planning
- Director of the Medical Ancillary Service
- Director of Education and Training. (JCAH, 1981, p. 93)

These representatives, like the QA coordinator, could assist departments on a part-time basis, making possible the coordination of many QA activities. Problems brought to the committee would be reviewed and delegated to the most appropriate discipline or department for QA intervention. QA activities and studies from each discipline or department would be reviewed and evaluated for thoroughness, appropriateness of methodology, and so on. Ultimately, the committee would approve reports when they were satisfactorily completed and then present them to the responsible governing authority, such as the Board of Trustees or the Joint Conference Committee for final acceptance by the organization. Members of the committee would need preparation for their roles and should have previous experience in QA or QA-related areas. As the committee's overall experience and knowledge grows, it can become more helpful to disciplines and departments with specific QA projects or needs. In this approach, the individual discipline or department completes the majority of the QA work. The approach does, however, provide assistance to disciplines or departments through appropriate guidance and redirection efforts.

The Psychiatric–Mental Health Nursing QA Plan

The psychiatric–mental health nursing QA plan is based on the goals of the QA program and is consistent with the departmental philosophy, goals, and objectives. In addition, the QA plan designates the sources and the methods to be used to identify problem areas, the process used in priority setting, the methods employed in investigating problems, the reporting mechanism employed for feedback to staff, the organizational QA program, the means for monitoring the plan, and the evaluation of the effectiveness of the plan. Exhibit 16–2 defines JCAH's guidelines for a facility-wide QA plan that can be adapted to a psychiatric–mental health nursing department plan.

The QA program in psychiatric–mental health nursing would not only look at problems in the care delivery system but would relate that care to established standards. The quality of care can be measured only when it is compared to predetermined, expected, and desired standards. The ANA's Standards of Psychiatric–Mental Health Nursing Practice can be used as a guideline in developing practice standards specific to the needs of each psychiatric–mental health nursing organization. The ANA further suggests a circular model for the QA process which identifies seven components (see Figure 16–1 and Exhibit 16–3). In addition to the seven components, evaluative monitoring must occur. This process ensures that the course of action chosen does, in fact, effect the change desired and in turn solves the problem and improves the quality of care provided.

For a detailed application of the QA modeling process to an institution that provides nursing care, see Figure 16–2.

IMPLEMENTATION OF PLAN

Once the departmental QA plan has been defined and initial establishment of standards of practice begun, the QA plan can be implemented. The psychiatric–mental health nursing administrator, in conjunction with the nursing staff involved in QA, implements the QA plan and assesses the quality of care being provided, identifies problems, seeks solutions, determines corrective actions, monitors outcomes and, ultimately, improves psychiatric–mental health nursing care.

Problem Identification

The QA focus of JCAH is frequently aimed at problem identification and resolution, especially those problems that have a positive impact on the quality of

Exhibit 16–2 Questions to Assist in the Evaluation of a Quality Assurance
Plan

Scope and Integration

Are all [job classifications] that provide patient care represented in QA activities?
Who is responsible for the administration/coordination of the overall QA program?

Problem Identification

What activities and data sources are used to identify problems?
Who conducts each of these problem identification activities?
How frequently is each activity conducted and reported?
To whom is each activity reported, and how is the information used?

Priority Setting

Who sets priorities for problem assessment and resolution?
Is there a mechanism for periodically updating priorities?
If priorities are not set centrally within the hospital, but rather on a departmental basis, is there a
    mechanism for central review and approval?

Problem Assessment

Who assesses identified problems?
Are predetermined, clinically valid criteria used to identify and assess problems?
To whom are results reported and how frequently?

Problem Resolution

Who is responsible for implementing action or resolution?
How frequently are results of action taken reported and to whom?

Problem Monitoring

Who is responsible for monitoring problem resolution?
To whom are monitoring results reported?

Evaluation

How frequently is the program evaluated?
Who conducts the annual evaluation?
Through what mechanism is the program evaluated?
To whom are the results reported?

Source: From *Quality assurance guide for psychiatric and substance abuse facilities,* (p. 82) by Joint Commission on the
Accreditation of Hospitals, 1981, Chicago: Author. © 1981 by JCAH. Reprinted by permission.

Figure 16–1 Model for Quality Assurance: Implementation of Standards

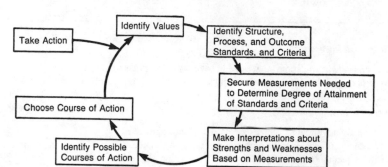

Source: From *A plan for implementation of the standards of nursing practice* by American Nurses' Association, 1977, Kansas City, Mo.: Author. © 1977 by ANA, p. 15. Reprinted by permission.

Exhibit 16–3 Model for Quality Assurance Process

1. *Identify Values.* . . . [A list] includes both those held by society (the clients) and those held by the profession . . . and scientific knowledge [as it] influences the formation of values. . . .
2. *Identify Structure, Process, Outcome Standards, and Criteria.* . . . This component is the identification of standards and criteria (outcome, process, and structure) for nursing care. . . . Structure standards and criteria are those which describe the purpose of the institution, agency or program, . . . organization characteristics, . . . qualifications of health professionals and other workers. Process standards and criteria focus on the nature, sequence of events, and activities in the delivery of nursing care. . . . Outcome standards and criteria pertain to the end results of nursing care, a measurable change in the state of the client's health. . . . Outcomes are the ultimate indicators of quality patient care. . . .
3. *Secure Measurements Needed to Determine Degree of Attainment of Standards and Criteria.* . . . Existing methods include direct patient observation, external and internal peer review, concurrent appraisal and introspective audit, UR, self assessment, teacher assessment, supervisor evaluation, and performance evaluation. . . .
4. *Make Interpretations About Strengths and Weaknesses Based On Measurements.* The measurement of the degree of attainment between the identified standards and criteria and the current level of nursing practice serves as the data base for interpretations. . . .
5. *Identify Possible Courses of Action.* . . .
6. *Choose the Course of Action.* . . . The important element here is that a plan for change is made. . . .
7. *Take Action.*

Source: From *A plan for implementation of the standards of nursing practice* by American Nurses' Association, 1977, Kansas City, Mo.: Author. © 1977 by ANA. Adapted by permission.

Figure 16–2 Use of Model in an Institution Which Provides Nursing Care

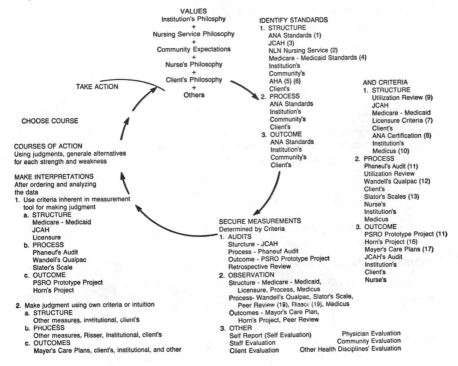

Source: From *A plan for implementation of the standards of nursing practice* by American Nurses' Association, 1977, Kansas City, Mo.: Author. © 1977 by ANA, p. 20. Reprinted by permission.

client care and clinical performance. The nurse-administrator has many valuable sources that can be used to identify problems within the psychiatric–mental health nursing setting. Some of these sources are—

- client care records
- client or visitor incident report forms
- client care monitoring (also known as individual case review performed on current cases)
- critical incidents
- client surveys
- aftercare reports
- staff meetings
- client "milieu" or unit meetings

- client complaints
- physician or other professional complaints
- direct observation
- peer review

Once suspected or actual problems have been identified, they need to be assigned priorities according to their possible impact on client care. Exhibit 16–4 provides a format in which the psychiatric–mental health nursing administrator can delineate problem areas, assign priorities to these areas, and thoroughly investigate them. Probable causes and alternative corrective actions would be determined, and selected corrective actions would be taken to resolve or correct the problem. Some possible problems in psychiatric–mental health nursing include the following:

- medication noncompliance
- client injuries in seclusion
- contraband in client care areas
- injuries during active sports
- falls
- medication errors
- suicide attempts
- destruction of property or destructive physical acting-out behaviors
- discharges against medical advice
- inadequate client precaution monitoring
- inappropriate use of seclusion or restraint
- inadequate nursing documentation on client record
- increased recidivism rate
- increased infections on children's or adolescents' unit

In determining the extent and the possible causes of suspected or actual problems, both concurrent and retrospective measures may be used. For example, if it is suspected that, during seclusion, clients are suffering injuries at a higher rate than previously, a QA study can be developed that would review the incident reports of previous seclusion room injuries for a designated period (retrospective). In addition, the records of clients injured during seclusion might also be retrospectively reviewed. At the same time, whenever a currently hospitalized client requires seclusion, a member of the psychiatric–mental health nursing QA program might interview staff members involved in the seclusion, observe seclusion techniques, and investigate reported client injuries immediately. This process

Exhibit 16–4 Identifying Departmental Problem Areas

Think about problems that might exist in your [department] and complete the following exercise on problem identification.

1. Note five problems that you suspect exist in your [department].
2. For each suspected problem, list all data sources that might help verify its existence.
3. For each suspected problem, note the ways in which [client] care might be affected adversely.
4. Note potential explanations for the existence of each problem.

Suspected Problems	Data Sources	Impact on Patient Care	Potential Explanations

Source: From *Quality assurance guide for psychiatric and substance abuse facilities* (p. 47) by Joint Commission on Accreditation of Hospitals, 1981, Chicago: Author. © 1981 by Joint Commission on Accreditation of Hospitals. Reprinted by permission.

would occur over a designated period of time and would be a concurrent activity. Information from these sources (e.g., incident reports, client records, personal interviews, direct observations) can provide the necessary data to identify the scope, the cause, and the magnitude of the problem.

With this information, all possible solutions can be explored, and the most appropriate corrective actions specified. Furthermore, investigation of seclusion injuries may isolate the problem to a specific unit on a specific shift; it may even identify one or two staff members who have been involved in the majority of the incidents. The injuries may be occurring because these staff members are new to the organization and did not attend the physical crisis intervention inservices. If this is the case, the employees can be scheduled to participate in the in-service training, giving return demonstrations. They may also be observed and coached on the job until their performance is more satisfactory. Additional refresher courses for all staff members may also be warranted. Incident reports can then be monitored over a period of time to determine if the corrective measure has been successful.

After the QA study has been completed, the entire process is documented with all supporting data and is then reported through the designated channels. The psychiatric–mental health nursing QA program needs to have a monitoring mechanism that provides for adequate evaluation to ascertain the degree of problem resolution for all problems addressed. Follow-up dates for the review of the problem areas need to be established upon completion of the study. The use of a tickler file or a flow chart can be helpful in tracking evaluative monitoring when several problems are being or have been addressed.

Use of the Psychiatric–Mental Health Nursing Audit

Another means of assessing the quality of care is through the use of an audit tool. An *audit* is "a methodical examination and review; the final report of an examination of accountability" (Davidson, Burleson, Crawford, & Chistofferson, 1977, p. 407). The psychiatric–mental health nursing audit, which provides specific, measurable criteria, based upon desired standards of care, is an excellent tool for measuring (evaluating) the quality of the psychiatric–mental health nursing care being given to the client population. Use of the audit process itself can be a valuable learning experience for the staff involved. It provides the staff members with an opportunity to set standards of care for specific client populations or client problems while assessing, determining, and evaluating their own achievement of such standards.

Role of Staff Development

The success of the QA program lies with the nursing staff. It is imperative that the nursing staff be aware of the standards of care they are expected to attain. Feedback about QA activities and the staff's role in the outcomes of these activities is essential. Staff development is a major component of QA. Many problems are related to the staff's knowledge of policies and procedures or the inadequacy of that knowledge. In either case, staff development personnel will have responsibility for providing educational programs to the staff for the resolution of indicated problems. Because staff development is a link between QA activity and the staff, staff development personnel should be included as active members of the QA program at both the departmental and the organizational level.

Risk Management and Quality Assurance

Risk management is concerned with the overall operations of the health care organization that place the client, staff, visitors, or the organization in jeopardy physically, mentally, or financially. As noted earlier, QA is concerned with the assessment and improvement of the care being provided. The focus of risk management is minimizing possible risks to clients, staff, visitors, and the organization. The focus of QA is the provision of maximum care. Exhibit 16–5 delineates the functions of both risk management and QA.

Exhibit 16–5 Functions of Risk Management and Quality Assurance

Risk Management	*Quality Assurance*
1. Protect financial assets of the hospital.	1. Is tied to the philosophy of the hospital.
2. Protect human and intangible resources.	2. Improves the performance of all professionals and protects the patients.
3. Prevent injury to patients, visitors, employees and property.	3. Focuses on the quality of patient care.
4. Loss reduction focusing on individual loss or on single incidents.	4. Sets the quality of care delivered against standards and measurable criteria.
5. Loss prevention to prevent incidents by improving the quality of care through continuing and ongoing monitoring.	5. Prevents future losses or patient injuries by continuous monitoring of problem resolution areas.
6. Review of each incident and the patterns of incidents through the application of the steps in risk management process: risk identification, risk analysis, risk evaluation and risk treatment.	6. Searches for patterns of non-compliance with goals, objectives, and standards. The following steps of the quality assurance process are applied: problem identification, problem assessment, implementation of corrective action, follow-up and reporting of findings.

Source: From ''Why risk management and quality assurance should be integrated'' by J.E. Orlikoff and G.B. Lanham, 1981, *Hospitals,* 55(15), p. 55. © 1981 by American Hospital Publishing, Inc. Reprinted by permission.

A necessary element of risk management is the safety and security programs of the organization. "Quality assurance requires individuals with clinical expertise, while risk management requires managerial expertise" (Orlikoff & Lanham, 1981, p. 54). Risk management focuses on prevention of problems, while QA focuses on improving care. Both have an impact on the quality of care provided, while approaching problems or potential problems from different directions. Figure 16–3 indicates the overlap of risk management and quality assurance.

Information generated by both programs can be very helpful to the success of each. It is desirable, then, to have psychiatric–mental health nursing representation, directly or through a liaison, involved with risk management programs. Review of incident reports by a risk manager may indicate a clinical issue that should be investigated by the psychiatric–mental health nursing QA program. For example, an increase in suicide attempts may be identified by risk management and referred to the psychiatric–mental health nursing QA liaison for further study. Likewise, a client may sustain a fractured wrist while playing volleyball during recreational therapy. Nursing would certainly need to contact the risk manager as soon as possible so that the organization's liability insurance carrier could be notified. Early response to risk situations can mean the difference between consumer protection and satisfaction on the one hand and legal action on the other. Cooperation and coordination are two key elements in the effective interface of risk management and quality assurance.

Figure 16–3 Overlap Functions of Quality Assurance and Risk Management

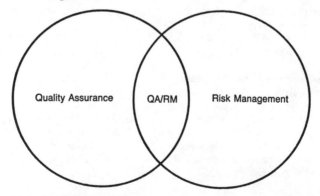

Note: QA/RM intersection of quality assurance and risk management is the area of least overlap between the two functions.

Source: From "Why risk management and quality assurance should be integrated" by J.E. Orlikoff and G.B. Lanham, 1981, *Hospitals,* 55(15), p. 55. © 1981 by American Hospital Publishing, Inc. Reprinted by permission.

EVALUATION OF THE QUALITY ASSURANCE PROGRAM

The effectiveness of the psychiatric–mental health nursing QA program needs to be evaluated at least annually. Through the review of the evaluative monitoring of QA studies, the effectiveness of corrective measures can be determined. If problems have not been resolved satisfactorily, additional steps must be taken. Persons involved in psychiatric–mental health nursing QA should review the QA plan as it relates to the organizational plan. Through feedback on QA activities, the group can identify the degree of goal attainment accomplished under the existing QA plan. If necessary, the plan should be modified to reflect the changes in organizational direction or departmental goals. When executed fully, the QA program can be a motivating influence for improving the quality of the psychiatric–mental health nursing care being provided to clients.

REFERENCES

American Nurses' Association. (1977). *A plan for implementation of the standards of nursing practice.* Kansas City, Mo.: Author.

Commission on Professional and Hospital Activities. (1981). *Quality assurance practicum for mental health and substance abuse facilities.* Ann Arbor, Mich.: Author.

Davidson, S.V., Burleson, B.C., Crawford, J.E., & Chistofferson, S. (1977). *Nursing care evaluation: concurrent and retrospective review criteria.* St. Louis, Mo.: C.V. Mosby.

Joint Commission on Accreditation of Hospitals. (1981). *Quality assurance guide for psychiatric and substance abuse facilities.* Chicago: Author.

Orlikoff, J.E., & Lanham, G.B. (1981). Why risk management and quality assurance should be integrated. *Hospitals, 55*(15), pp. 54–55.

SUGGESTED READING

Apostoles, F.E., Little, M.E., & Murphy, H.D. (1977). Developing a psychiatric nursing audit. *Journal of Psychiatric Nursing and Mental Health Services, 15*(5), 10–11, 13.

Chapter 17

Documentation Systems in Psychiatric–Mental Health Nursing

An integral component of any quality assurance program is the documentation system used by the psychiatric–mental health organization. This documentation not only records the client's progress, but also provides material for monitoring the quality of care provided, identifying problem areas, and orchestrating changes to correct previously identified problem areas. With the increasing emphasis on the justification and containment of health care costs, documentation of patient care must be more detailed, individualized, and objective.

The selection or change of a documentation system will, most likely, not lie solely with the psychiatric–mental health nursing administrator, but will be the result of a committee decision. Such a committee would be composed of clinical department heads and some medical staff who are involved in the documentation process. Regardless of the committee's composition, the nurse-administrator must be an equal participant in any selection, review, or change in a documentation system so that the most accurate method of documenting the nursing process in the delivery of quality client care is ensured.

ASSESSMENT PROCESS AND SELECTION OF A SYSTEM

In the review process for the selection or revision of a documentation system, the committee should assess the various types of systems available in view of the needs of the organization, staff, and clients. The organization's structure, number of disciplines involved in documentation, philosophies of the organization and of the individual disciplines, as well as other factors, should be considered when a documentation system is being selected. The client population characteristics should also be a part of the decision process, because the type of the treatment offered may dictate certain documentation needs. For example, an organization that offers primarily one-to-one therapy sessions for clients with chronic schizophrenia needs a different documentation system from one that includes short-term inpatient acute treatment.

Types of Documentation Systems

Traditional or Source-Oriented Documentation Systems

Once the committee has defined the organization, staff, and client needs in regard to a documentation system, the committee is ready to review systems in view of these needs. The types of documentation systems fall into two main categories, with variations within each category. In the traditional or source-oriented system, each discipline generally charts separately on one client in separate areas of the medical record. Although this system may facilitate each discipline's review of the client's progress in relation to that discipline, there is no documented blending of client information to create an overall picture of the client's progress and current status. Verbal exchange of information must serve to consolidate treatment approaches. Within this system, formats may vary between disciplines, depending upon the collaborative nature of the organization.

Focused Documentation Systems

The term *focused documentation systems* refers to documentation systems that require that charting be done according to certain pre-identified issues—problems, topics, goals. In each system, documentation focuses on specific identified issues (i.e., problems, topics, goals, etc.) through the course of the client's treatment. All disciplines chart in the same section of the medical record. This practice provides a continuous picture of the client's progress in general, as well as in relation to specific identified areas.

Inasmuch as all focused documentation systems follow the same general format, the problem-oriented documentation system is used as a sample of this type of system. Components, techniques, and formats used within this type of focused documentation system can be applied to any focused documentation system by a change of the identified focus. The problem-oriented documentation system was the first of its type to be used extensively. It continues to be frequently used in a variety of psychiatric–mental health settings. It was developed "to actualize the concept of a health care system which focuses on the total [client] and encompasses all phases of health care . . . using all health professionals to their highest potential" (Harris, 1978, p. 35).

There are four components to this and all focused documentation systems: "(a) defined data base, (b) complete problem [topic/goal/etc.] list, with numbered and titled problems [topics/goals/etc.]; (c) [initial] treatment plans, with correspondingly numbered and titled entries; and (d) progress notes, numbered and titled according to problem [topic/goal/etc.]" (Woody & Mallison, 1973,

p. 1169). The data base is composed of all client information necessary to identify focus areas, to determine appropriate treatment plans, and to delineate goals or outcomes. Information is gathered not only on admission but throughout the course of treatment and serves as a foundation upon which to base treatment.

In order to develop a problem (topic/goal/etc.) list, the organization must identify its specific focus. According to Holmes (1980), a *problem* can be defined as "some aspect of the [client's] health or environment that produces or threatens to produce functional disability, morbidity, or increased risk of mortality" (p. 42). However, not every problem/topic/goal is included on this list. If a focus is major, ongoing, or apt to have an impact on treatment or its course, it should be included on the identified list.

Treatment plans, both initial and revised, must address all items on the list of previously identified items. These plans must be tailored to the individual client to reflect the client's strengths and weaknesses. Generally, these plans should also include assignment of treatment responsibilities, patient involvement, discharge planning, and specific areas of needed client education. If an organization chooses to follow the original problem-oriented documentation system, the plans would also be grouped according to "(1) diagnosis, (2) therapeutic measures, (3) parameters to monitor the progress of therapy, [and] (4) patient education" (Ryback, 1974, p. 14).

Under this type of documentation system, progress notes can be divided "into three types: narrative notes, flow sheets, and discharge notes" (Woody & Mallison, 1973, pp. 1171–1172). The types of notes used are based on previously defined organizational and departmental needs. All disciplines chart on the same forms in the client's record and indicate, through a preestablished mechanism, the focus of each individual note. The format for the actual charting varies, but it is often the so-called SOAP format (subjective, objective, assessment, plan). Similarly, the formats for any necessary flow sheets and the discharge note would depend upon each organization's requirements and should be detailed within the organization's and the department's policies and procedures.

Open Treatment Record

An additional variant on any documentation system is the use of an open treatment record. By definition, this process allows and encourages clients to read and to review their personal treatment records. Practiced in an in-patient psychiatric–mental health setting, this would seem a logical option, inasmuch as "sharing responsibility with the [client] is a fundamental concept of a therapeutic community" (Simonton, Neuffer, Stein, & Furedy, 1977, p. 25). In one psychiatric hospital, this process was piloted successfully, and several advantages were identified. The process increased the client's knowledge of, and involvement in, the treatment plan and reinforced the client's own progress *with* the client himself/

herself. One main disadvantage that was discovered was selective charting. Certain client information was communicated verbally, rather than being documented. It was also discovered that staff members must be available when clients review their charts and that these staff members must be able to answer and to clarify the majority of the client's questions (Simonton et al.). The inclusion of this process as a component of an overall documentation system would depend upon the philosophy and mission of the particular psychiatric–mental health organization.

Nursing Care Plans

In psychiatric–mental health organizations with comprehensive treatment plans developed by the patient and the treatment team, a separate nursing care plan may not be routinely needed. However, nursing care plans may be helpful in further delineating the nurse's treatment role. These plans would incorporate guidelines similar to those used in other nursing practice areas, with the major emphasis on the need for measurable criteria. The abstract nature of psychiatric–mental health nursing care makes it increasingly important for nursing diagnosis, goals, objectives, interventions, and evaluative criteria to be specific, behaviorally oriented, and measurable. Any source of ambiguity in the above serves to decrease the continuity and consistency of care by allowing for varying interpretations throughout the nurses' implementation of the treatment plan.

SELECTION AND PLANNING IMPLEMENTATION

After a review of the available documentation systems, the committee should select one system that can be tailored to the organization. Keeping in mind the pre-identified needs and the strengths and weaknesses of each system, the committee should also consider the impact of the regulatory agencies that will be reviewing the organization's documentation. For example, the JCAH expects that a documentation system will

> (1) serve as a basis for planning for continuity of [client] care; (2) . . . provide a means of communication among fellow professionals involved in [client] care; (3) . . . furnish documentary evidence of ordered and supervised treatments, observations of the [client's] behavior and responses to treatment; (4) . . . serve as a basis for review, study, and evaluation of care rendered to the client; (5) . . . assist in protecting the legal rights of the client, the facility, and the professional staff; and (6) . . . provide data for research and education. (Ryback, 1974, p. 3)

Hence, the documentation system chosen should provide a framework for the achievement of these actions, if accreditation is sought. A system that does not help the organization in this aspect of the provision of comprehensive quality care can impede the organization's and the department's progress and growth.

Once an appropriately designed documentation system has been selected, the committee begins to plan for its implementation. As is the case with any organizational change, resistance can be expected. However, if the committee recognizes and anticipates major sources of resistance, it can make plans to overcome potential problems. Often, complaints are attributable to the time requirements of a more detailed documentation system.

Recognizing the roots of the problem, the committee can make plans to confront this issue realistically. Frequently, documentation has been done only for legal reasons and is task-oriented, not focused on implementing the nursing process in its entirety (Harris, 1978). It must be emphasized that documentation is an integral component of treatment and reinforces the entire nursing process. When the system is viewed as an important communication process that clearly and logically follows the client's course of treatment, it will be accepted.

Another major area of resistance arises from the control certain disciplines exert over the management of client care and client records. This control often concerns not only the type of documentation system used, but also how it is used. It often results from a discipline's need to maintain its autonomy. The discipline exercising control should have that control dispersed among all the disciplines, so that the provision of quality care can be shared and facilitated by all mental health professionals. Often the findings of regulatory agencies support a change to an improved documentation system.

A final area of resistance may lie within the nursing department itself. The staff nurse may hesitate to make nursing decisions that affect client care because either nursing management does not support such decisions or physicians undermine the nurse's actions. If this is the situation, client-centered care is not being practiced. This circumstance makes it extremely difficult for the organization to initiate a client-centered documentation system. The department must change its philosophy and practice, and foster staff nurses who are responsible and who readily accept accountability for their client care actions (Harris, 1978).

Once the potential resistances have been addressed and included in the planning process, the organization can begin to implement the actual change through mechanisms similar to those involved in other major organizational changes. Pilot projects, in-service training, and evaluative mechanisms can enable the organization to revise successfully the documentation system over a specified period of time.

Once a documentation system is in place, the work of the committee continues. Although the original committee may disband, other persons will be needed to initiate, to maintain, and to monitor the system. Feedback from documentation audits will enable all levels of the staff to focus upon problem areas in the system and to work toward their resolution. Continuing education will disseminate audit results, addressing problem areas with existing staff, as well as orienting new staff. By creating a climate conducive to change and supporting the change in systems once it is accomplished, the organization and the department will have established a documentation system that not only meets the organization's needs but functions as an integral component of the quality assurance (QA) program.

Importance of Charting

"With the increased emphasis on the responsibility and accountability of nurses in their practice and with the ensuing interest in third party payment for nursing services, documentation of practice has become highly significant with written documentation of nursing practice readily demonstrating adherence to established standards" (Holmes, 1980, p. 40). However, "the combined phenomena of too few nurses for too many patients, a fear of committing themselves on paper, and the traditional priority given to actually completing treatments and medications, all interfere with and inhibit the documenting process" (Barbiasz, Hunt & Lowenstein, 1981, p. 22). In order to reverse this type of situation, the practice of charting should receive recognition and support commensurate with its importance within the department. If accurate charting that is nursing-process oriented is valued by the department but is not rewarded, departmental expectations and standards cannot be met. The nursing department must incorporate recognition of quality charting into its reward system, either as an element within a merit raise system, by public recognition, or by some other acceptable means that provides the staff with the positive reinforcement they need to document continuously on a quality level.

Charting Early in the Shift

Another mechanism that may aid in the improvement of charting, which suffers from a reported "lack of time," is documentation that is performed early in the shift. This system requires that a nurse thoroughly assess each client at the beginning of the shift and record this assessment in the chart. This assessment adds information to the basic comprehensive client assessment that was done upon admission and provides an excellent picture of the client's current status. Thereafter, the nurse reassesses each client at specific time intervals during the shift and records observations on flow sheets applicable to that unit or service. Should changes in the initial assessment occur, they are recorded in the client's chart in a specified format.

In addition to being a more efficient use of time, early charting has shown several positive outcomes. "Other nurses read the charts for pertinent information and are, at times, complimentary. . . . Professional dialogue among nursing peers is increased. . . . Doctors using the charts ask fewer questions. . . . Symptoms are found early, interventions are started promptly, and a [client's] well-being is directly and positively affected by implementation of this system" (Rexilius, 1981, p. 53). Finally, any person reading the medical record obtains a current status report on the client without needing a verbal explanation from the nurse (Rexilius).

This system is applicable to most psychiatric–mental health organizations because of the nature of the client population. In most psychiatric–mental health settings, the client's improvement may be minimal from shift to shift and only slightly perceptible over time. Through this charting mechanism, the nurse is free to use additional time interacting with clients after the initial shift assessment. Changes in clients' conditions can be more accurately associated with treatment components, because they are recorded immediately upon observation. Medication adjustments can be made more promptly as a result of consistent observation of client responses. Through this process of charting, psychiatric–mental health nurses can be more responsive to the individual client's needs and, thus, be able to provide improved quality care.

Computer Use in Charting

As complexity in client care in psychiatric–mental health nursing increases, more and more organizations will be using computers to improve documentation of client care. For nurses, this practice again introduces the issue of accountability in records. To be entered into the computer, documentation must be concise and objective. This change can benefit documentation within psychiatric–mental health nursing, as increased objectivity and conciseness in nursing notes lead to accurate revisions of initial treatment plans and early recognition of the attainment of discharge criteria. "The challenge for nursing managers is to provide the tools and support that nurses need to become proficient with the computerized system while helping them retain the uniqueness of nursing" (Gluck, 1979, p. 24). As a major system change, the introduction of such computers may result in staff resistance and the need for extensive educational programs. Through advanced planning and supportive efforts, the staff's adaptation to this documentation process can be facilitated.

Importance of Supportive Forms

In addition to the forms on which routine charting is recorded, there are myriad supportive forms (such as flow sheets, medication sheets, kardexes) that are used to provide additional information necessary for the planning of comprehensive quality care. The forms proposed or currently being used should be reviewed to determine whether they are applicable to the psychiatric–mental health nursing department. Often, forms applicable to other nursing specialities are used in psychiatric–mental health nursing without modification or consideration of the role they play in the nurse's provision of quality care. Therefore, the content and format of each form should be tailored to meet the needs of the individual psychiatric–mental health nursing department or unit or service. Such individualized forms need not be developed by the department but may be found through a literature search or through networking with other psychiatric–mental health nursing administrators. By using forms that are more appropriate to the particular client population and psychiatric–mental health nursing department, the nursing staff will be able to document more effectively and efficiently.

EVALUATION OF SYSTEM

Evaluation of an organization's documentation system must be done on a regular basis. Such evaluation may occur independently, or it may be part of an overall QA annual review. The goals and objectives of the system must be compared with the outcomes achieved by that system. Ongoing QA activities, such as audits, often identify problem areas that require attention. The committee responsible for the monitoring of the documentation system then needs to develop approaches to identify the causes of the problems, to determine plans for resolution of the problem areas, and to monitor the outcomes of the corrective actions. The specific mechanisms or protocols used to complete this evaluation process are similar to those used in other areas of nursing, but they need to be adapted for use with psychiatric–mental health client populations.

REFERENCES

Barbiasz, J.E., Hunt, V., & Lowenstein, A. (1981). Nursing documentation: A format not a form. *The Journal of Nursing Administration, 11*(6), 22–26.

Gluck, J. (1979). The computerized medical record system: Meeting the challenge for nursing. *The Journal of Nursing Administration, 9*(12), 17–24.

Harris, R.J. (1978). Facilitating change to the problem-oriented medical record system. *The Journal of Nursing Administration, 8*(8), 35–38.

Holmes, A.M. (1980). Problem-oriented medical records, nursing audit and accountability. *Supervisor Nurse, 11*(4), 40, 42–43.

Rexilius, B. (1981). Why not chart first. *Supervisor Nurse, 12*(2), 52–53.

Ryback, R.S. (1974). *The problem oriented record in psychiatry and mental care.* New York: Green & Stratton, Inc.

Simonton, M.J., Neuffer, C.H., Stein, E.J., & Furedy, R.L. (1977). The open medical record: An educational tool. *Journal of Psychiatric Nursing and Mental Health Services, 15*(12), 25–30.

Woody, M., & Mallison, M. (1973). The problem oriented system for patient-centered care. *American Journal of Nursing, 73*(7), 1169–1175.

Chapter 18

Research as a Component of an Administrative Program in Psychiatric–Mental Health Nursing

Research in psychiatric–mental health nursing is a desirable component of the nurse-administrator's program for the department. The rationale for this statement is derived from the standards for the profession. This point of view is expressed in the Standards of Psychiatric and Mental Health Nursing Practice, Standard XI: "The nurse contributes to nursing and the mental health field through innovations in theory and practice and participation in research" (ANA, 1982, p. 19). In addition, the importance of research is supported in Standard XI of the ANA's Standards for Nursing Services (1977): "A nursing service supports research in the health care field" (p. 7).

Even if research were not mandated by these professional standards, the psychiatric–mental health nursing administrator's responsibility to the profession, as well as for the provision of quality care, makes research a desirable component of the nurse-administrator's administrative program. Research is important for the development of a knowledge base unique to psychiatric–mental health nursing; this knowledge base is necessary for the growth of the profession and for the improvement of the quality of psychiatric–mental health care provided (Fawcett, 1980). Nursing needs to be involved in the development of this knowledge base because the only way "to generate, refine or enlarge the knowledge needed by nursing [is] . . . through scientific research" (Fawcett, 1980, p. 37).

The ANA recognized the importance of nursing research when, in 1974, it issued the following statement: "All professional nurses should foster the initiation, dissemination, and utilization of research as an accepted and integral part of nursing practice, nursing services and nursing education" (Sweeney & Olivieri, 1981, p. 22). Conway (1978) states, "the most important task for a science-based practice is the constant assessment of current knowledge and the testing of beliefs about efficacious methods of applying that knowledge" (p. 27). This knowledge can only be improved by the use of clinically based research (Sweeney & Olivieri).

ORGANIZATIONAL AND DEPARTMENTAL ASSESSMENT

A thorough assessment of the organization, the department, and the staff must be completed before the initiation of a planning process for the introduction of research into the clinical setting. In order to do this assessment in a knowledgeable fashion, familiarity with basic research terms is desirable.

Definition of Research Terms

All research terminology need not be reviewed here. However, a knowledge of the following terms is helpful to promote an understanding of the research process and its application to psychiatric–mental health nursing.

A *proposition* is a "statement of the presumed or validated knowledge about one or more concepts" (Fawcett, 1980, p. 26). When a proposition contains operationally defined concepts or states relations that are observed, it is a *hypothesis*. A hypothesis for psychiatric–mental health nursing might state:

> Manic depressive clients who receive medication information about lithium before discharge demonstrate better medication compliance than manic depressive clients without this information.

"A *theory* is a set of interrelated constructs (concepts), definitions, and propositions that present a systematic view of the phenomena by specifying relations among variables, with the purpose of explaining and predicting the phenomena" (Sweeney & Olivieri, 1981, pp. 28–29). "The purpose of theory is to explain relevant events in the world, and in practice [and] . . . to provide knowledge which can be used to guide and direct the actions of members of that discipline" (Fawcett, 1980, p. 37). Theory has a reciprocal relationship with research; it directs research while the results of research activities impact the development of theory (Fawcett).

Types of Research

Within research, there are various types. The type selected depends upon the amount of information known about a particular topic. This progression includes descriptive research, correlational research, predictive research, and replicative research (Fawcett, 1980, p. 37). "*Descriptive* studies examine the specific characteristics of an individual, group, situation, or event [and] are required when nothing or very little is known about the particular phenomenon" (Fawcett, p. 37). In psychiatric–mental health nursing, descriptive studies might be done to determine characteristics about a particular client population being served—such as battered spouses or schizophrenic clients, who are able to function in society with minimal support.

Correlational research is "appropriate when the essential characteristics of the study variables have been identified. The goal of these [correlational] designs is to explain relationships among variables" (Fawcett, 1980, p. 37). A study that addresses the relationship between nursing assignment systems (e.g., primary, team, etc.) in psychiatric–mental health and client satisfaction with nursing care would be a correlational study. *Predictive* research occurs "when relations among concepts have already been explained and causal inferences are not of interest" (Fawcett, p. 37). Using various groups, a predictive study would examine "the type of information that has the strongest causal effect in reducing clients' distress [before and] after" (Fawcett, p. 37) electroconvulsive therapy. *Replicative* studies are "necessary to establish the generalizability of research findings to various settings and groups of people" (Fawcett, p. 37). Replication of an inpatient study in an outpatient setting would begin to establish the generalizability of identified psychiatric–mental health nursing interventions.

Methods of Incorporating Research into a Clinical Setting

In addition to the various research designs, there are several methods of incorporating research into clinical practice. These methods may be of a popularizing, an empirical, or a theoretical nature. "The *popularization* method translates technical research into a . . . form easily used by practitioners" (Fawcett, 1980, p. 38). Through this method, however, the accuracy of the research is often lost to the point that the translation is of minimal value. "The *empirical* method requires the [psychiatric–mental health] clinician to read research reports and case histories on a regular basis and to apply relevant findings or conclusions whenever a practice problem is presented" (Fawcett, p. 38). This, also, is often not helpful inasmuch as relevant findings applicable to the clinician's setting may be few. For example, nursing interventions that increase medication compliance with schizophrenic clients in inpatient settings may not be applicable for a clinician working in an outpatient clinic.

Assessment Process

After a review of nursing research literature, the nursing department needs to be assessed to identify the most appropriate means of incorporating research into a particular psychiatric–mental health setting. Any research program must, of course, be consistent with the resources and goals of the organization, the department, and the staff. Any inconsistency between the program and these important aspects results in continued difficulties during the planning and implementation phases.

Feasibility Study

In order to determine the readiness of the organization and the department for the implementation of a psychiatric–mental health nursing research program, a feasibility study should be conducted. This study may be done by in-house persons or by an outside consulting firm. Regardless of who conducts this study, there are evaluative criteria that determine whether the research climate is ready for the implementation of a research program (see Table 18–1). If certain criteria are not met, these should be further developed before the implementation of any nursing research program (Egan, McElmurry, & Jameson, 1981). The first criterion to be examined is *subject participation*. The investigators must determine whether there are sufficient research problems to support the development of a full scale research program. Within psychiatric–mental health nursing, little research has been conducted. Therefore, there are multiple research practice problems that could be investigated. In addition, there must be willing participants. The investigators must also determine whether psychiatric clients fully understand consent forms, and if not, what precautions would be recommended to protect these clients' rights.

The second criterion to be assessed is the *availability of professional participants*. In assessing this area, the investigators determine whether persons are present on staff, or available for consultation, who have the "preparation, abilities, experience and interest" (Egan et al., 1981, p. 27) to be active in the research program. In psychiatric–mental health nursing, few people on the staff may qualify in all these areas. However, these persons could be encouraged and developed as well as using outside consultants or educators to support their efforts.

Certain *market factors* must be in place before implementing a research program. These would include such items as receptivity and demand for the knowledge created by the research, and the allowance of staff time for the work required by the research project. If the organization or the department does not value nursing research, this lack of interest must be dealt with before any additional planning so that a climate is provided in which research can flourish. This factor is also related to the criterion of *organizational systems*. An assessment of these systems examines the relationship of organizational administration to the study of psychiatric–mental health nursing problems. Again, if there are no supports in this area, they must be developed before any future implementation.

Economic factors must also be examined. This examination includes an assessment of the costs and benefits of the program to both the department and the organization. Because health care systems are subject to constant demands for improved cost-effectiveness, cost is an important area to be investigated. Program costs should be realistic; some costs can often be defrayed through improvement in quality care, decrease in risks presented to the clients, publications, public relations for the organization, and so forth. Through these efforts, the program can demonstrate its cost-effectiveness.

Table 18–1 Sources of Information for Assessing Eight Conditions Affecting Research Climate in Hospitals

Condition	Internal Measures	External Measures
1. Subject participation	Nursing personnel Nursing audit studies Policies regarding consent for release of data Existing data bases Programs regarding advisement of patient rights	Professional association Priorities for funding research Patient Rights guidelines
2. Professional participation	Nursing personnel	Professional recommendations regarding level of preparation for researchers Prototype nursing research programs
3. Market factors	Hospital departments Hospital mission statements Nursing personnel	Public policies regarding health research and evaluation Prototype nursing research programs
4. Organizational systems	Nursing department and hospital organization Audit procedures	Prototype nursing research programs
5. Economic factors	Hospital departments Summary of educational programs' use of hospitals for research projects Nursing department's criteria for the approval of research projects Policies regarding incentives for personnel participation in systematic studies	Prototype nursing research programs Medical center resources Potential sources for private and public funding
6. Legal/statutory	Institutional and departmental standards for service, education, and research Protocols and guidelines for use of humans in research Institutional research review committee Quality assurance program	Professional standards Hospital accrediting standards and regulations State laws Medicare certification regulations Ethical guidelines for practice and research

Table 18–1 continued

Condition	Internal Measures	External Measures
7. Facilities and resources	Hardware, software, library space, and consultants	Medical center resources Prototype nursing research programs
8. Contributions to the research endeavors of educational institutions	Rate review formulations Summary of present contributions Present system for approval of studies Nursing personnel	Participating educational programs

Source: From *Practice based research: Assessing your department's readiness* by E.C. Egan, B.J. McElmurry, & H.M. Jameson, 1981, *Journal of Nursing Administration 11*(10), 28. © 1981 by J.B. Lippincott Co. Reprinted by permission.

The investigators must examine the *legal and statutory provisions* that can have an impact on such research programs. These would include the "standards and regulations regarding nursing research, nursing service, and the use of human subjects" (Egan et al., 1981, p. 27). Even if the psychiatric–mental health nursing administrator does not anticipate the immediate inclusion of human subjects, this possibility must be anticipated in order to provide the groundwork for the future growth of the program into these areas.

Basic to the success of any proposed program is the existence of supportive *facilities and resources*. In terms of the research program, this support would include such items as "data banks, library services, hardware, software, consultants, [and] support personnel" (Egan et al., 1981, p. 27). Without these, however, the program can function at a diminished rate, and some programs may not initially need extensive supportive services. However, these issues should be included in the feasibility study report in order to prepare the foundation for the future expansion in technology needed by a growing program.

The final criteria to be examined are those concerned with whether the psychiatric–mental health nursing research program would *"contribute to the research endeavors of educational institutions"* (Egan et al., 1981, p. 28). This question addresses both past and future support for nursing students' efforts in the research area. The enhancing of this aspect of the research program can work to strengthen the department's ties with educational institutions and may, in turn, improve the department's recruitment of nurses from those institutions (Egan et al.).

Interview of Administrators to Determine Perspective

In addition to conducting the feasibility study, the investigators should also interview nursing and hospital administrators to determine their perspectives of the research program proposal. Nursing staff should also be surveyed to identify their interests, skills, and previous experiences in nursing research. Early involvement of the nursing staff in this initial assessment at the beginning stages of planning can facilitate their continuing contributions for the remainder of the implementation process. It is hoped that this involvement will also serve to decrease resistance as staff members recognize that they have been involved since the beginning and that their input has been considered valuable.

The psychiatric–mental health nursing administrator has an important role in this phase of the process. The presence of a departmental research component, while having been mandated by professional organizations, lies within the responsibility of the nurse-administrator, who has control over the sophistication level of the program as well as the rate with which it is implemented. By playing devil's advocate, the nurse-administrator can question and challenge surveyor findings to ensure that the basis for the program is well constructed, and can compare the findings with basic criteria needed for a research program (see Table 18–2). Through examination of all the preresearch criteria affecting the department and organization, guidelines are determined for future actions. These may range from the beginning of support relationships—both within and without the organization—to the initial search for relevant research problems. A foundation should be present before the implementation of a nursing research program.

PLANNING FOR PROGRAM IMPLEMENTATION

Planning for the implementation of a nursing research program requires much the same careful and thorough approach as does the assessment process. The areas previously assessed must meet all the appropriate criteria in order to provide the foundation for a psychiatric–mental health nursing research program. Again, this foundation must be prepared before additional planning is done. However, even after careful and thorough planning, resistance to the psychiatric–mental health nursing research program often surfaces. To meet this resistance, strategies for facilitating the program's implementation must be incorporated into the initial planning process.

Resistance to Research

Sources of Resistance

Among the sources of staff resistance to research, the following are frequently identified and are listed by Padilla (1979):

- [The] perception of many nurses that research is an activity outside the normal responsibility of a nursing service.

Table 18–2 Criteria for Assessing Readiness for a Practice-Based Research Department

Condition	Criteria
Subject participation	Sufficient numbers of research topics to maintain a studies program over time
	Acceptability of participation in research studies by patients
Professional participation	Nucleus of personnel with some experience and interest in research
	Presence of incentives for personnel to participate in research
Market factors	Organizational expectations for systematic investigation into unsolved problems
	Acceptability of systematic studies in nursing
Organizational systems	Complementarity of a research program with established structure and functions
Economic factors	Presence of various mechanisms for funding systematic studies
	Identifiable benefits to be accrued from systematic studies
Legal/statutory provisions	Presence of mechanisms to assure protection of human subjects
	Presence of mechanisms and guidelines for approval of research projects
Facilities and resources	Availability of essential facilities and resources necessary for the conduct of systematic studies
Contributions to educational research endeavors	Presence of systems, procedures, and support for student research
	Identifiable study topics appropriate for students

Source: From *Practice based research: Assessing your department's readiness* by E.C. Egan, B.J. McElmurry, & H.M. Jameson, 1981, *Journal of Nursing Administration, 11*(10), 29. © 1981 by J.B. Lippincott Co. Reprinted by permission.

- Lack of understanding of the research process and techniques.
- Lack of institutional support for nursing research.
- Lack of client support. (p. 48)

Hefferin, Horsley, and Ventura (1982) expand this list and add the following:

- Research language not understood.
- Findings not transferable to practice.

- Workload too heavy to pursue research activity.
- Research participation not valued by nursing administration.
- Statistical analysis not understood.
- Lack of funds to support research activities.
- Physicians would not cooperate.
- Research participation not rewarded.
- Nurses unwilling to change or try new ideas.
- Nurses not interested in research activity.
- Lack of contact with outside resources, consultants, etc.
- Researchers with expertise not available to the staff.
- Research activity not seen as beneficial to staff growth.
- Nurses' inability to identify researchable problems/areas.
- Insufficient research yet available for current problems.
- Insufficient research articles in practice journals.
- Cannot judge value of research for use in clinical areas.
- No systematic means for sharing research with units. (p. 36)

Strategies to Decrease Resistance

Not all these sources of resistance are relevant to a particular psychiatric–mental health organization; however, the appropriate planning committee should identify those that are most likely to occur and then develop strategies to address each. Methods that have proven helpful in decreasing resistance include these cited by Krueger (1978):

- Identify persons or departments who have "always done it this way" and whose system or procedures might be thrown out of balance if change were instituted.
- Discuss plans early with those who might see the proposed change as a threat.
- Avoid direct pressure for change by working to decrease the strength of inhibiting forces prior to change.
- Emphasize that the proposed change is favored by prestigious people in the profession whose judgment would be respected.
- Indicate the benefit of the proposed change to those whose equilibrium may be affected by it.
- Present ideas to decision makers and/or informal leaders and let their commitment help to influence others.

- Introduce change through a pilot project on select units with the idea that it will be examined if not producing the desired results.
- Take the time to gain commitment of those who will be involved in change. (p. 8)

Through the use of the above strategies, the staff can be assisted to accept changes necessitated by the psychiatric–mental health nursing research program. A plan that includes addressing potential sources of resistance will be proactive and provide the department with a better foundation for the implementation of the anticipated changes.

Consent to Participate in Research

Another research aspect pertinent to psychiatric–mental health organizations that warrants particular attention is consent for participation in research. It is imperative that all persons involved in nursing research be informed of their specific role in the research program and voluntarily agree to participate. This requirement would include the participation of the staff as well as the clients. Hodgman (1981) indicates that all hospitalized persons are considered to be vulnerable in regards to research involvement. Moreover, persons who are mentally or emotionally ill are more vulnerable because of their inability, at times, to interpret reality correctly. Hence, the psychiatric–mental health client who is emotionally (and, perhaps, physically) involved in nursing research may be placed at great risk. Protection of clients is a prime consideration; therefore, policies and procedures must provide guidelines for client participation, consent for that participation, and resolution of legal and ethical concerns.

The psychiatric–mental health nursing staff should also expect to be well informed about any research process in which they are to participate. By reviewing the ANA's *Human Rights Guidelines for Nurses in Clinical and Other Research*, each nurse can have a clearer understanding of the role nurses should assume in the nursing research process. As a professional, any nurse is expected to be knowledgeable of the demands research makes on the participants—both the nurse and the subject-client. Through preparation, the nurse can do much to facilitate and to ensure the reliability and validity of the research. (See Chapter 4, section on research.)

Organizational and Departmental Mechanisms

Within the organization and department, mechanisms that support the overall psychiatric–mental health nursing research program must also be included in the planning process. One mechanism that facilitates nursing's involvement is the incorporation of research activities into the reward system of the department. Two examples of this incorporation include providing work time for nursing research when done by interested nurses and tangible recognition and rewards for nurses who are involved in research. These efforts clearly indicate to the staff that the psychiatric–mental health administration strongly supports and encourages nursing research. This awareness of support also provides additional incentives for further research interest within the department (Davis, 1981).

Further consideration must be given to other supportive mechanisms. These would entail mechanisms that review nursing research protocols, approve nursing research topics in terms of their scientific merit and protection of subjects, provide support services to facilitate the conduction of nursing research, encourage other departments to develop positive attitudes toward nursing research, and that use the generated data (Egan et al., 1981). By reviewing the steps in the nursing research process (see Exhibit 18–1), sufficient and appropriate staff and mechanisms within the department can be developed to address each step of the research process systematically. These steps can be used to provide a framework for the planning process which would comprehensively support nursing research efforts at every point.

Funding is an important aspect of any program planning. The funds for the staff incentive program, as well as those for the program itself, need to be incorporated in the nursing budget. A separate cost center for nursing research may be established. This strategy may not be as effective during times of fiscal restraint; however, in those situations, funds for research activities may be included in the operational budget. The psychiatric–mental health nursing administrator should meet with the organization's administrator and financial officers to identify the costs and the sources of potential funding. Such sources may include grants,

---

Exhibit 18–1 Steps in the Research Process

---

1. Formulate the problem.
2. Review the literature.
3. Formulate the framework of theory.
4. Formulate hypotheses.
5. Define the variables.
6. Determine how variables will be quantified.
7. Determine the research design.
8. Delineate the target population.
9. Select and develop method for collecting data.
10. Formulate method of analyzing the data.
11. Determine how results will be interpreted (generalized)
12. Determine method of communicating results.

Source: From *An introduction to nursing research: Research, measurement, and computers in nursing* by M.A. Sweeney & P. Olivieri, p. 48, 1981, Philadelphia: J.B. Lippincott Co. © 1981 by J.B. Lippincott Co. Reprinted by permission.

endowments, or research funds provided for the entire organization. Even when the departmental research efforts are limited to small projects completed on a yearly basis, funding must be allocated for portions of staff salaries and support services (e.g., typing, computer time, supplies). As the nursing research program grows, the budget will also increase proportionately.

IMPLEMENTATION OF A NURSING RESEARCH PROGRAM

The implementation of a nursing research program in a psychiatric–mental health setting is similar to the implementation of research programs in other health care organizations. Nevertheless, when a nursing research program is incorporated into a nursing department, it must be designed to be applicable and useful to that department. This design requirement can be accomplished by ensuring that the nursing research problems investigated are relevant to the nursing practice environment, by facilitating the nursing staff's involvement in the research, and by addressing the particular problems of the client population in obtaining consent to participate in research protocols.

Nursing Audits

One mechanism for the introduction of nursing research concepts to the nursing staff is through the application of nursing audits. Within the psychiatric–mental health setting, nursing audits and the problem-oriented record are similar to the research process and so they would assist the department in making a transition to the incorporation of nursing research thinking into everyday practice (see Table 18–3).

Audits—generally a component of a QA program—"prepare nurses for involvement in research, since evaluation of the outcomes of nursing care is the first step in the research process" (Padilla, 1979, p. 46). Through the following processes, research techniques could be incorporated into the nursing audit.

- Operational definitions of client outcome criteria would be based on literature searches.
- The reliability of the auditors would be determined on a random sample of records and an acceptable level of reliability determined.
- In the analysis of audit findings, aspects of research dealing with problem identification would be incorporated. The reasons a given outcome criteria was not met would be determined after consideration of alternative explanations. From the alternative explanations, the correct problem would be identified on the basis of expert clinical judgment and a review of research findings in that clinical area.

Table 18–3 Processes Used for Patient Care Evaluation

Basic Questions for Problem Solving	Nursing Process	Problem-Oriented Medical Record	Nursing Audit	Nursing Research
What is the problem/ question?			Select population	
			Determine outcome criteria	
	Assess patient status	Define data base: Historical data Demographic data Physiological data Laboratory data	Audit outcome criteria	Evaluate preliminary data pilot study/audit of outcome criteria/clinical experiences
What and how are solutions/ answers sought?	Define problem	List problems	Analyze audit findings Identify deficiencies	Define problem and population
	Plan intervention	Identify plans Diagnostic plan Therapeutic plan Education plan	Select corrective intervention	Review literature Select framework State hypothesis Operationally define variables Test manipulations & tools Select design Define sample Define data collection procedure
	Implement intervention	(assumed)	Implement corrective intervention	Implement study and collect data

Table 18–3 continued

Basic Questions for Problem Solving	Nursing Process	Problem-Oriented Medical Record	Nursing Audit	Nursing Research
Do the answers resolve the problems in question?	Evaluate intervention	Evaluate process with: Subjective patient data Objective data Assessment of status of problems Plans for continuing clinical actions	Evaluate corrective intervention	Analyze data
			Revise outcome criteria	Interpret and communicate results

Source: From "Incorporating research in a service setting" by G.V. Padilla, 1979, *Journal of Nursing Administration, 9*(1), p. 45. © 1979 by J.B. Lippincott Co. Reprinted by permission.

Finally, the problem would be defined in specific, measurable, and answerable terms.

- The corrective intervention selected would be based on research findings published in scientific journals and should fit a conceptual framework.
- In implementing the corrective intervention, factors which contribute to validity and reliability of such aspects of research methodology as design, subject selection, rater, and data tools would be considered.
- In evaluating corrective techniques, appropriate statistical techniques could be used to extract valid results. (Padilla, p. 47)

Through these adaptations, a currently used audit system can serve as an effective transition vehicle to a research program.

Supporting the Research-Oriented Nurse

A crucial component of the initial implementation process of any nursing research program is the support of the nurses interested in research. If nurses are not supported during their initial expression of interest, their interest may not continue. Supportive efforts indicate to all involved that research activities are rewarded and encouraged.

Research Support Group

One mechanism which aids in the support of the staff is the research support group. This group can function in a variety of ways. It can be used as an initial source of information to provide basic research education to those newly interested; or it can serve as an ongoing support mechanism for those nurses actively involved in nursing research. Most likely, the group itself will undergo a transition inasmuch as members' needs change and other vehicles, such as videotapes, can be used to provide basic information. Whatever the purpose, this group can provide support and direction to nurses functioning at a variety of levels in the research program (Davis, 1981).

Other Support Techniques

In addition to the reward system and a research group, many other mechanisms can be used to support the nurse with research interests. Four mechanisms suggested by Larson (1978) should be noted:

(1) Nurse researchers who are conducting research in the organization can be asked to discuss their research with the staff.
(2) A file of research publications (articles and texts) can be developed and made available to staff.
(3) The nursing department should make an effort to be on the mailing lists of local organizations who present nursing research findings.
(4) The announcements of such presentations should be made available to all nursing staff members.

Through these techniques and many others, research-oriented nurses can be supported, and an environment can be developed that is receptive to nursing research.

Role of the Clinical Nurse Specialist

The psychiatric–mental health clinical nurse specialist has, as part of the generally defined role, the responsibility to foster and to conduct nursing research. Should the clinical nurse specialist choose not to conduct research directly, the nursing staff's nursing research interests can still be fostered by the support of the clinical nurse specialist. The nursing staff should be encouraged to use professional publications to determine other approaches to the client care problems they identify. Also, when certain problems continue to be manifested, the clinical nurse specialist can aid the staff in testing approaches to the problem by ''(1) looking in the literature to see what else has been done; (2) defining the problem in concrete and measurable terms; (3) constructing the intervention to be tested; (4) deciding how to evaluate the effectiveness of this intervention; and (5) looking at ways of collecting and analyzing the data" (Fife, 1983, p. 13). Through these efforts, the clinical nurse specialist can do much to support the nursing administration's efforts and can foster a research-oriented environment.

Reviewing Research Proposals

Much has been written on the review process for research proposals. Guidelines exist within various professional organizations and regulatory agencies. Research committees often serve to review research proposals and protect the rights of participants in the proposals. The membership of these committees varies, but they should include persons with experience in this process.

The psychiatric–mental health nursing administrator may not be expected to be an expert in this area, but, as the person ultimately accountable for programs within the nursing department, the administrator can be expected to have knowledge of the review process. If assistance is needed in this area, resources may exist within the organization or an outside consultant may be contacted. Criteria do exist that can serve as guidelines to the nurse-administrator in the review process. Exhibit 18–2 identifies these criteria. In addition to using these criteria, the nurse-administrator reviewing a nursing research proposal must ask certain "questions" to determine internal consistency. Table 18–4 details this perspective in the

---

Exhibit 18–2 Criteria for Reviewing Research Proposals

Research Proposal
Purpose and significance of the study
Methods used to collect and analyze data
Copies of questionnaires
Criteria used to select participants

Protection of Participants' Rights
Explanation of how participants' rights will be protected
Copy of participant consent form
Plan for disposal of raw data once study is completed

Institutional Involvement
Specific involvement of institutional personnel and/or materials
Projected duration of research activity

Researcher's Qualifications and Requirements
Résumé listing education and experience
Procedure for processing the research request

Source: From "Evaluating research requests: A model for the nursing director" by E.E. Gulick, 1981, *Journal of Nursing Administration, 11*(1), p. 27. © 1981 by J.B. Lippincott Co. Reprinted by permission.

Table 18–4 Internal Consistency Guide

Problem Statement	Theoretical Framework	Method(s)	Data Analysis Plan	Outline of Findings	Targets for Recommen-dations
In one sentence, state the problem to be studied.	Outline the theory or theories that will be used to underpin study, or list the assumptions.	If experimental—specify the design; if nonexperimental—specify kind. Also, list major variables, instruments, or other data collection techniques.	What will collected data look like? Will analysis be statistical or not? Will it be nonparametric or parametric? What specific tests will be used?	Will findings be at a level of trends because small convenience sample used? Will findings be directly applicable to care; are they at a basic level; or are they exploratory in nature?	Theory/research: Possible implications for future research and theory testing or modification.
Objectives: Describe broad objectives, specific aims, or even the hypotheses: 1. 2. 3. etc.	Previous research: Outline types of research or specific studies that lead to this study; or outline the literature to be reviewed.	Sampling design: Describe whether sampling is random or convenience; report other sampling design specifications, such as how many groups, numbers in each group, methods of selection and assignment.			Practice: Action, research, and demonstration projects have direct practice implications. State possible recommendations.

Source: From "Developing staff research potential, part 2: Planning and implementation of studies" by J.S. Stevenson, 1978, *Journal of Nursing Administration, 8*(6), p. 10. © 1978 by J.B. Lippincott Co. Reprinted by permission.

review process. Through knowledge of these, and other guidelines, the nurse-administrator can support the work of nurses in the review process and provide an administrative perspective to this clinically based activity. Without this input, valuable resources and support may be delayed because of communication problems.

Whatever mechanisms are available or are used by the psychiatric–mental health nursing administrator, the ultimate responsibility for the initial development of the research component lies with this administrator. The tone set by this person will also set the tone for many of the nursing staff and can facilitate or impede the incorporation of nursing research within a particular setting. Through effective planning and implementation, an environment can be fostered in which nurses feel comfortable in seeking answers to nursing research questions.

EVALUATION OF A NURSING RESEARCH PROGRAM

Like that of any program, the outcomes of the nursing research program should be compared annually with the stated program goals and objectives. Modifications in the approach or in the components of the program must be made to bring actual outcomes into congruence with expected outcomes. In addition, the cost of research must often be justified when budgets are scrutinized. Nursing research outcomes must be related to the cost-effectiveness of quality client care and must demonstrate the cost-containment impact of nursing research findings. In doing so, one must be certain to include such nontangible cost benefits as increased visibility of the organization and the staff in the community and the increased client population due to the organization's reputation for being a leader in health care innovations. Research can do much to strengthen a department's and an organization's standing—financially and in terms of reputation. Through ensuring that an effective nursing research program is maintained within the department, the psychiatric–mental health nursing administrator contributes to the organization's improved status.

REFERENCES

American Nurses' Association. (1977). *Standards for nursing services*. Kansas City, Mo.: Author.

American Nurses' Association. (1982). *Standards of psychiatric and mental health nursing practice*. Kansas City, Mo.: Author.

Conway, M.E. (1978). Clinical research: Instrument for change. *Journal of Nursing Administration*, *8*(12), 27–32.

Davis, M.Z. (1981). Promoting nursing research in the clinical setting. *Journal of Nursing Administration*, *11*(3), 22–27.

Egan, E.C., McElmurry, B.J., & Jameson, H.M. (1981). Practice based research: Assessing your department's readiness. *Journal of Nursing Administration*, *11*(10), 26–32.

Fawcett, J. (1980). A declaration of nursing independence: The relationship of theory and research to nursing practice. *Journal of Nursing Administration, 10*(6), 36–39.

Fife, B. (1983). The challenge of the medical setting for the clinical specialist in psychiatric nursing. *Journal of Psychosocial Nursing and Mental Health Services, 21*(1), 8–13.

Gulick, E.E. (1981). Evaluating research requests: A model for the nursing director. *Journal of Nursing Administration, 11*(1), 26–30.

Hefferin, E.A., Horsley, J.A., & Ventura, M.R. (1982). Promoting research-based nursing: The nurse administrator's role. *Journal of Nursing Administration, 12*(5), 34–41.

Hodgman, E.C. (1981). Research policy for nursing services: part 2. *Journal of Nursing Administration, 11*(5), 33–36.

Krueger, J.C. (1978). Utilization of nursing research: The planning process. *Journal of Nursing Administration, 8*(1), 6–9.

Larson E. (1978). The inquisitive nurse: Bringing research to the bedside. *Nursing Administration Quarterly, 2*(4), 9–21.

Padilla, G.V. (1979). Incorporating research in a service setting. *Journal of Nursing Administration, 9*(1), 44–49.

Stevenson, J.S. (1978). Developing staff research potential, part 2: Planning and implementation of studies. *Journal of Nursing Administration, 8*(6), 8–12.

Sweeney, M.A., & Olivieri, P. (1981). *An introduction to nursing research: Research, measurement, and computers in nursing*. Philadelphia: J.B. Lippincott Co.

Chapter 19

Policies and Procedures

ASSESSING NEEDS

Well-defined policies and procedures addressing overall work activities contribute to the smooth functioning of any organization. Policies and procedures provide consistency and direction to the staff as they carry out their daily work. Among the responsibilities of the psychiatric–mental health nursing administrator is the assurance that appropriate and comprehensive policies and procedures are furnished to staff members so they can provide care in the most efficient, safe, and professional manner. Brown (1979) defines *policy* as the "basic principles or guidelines that govern and direct an organization's activities and upon which its procedures are founded." He defines *procedure* as "operational rules, regulations, and methods based on policies established to provide consistency and direction to organizational activities."

Rowland and Rowland (1980), in their description of administrative duties, state that the nurse-administrator "plans and conducts conferences and discussions with administrative and professional nursing staff to encourage participation in formulating departmental policies and procedures . . . and interpret new policies and procedures" (p. 82). These remain as duties for the psychiatric–mental health nursing administrator as well. Adequately and thoroughly documented policies and procedures, when followed by the staff, provide clear definitions of assignments, delineate roles and responsibilities, standardize methods, increase consistency of treatment, and reduce errors. In addition, tasks are simplified so that they are more easily understood and the efficiency and effectiveness of staff are enhanced. The policies and procedures manual is a valuable communication tool that, when presented in a comprehensive, clear, and concise format, can alleviate the frustration of staff members who may be confused about the proper and acceptable way to perform their jobs. Policies and procedures, then, state the standard of performance expected of the staff, and, along with job descriptions, define the responsibility and authority accorded each position in the department. Although the nurse-administrator may not assume personal responsibility for the development and implementation of all departmental policies and procedures, approval of such delegated activities rests solely with that administrator.

Occasionally psychiatric–mental health nursing administrators are required to initiate a new mental health service that requires development of policies and procedures beginning at the ground level. Usually, however, some basic policies and, perhaps, procedures are already in place; then additions, deletions, and revisions are periodically needed to keep the policies and procedures current. In assessing policy and procedure needs (whether starting from scratch or refining existing policies and procedures), consideration is given to those areas mandated by law, those identified by accrediting and regulatory bodies, and those specific to all aspects of the type of psychiatric–mental health care being provided. Each clinical unit—because it has unique program elements—requires policies and procedures pertinent to that particular area. For example, an acute inpatient adult psychiatric unit would need different policies and procedures for many aspects of care than would a long-term children's unit. A behavior modification privilege system, which may be a key treatment method on an inpatient adolescent unit with an average length of stay of 60 days, would be inappropriate and unusable in a psychiatric crisis center where adult clients are seen for assessment, crisis intervention, and referral (see Exhibit 19–1).

In assessing the policy and the procedure needs of the area, attention must be paid to the audience being addressed and the practice area involved. Furthermore, development of policies and procedures cannot be adequately undertaken without discussion of the practice concerns of the persons providing psychiatric–mental health care. Active involvement of the staff is essential for the development of useful policies and procedures. Whether accomplished through a committee or as an assigned task, policy and procedure development or revision requires a commitment from the nurse-administrator to provide sufficient staff and materials to accomplish the job.

PLANNING POLICIES AND PROCEDURES

The policies governing an organization's operations are usually stated in broad terms so that departments or divisions can establish procedures pertinent to their needs without having to modify policies frequently. The statement of departmental policies, like that of organizational policies, should be broad enough to be understood while remaining a fairly stable statement. Policies, by their nature, do not need revisions as often as do procedures. Basic principles rarely change; however, methods need more frequent modification.

Depending on the organization, the psychiatric–mental health nursing administrator may assign policy and procedure development and revision to an indi-

Exhibit 19–1 Policy and Procedure Concerns: Acute Psychiatric Setting

The following list of concerns is a partial list of those that should be included in the policies and procedures manual for an acute psychiatric–mental health inpatient setting

- Abuse of clients (suspected/actual)
- Admission, transfer and discharge
- Client confidentiality
- Client rights
- Department/division job descriptions
- Department/division philosophy
- Diagnostic studies
- Discharge against medical advice
- Documentation in the clinical record
- Electroconvulsive therapy
- Elopement (escape) precautions
- Harmful/dangerous articles ("sharps")
- Illegal and illicit contraband
- Incident reporting
- Infection control measures
- Interdisciplinary treatment planning
- Involuntary (court ordered) admissions
- Medication administration
- Photographing, fingerprinting, audiovisual recording of clients
- Physical management of acting-out client
- Privilege systems
- Psychosocial nursing assessment
- Searches—client's room, belongings, or body
- Suicide precautions
- Staffing
- Therapeutic client activities
- Use of restraints
- Use of seclusion
- Voluntary admissions

vidual person or to a group. In many organizations a policy and procedure committee, with a chairperson appointed by the nurse-administrator, has functioned efficiently. Members of the committee should represent management, staff education, and the staff at the nursing unit level. This type of committee provides an opportunity for input from several levels of the staff, thus focusing on actual practice situations. Another effective mechanism that can be used to get staff involvement is to circulate proposed policies and procedures before their implementation or revision and to ask the staff for feedback before their adoption. The nurse-administrator may chair the policy and procedure committee or may be a liaison or resource person to either the committee or the person responsible for the policies and procedures manual. Involvement of the psychiatric–mental health nursing administrator in the policy and procedure process can give staff members another means of access to that administrator. Regardless of the involvement, final approval for departmental or division policies and procedures rests with the nurse-administrator.

Manual Format

When planning policies and procedures, a decision must be made about the format of the manual. Several options are available. Policies and procedures can be incorporated in separate manuals—one book for policies, another for procedures. However, both can be included in one handbook under separate sections—usually, policies in the front of the manual and procedures in the back. Another option is the integration of policies and procedures, which provides a centralized source of information. Rowland and Rowland (1980), however, see some objections to this format. "Some manuals contain a combination of policies and administrative procedures. Others are limited to policies only. When the two are mixed, it is often difficult to be sure what is policy and what is procedure, and the manual may become bulky with lengthy instructions and sample forms. But whatever works best for the individual department should be included" (p. 115). A way to avoid confusion of policy and procedure in the use of an integrated manual is to establish a page format that includes a space at the beginning of the procedure for the policy statement related to that procedure (see Exhibit 19–2).

Policies are established by management and are the basic guidelines from which procedures are then developed. In some instances policies may be found in memoranda and other communications that were not formally placed in a policies and procedures manual. Before developing policies and procedures, then, the person responsible for the project needs to locate all the documents available that relate to the topics under review. Informal, unwritten policies need to be searched out for consideration in the final format of the document.

Persons responsible for the development of a policies and procedures manual will find the task to be manageable if they use a systematic approach. The steps listed below can provide that approach:

1. Develop major section headings for the manual; it will make the task manageable and orderly.
2. Assign section numbers to each major section of the manual.

Exhibit 19–2 Integrated Policy and Procedure Manual Excerpt

KINGSWOOD HOSPITAL	POLICY TITLE: ACUTE SUICIDE PRECAUTIONS
10300 W. EIGHT MILE RD.	
FERNDALE, MI 48220	
NURSING DEPARTMENT	SECTION: 19 NUMBER: 02a

POLICY:

Persons assigned to Acute Suicide Precautions (A.S.P.) by the physician, or Nursing Acute Suicide Precautions (N.A.S.P.) by the nurse, are those who demonstrate behavior (verbal/nonverbal) indicative of serious and/or imminent suicidal potential. Assigning persons to this status accomplishes the following:

1. Provides *constant* supervision to protect the patient from self-injury.
2. Provides the opportunity to gather more data with which to assess lethality in an ongoing fashion.
3. Communicates the need for *constant* supervision to all clinical disciplines involved in care of the patient.
4. Provides *at all times* external control to assist the patient to regain control over suicidal impulses.

PROCEDURE:

I. Acute Suicide Precautions (A.S.P.) is ordered by a physician or may be instituted by the Nurse in Charge (N.A.S.P.) for a patient who is judged to be in imminent danger of suicidal behavior in the following manner:

    A. Initiated by the physician's order or by written order by the Nurse in Charge if the physician cannot be contacted.

    B. Communicated as follows:

        1. To the Nursing Supervisor

        2. Should be included on the 24 Hour Condition Report and reflected in acuity assessment.

        3. The nurse is to document in the progress notes the behavior responsible for instituting the precaution.

        4. Should be communicated to all nursing staff on the unit on all shifts through oral/written report.

        5. Should be communicated to all clinical disciplines involved in care of the patient by notification of Department Heads (Social Service/Psychology/Education Secretary, O.T./R.T. Department Head).

II. The following care will be provided for patients on A.S.P./N.A.S.P.:

    A. Patient must be *accompanied* by a member of the Nursing Staff, assigned agency nurse staff, or medical staff member *at all times*. The designated staff person must be physically present during all activities so that immediate verbal and physical intervention is possible to prevent self harm.

Exhibit 19–2 continued

    1. The staff person is present during toileting, bathing, sleeping, etc.
    2. Physical barriers such as closed doors are never permitted when so accompanied.
    3. Physical distance may not interfere with the staff's ability to immediately intervene if necessary.

B. Patient's room should be near the nurse's station for close supervision.
C. Patient is not allowed off the unit, including the dining room and regularly scheduled activities, without a specific physician's order, and then only with 1:1 supervision.

    1. Patients on (N.)A.S.P. are not allowed to participate on hospital outtrips.
    2. If a physical exam is required, the internist is required to perform this on the unit.
    3. If a medical consult is ordered by the physician, or if an emergency arises requiring outside services, two staff members will be assigned to accompany the patient to the designated caregiver.

D. When placed on (N.)A.S.P., the patient will have a personal and a room search completed and documented following procedure. Periodically the Nurse in Charge may at his/her discretion have a unit, personal and/or room search completed and documented to maintain a safe environment.
E. Follow procedure for provision of general safety for all psychiatric patients.

    Belts and shoelaces will be collected by the staff assigned to the patient and returned when the precaution is discontinued. This will be explained to the patient in a supportive manner.

F. If a patient on (N.)A.S.P. has submitted a "Notice of Intent to Terminate Formal (Informal) Voluntary Agreement", the patient's physician will be notified by an R.N. since commitment proceedings may need to be instituted by the physician.
G. Transfers for adult patients to 5L are not allowed.
H. No passes or L.O.A.'s are allowed.
I. O.T./R.T. and educational activities are allowed with 1:1 supervision and physician's order.
J. Attending Group Therapy is a decision to be made jointly with the Group Therapist and Nurse in Charge. If the decision is made to allow attendance, a staff person will be immediately available if there is only one Group Leader. If the group is co-led, one therapist will agree to be available to escort the patient if return to the unit becomes necessary.
K. In the event of seclusion, at least one staff member will stay with the patient for 1:1 supervision to ensure the patient's safety.
L. In the case of N.A.S.P.:

    1. The order may not be discontinued until an assessment is completed by the physician who has assessed the patient within 24 hours.
    2. A written order by the physician to discontinue N.A.S.P. is necessary if in the physician's judgment the precaution is no longer necessary.

III. Documentation

A. The patient will be provided an explanation of the precaution which is to be documented in the progress notes.
B. The patient's verbal/nonverbal response to the explanation, degree of understanding, and ongoing reaction is to be documented.

Exhibit 19–2 continued

> C. *Documentation* by the assigned nursing staff person will be completed in progress notes at least *hourly*. Care will be made to document the patient's mood, verbal and nonverbal behavior indicative of status of suicidal potential (i.e., patient's statements related to depression, suicide, activity pattern, sleep pattern, eating, sudden mood or behavior changes, etc.).
>
> D. Reporting any suicidal threats, gestures or sudden mood or behavior changes will be done immediately for assessment by the Nurse in Charge who will determine the appropriate action.
>
> PROCEDURE APPROVED: _____ REVIEWED/REVISED: ___6/84___
>
> ORIGINATED: ___1977___   ___ ___ ___
>
> *Source:* Reprinted from *Nursing Policy and Procedure Manual* with permission of Kingswood Hospital, Ferndale, Mich.

3. Sort out policies by section and the assigned numbers within each section.
4. Finally, develop an index, listing all the subjects in the manual (see Exhibit 19–3).

Procedure Development

When the manual format has been established, procedures can be developed for corresponding policies. Researching the subject under question is important. Besides collecting all existing documentation on the issue, the policy and procedure committee, representatives of the committee, or the policy and procedure coordinator begin discussions with staff members involved in the actual work situation, obtain input from recent psychiatric–mental health nursing literature on the subject, review existing policies and procedures, and interview nurses with expertise in the area under review. After this approach, legal issues that need to be clarified are referred to the organization's legal department for an opinion and direction. All information is then evaluated and an outline is prepared that lists all the supplies necessary, if applicable, and the steps involved in the procedure. From this outline, the procedure is then written. Procedures include step-by-step directions that sequentially lead staff members from the initial phase of the procedure to its conclusion Steps are written as clearly and concisely as possible to avoid confusion.

Cross References

All organizations have policies and procedures that cross into areas other than nursing. Even within the department, policies and procedures may be closely related or flow one into another. In these instances, cross references can be made in

Exhibit 19–3 Policy and Procedure Manual Index and Table of Contents

8.01—INTRODUCTION

    8.01.01 Philosophy of Psychiatric Nursing
    8.01.02 ANA Standards
    8.01.03 Environmental Policy

8.02—ABBREVIATIONS

8.03—ABORTION, CONTRACEPTION & STERILIZATION

8.04—ADMISSIONS, TRANSFERS & DISCHARGES

    8.04.01 Admission Policy & Procedure
    8.04.02 Nursing Admission Interview
    8.04.03 Nursing Assessment (Adult & Adolescent) Screening
              Immunization History
    8.04.04 Inter-Ward Transfer Policy & Procedure
    8.04.05 Discharge/Transfer Summary
    8.04.06 Property of Discharged Patients

8.05—CHARTING

    8.05.01 Charting Policy & Procedure
    8.05.02 Observation & Charting
    8.05.03 Retrospective Charting
    8.05.04 Goal Directed Charting

8.06—COMMUNICATION

    8.06.01 Privileged Communication
    8.06.02 Michigan Department of Mental Health Rules
    8.06.03 Incident Report
    8.06.04 Hospital Paging Policy & Procedure

8.07—DEATH

    8.07.01 Death of Patient
    8.07.02 Department of Mental Health Rules
    8.07.03 Post Mortem Care

8.08—DEPARTMENTAL POLICIES

    8.08.01 Organizational Plan & Chart
    8.08.02 Staffing
    8.08.03 Patient Assignments
    8.08.04 Petty Cash

8.09—DIAGNOSTIC STUDIES

    8.09.01 CAT Scans
    8.09.02 Dexamethasone Suppression Test
    8.09.03 Electroencephalograms & Echo-Electroencephalograms
    8.09.04 Internal Medicine Consults
    8.09.05 Laboratory Studies
    8.09.06 Physical Examination & Laboratory Tests
    8.09.07 Radiology

Exhibit 19–3 continued

8.10—DIETARY SERVICES
    8.10.01 Dining Room Policy & Procedure
    8.10.02 Dining Room & Special Diet Responsibilities

8.11—PRAYER ROOM

8.12—EMERGENCY PROCEDURES
    8.12.01 Ambulance Service
    8.12.02 Resealing The Emergency Box
    8.12.03 Emergencies Arising Inside the Hospital—CODE BLUE
            Emergency Lighting—See Safety, Security & Emergency Policies and Procedures
            PBX—See Safety, Security & Emergency Policies & Procedures
            Medical Emergency Manual—See Manual in front of the Nursing Manual
    8.12.04 First Aid Kits

8.13—INFECTION CONTROL
    8.13.01 Infection Control
    8.13.02 Communicable Disease Reporting
            Communicable Disease List
    8.13.03 Handwashing
    8.13.04 Reporting & Containing Infections
    8.13.05 Isolation—Enteric Precautions
    8.13.06 Respiratory Isolation
    8.13.07 Strict Isolation
    8.13.08 Isolation—Wound & Skin Precautions
    8.13.09 Isolation & Gowning Techniques
    8.13.10 Refrigeration
    8.13.11 Infection Control Officer
    8.13.12 Infection Control—Employee Health
    8.13.13 Sterile Supplies & Equipment

8.14—JOB DESCRIPTIONS
    8.14.01 Director of Nursing
    8.14.02 Assistant Director of Nursing
    8.14.03 Clinical Coordinator
    8.14.04 Clinical Specialist
    8.14.05 Day Supervisor
    8.14.06 Evening Administrator
    8.14.07 Head Nurse
    8.14.08 Charge Nurse
    8.14.09 Staff Nurse
    8.14.10 LPN
    8.14.11 Mental Health Worker
    8.14.12 Psychiatric Worker
    8.14.13 Nursing Office Secretary
    8.14.14 Unit Clerk

Exhibit 19–3 continued

8.15—MEDICATIONS
 8.15.01 Medication Policy
 8.15.02 Medication Procedure
 8.15.03 Medication Error Policy & Procedure
 8.15.04 Administering Medication
     Needle Injections
     Oral
     Rectal
     Topical
 8.15.05 Prescription Pads
 8.15.06 Controlled Substances Policy & Procedure
     Disposal of Needles & Syringes—See Patient Safety

8.16—PASSES/LEAVE OF ABSENCE(S)
 8.16.01 Statement of Passes & LOA Policy
 8.16.02 AWOL Patients Policy

8.17—PATIENT ACTIVITIES
 8.17.01 RT Equipment In Absence of RT Person
 8.17.02 Use of OT Skills Room

8.18—PATIENT POLICIES

8.19—PATIENT PRECAUTIONS
 8.19.01 Elopement
 8.19.02 Suicide Precautions
 8.19.02a Acute Suicide Precautions
 8.19.02b General Suicide Precautions
 8.19.03 Seizure Precautions
 8.19.04 Close Nursing Observation

8.20—PATIENT RIGHTS
 8.20.01 Summary
 8.20.02 US Mail, Visitors, Packages, Telephones
 8.20.03 Patient Abuse

8.21—PATIENT SAFETY
 8.21.01 Search & Room Check Policy
 8.21.02 Search & Room Check Procedure
 8.21.03 Sharps
 8.21.04 Sharps List
 8.21.05 Use of Toaster
 8.21.06 Discarding of Used Disposable Needles & Syringes
 8.21.07 Razors

8.22—PERSONNEL POLICIES
 8.22.01 Dress Code

Exhibit 19–3 continued

8.23—PHYSICAL NURSING CARE

    8.23.01 Ace Bandage, Applying
    8.23.02 Assisting Patient Into a Chair
    8.23.03 Administration of Oxygen
    8.23.04 Assisting With Physical Examination
    8.23.05 Assisting Patient to Walk
    8.23.06 Bedmaking
    8.23.07 Enema
    8.23.08 Sitz Bath
    8.23.09 Catheterization of Male
    8.23.10 Catheterization of Female
    8.23.11 Cold Compresses
    8.23.12 Vital Signs
    8.23.13 Daily Blood Pressures
    8.23.14 Personal Hygiene of Patients

8.24—PHYSICIANS ORDERS

    8.24.01 Noting Doctors' Orders

8.25—SECLUSION & RESTRAINT

    8.25.01 Policy & Procedure
    8.25.02 Use of Restraints
    8.25.03 Manual Restraint

8.26—TRANSPORTATION OF PATIENTS

    8.26.01 Cab Service
              Ambulance Service—See Emergency Procedures

8.27—TREATMENT PLANNING

    8.27.01 Nursing Care Plan
    8.27.02 Policy For Special Nursing Procedure
    8.27.03 Treatment Care Planning Policy & Procedure

8.28—ADOLESCENT/YOUNG ADULT PROGRAM

    8.28.01 Drug Abuse Protocol
    8.28.02 Personal Belonging Policy

Source: Reprinted from *Nursing Policy and Procedure Manual* with permission of Kingswood Hospital, Ferndale, Michigan.

the index or on the policy and procedure itself. This gives the reader another resource in which further information on the subject can be found. In some organizations each department is assigned a policy and procedure manual number so cross referencing between departments can be facilitated (see Table 19–1).

Preparing Final Draft for Approval

After the manual and page formats have been decided, the section numbers assigned, and policies numbered and placed in each section, procedures are

Table 19–1 Use of Departmental Number in Manual for Cross Referencing

Subject	Number	Also Related
Damage to hospital property by patients	1.61	
Day care services	1.05	
Death of a patient	1.21	7.00; 8.00
Dental care	1.35	7.00; 8.00
Discharge against medical advice	1.14	8.00
Disclosure of medical record information from patient charts	1.20	1.19; 6.00; 7.00; 8.00
Disclosure of medical records	1.19	6.00; 7.00; 800
Disease report to Oakland County Health Department	1.56	1.57
Elopements	1.14	8.00
Emergency services	1.24	1.25; 8.00
Employee medical care	1.25	1.57; 8.00
Federal Rehabilitation Act of 1973	1.48	
Fingerprinting of patients	1.13	1.11
Food-borne outbreaks	1.22	5.00; 8.00
Food service	1.23	2.00; 4.00; 5.00
Formal voluntary admission	1.04	1.02
Guidelines for use of psychotropic drugs	1.60	

Note: Sample of Portion of Index

Source: Reprinted from *Administrative Manual* with permission of Kingswood Hospital, Ferndale, Michigan.

---

developed. Policies that have been informally in place are rewritten in a policy format. Included with the policy are procedures related to the policy. Using the outline developed from researched information, a written draft is formulated, carefully attending to the sequence of events and sentence structure. Staff members who are experts in the area can critique the policy and procedure before the draft is made final. The draft is then sent to the psychiatric–mental health nursing administrator for final approval before being reproduced and distributed.

IMPLEMENTING DISTRIBUTION

Upon approval of the psychiatric–mental health nurse administrator, the policy and procedure is ready for reproduction and distribution. Because most policies and procedures manuals are quite comprehensive, it is not usually feasible for each staff member to have a personal copy. Copies should be distributed to key administrative, management, and staff development personnel as well as to each unit. If staff members are expected to use the policies and procedures manual it needs to be easily accessible to them. Whenever revisions, additions or deletions are made, a memo explaining the changes, along with replacement pages, should be sent to each person with a copy of the manual. Explanations of new or revised policies and procedures can be shared with the nursing management team before implementation. After this discussion, the policies and procedures can then be implemented by the nursing management team. In some instances, policy and procedure additions or revisions can be handled through unit staff meetings. Where a major change is involved or a complicated procedure is initiated, in-service training for staff members may be required. In any event, the staff must be informed of all policy and procedure changes in a timely fashion. If staff members are unaware of the current policies and procedures, they certainly cannot follow them.

EVALUATION OF EFFECTIVENESS

After policies and procedures have been implemented, follow-up evaluation of their effectiveness is needed. All policies and procedures should be reviewed on a regular basis, usually once a year. At that time changes can be made to reflect current practice and staff needs. Circumstances may change that require a modification in a procedure. If the policies and procedures manual is not kept up-to-date, it becomes confusing and often useless to the staff. New personnel also need current policies and procedures manuals; their familiarity with the departmental procedures is often minimal. An up-to-date policies and procedures manual can be a useful resource tool for the staff, reducing confusion and anxiety and enhancing the quality of care provided to clients.

REFERENCES

Brown, B.L. (1979). *Risk management for hospitals: A practical approach*. Rockville, MD: Aspen Systems.

Rowland, H.S., & Rowland, B.L. (1980). *Nursing administration handbook*. Rockville, MD: Aspen Systems.

SUGGESTED READING

Beis, E.B. (1984). *Mental health and the law*. Rockville, MD: Aspen Systems.

Griffith, J., & Ignatavicius, D. (1984). Procedure development: A simplified approach. *Journal of Nursing Administration, 14*(9), 27–31.

Sisk, H.L. (1973). *Management and organization*. Cincinnati: South-Western Publishing Co.

Travis, A.B. (1984). *The handbook handbook*. New York: R.R. Bowker Co.

Index

About the Authors

CHRISTINA L.S. EVANS, RNC, MSN, CNA is the Assistant Director of Nursing at Kingswood Hospital, Ferndale, Michigan (a private nonprofit psychiatric hospital). Previous to this position, she has held various management positions in psychiatric nursing (clinical specialist/supervisor, evening administrator, relief midnight supervisor) as well as the clinical positions of clinical specialist, clinical nursing instructor, and staff nurse. She received a BSN and a MSN (major: nursing administration; minor: psychiatric nursing care of children) from Wayne State University, Detroit, Michigan. She is certified by the American Nurses' Association as a Nurse Administrator and a Psychiatric–Mental Health Nurse. Currently, Ms. Evans is the Chairperson of the Division on Psychiatric–Mental Health Nursing Practice and the Membership Committee of the Michigan Nurses' Association. In addition, she chairs a divisional support group for the Directors of Nursing of State Psychiatric Facilities and has been supporting the development of additional support groups for various levels of psychiatric nurse managers. She also serves as a Director on the Board of the Detroit District Nurses' Association, and as a member of the Greater Detroit Area Association of Nurse Administrators, the ANA Councils of Nurse Administrators and Continuing Education.

SHARON K. LEWIS, RN, MA, CNA, is Administrative Assistant for Professional Services at Kingswood Hospital, Ferndale, Michigan. Prior to her current administrative position, Ms. Lewis was Assistant Director of Nursing and then Director of Nursing at Kingswood Hospital. She has had extensive experience in psychiatric–mental health nursing and progressive management experience in both general hospital and private psychiatric settings. She is a graduate of Providence Hospital School of Nursing, Southfield, Michigan, and received her BA and MA degrees from the University of Detroit, Detroit, Michigan. Ms. Lewis is past president of the Oakland District Nurses' Association and is currently serving as First Vice Chairperson of the Michigan Nurses' Association Division of

Psychiatric–Mental Health Nursing Practice. She is on the Board of Directors of the Greater Detroit Area Association of Nurse Administrators serving a second term as Chairperson of the Program and Education Committee. She also serves on the Advisory Committee of the Schoolcraft College Nursing Program. Ms. Lewis has given seminars on various psychiatric–mental health nursing and nursing management topics for hospital nursing staff as well as through continuing education programs of local universities.